T0195543

Molecular Pathology

Editor

LAUREN L. RITTERHOUSE

SURGICAL PATHOLOGY CLINICS

www.surgpath.theclinics.com

Consulting Editor
JASON L. HORNICK

September 2021 • Volume 14 • Number 3

ELSEVIER

1600 John F. Kennedy Boulevard • Suite 1800 • Philadelphia, Pennsylvania, 19103-2899

http://www.theclinics.com

SURGICAL PATHOLOGY CLINICS Volume 14, Number 3
September 2021 ISSN 1875-9181, ISBN-13: 978-0-323-79466-4

Editor: Katerina Heidhausen
Developmental Editor: Diana Ang

© **2021 Elsevier Inc. All rights reserved.**

This periodical and the individual contributions contained in it are protected under copyright by Elsevier, and the following terms and conditions apply to their use:

Photocopying
Single photocopies of single articles may be made for personal use as allowed by national copyright laws. Permission of the Publisher and payment of a fee is required for all other photocopying, including multiple or systematic copying, copying for advertising or promotional purposes, resale, and all forms of document delivery. Special rates are available for educational institutions that wish to make photocopies for non-profit educational classroom use. For information on how to seek permission visit www.elsevier.com/permissions or call: (+44) 1865 843830 (UK)/(+1) 215 239 3804 (USA).

Derivative Works
Subscribers may reproduce tables of contents or prepare lists of articles including abstracts for internal circulation within their institutions. Permission of the Publisher is required for resale or distribution outside the institution. Permission of the Publisher is required for all other derivative works, including compilations and translations (please consult www.elsevier.com/permissions).

Electronic Storage or Usage
Permission of the Publisher is required to store or use electronically any material contained in this periodical, including any article or part of an article (please consult www.elsevier.com/permissions). Except as outlined above, no part of this publication may be reproduced, stored in a retrieval system or transmitted in any form or by any means, electronic, mechanical, photocopying, recording or otherwise, without prior written permission of the Publisher.

Notice
No responsibility is assumed by the Publisher for any injury and/or damage to persons or property as a matter of products liability, negligence or otherwise, or from any use or operation of any methods, products, instructions or ideas contained in the material herein. Because of rapid advances in the medical sciences, in particular, independent verification of diagnoses and drug dosages should be made.

Although all advertising material is expected to conform to ethical (medical) standards, inclusion in this publication does not constitute a guarantee or endorsement of the quality or value of such product or of the claims made of it by its manufacturer.

Surgical Pathology Clinics (ISSN 1875-9181) is published quarterly by Elsevier Inc., 360 Park Avenue South, New York, NY 10010. Months of issue are March, June, September, and December. Business and Editorial Office: Elsevier Inc., 1600 John F. Kennedy Blvd., Ste. 1800, Philadelphia, PA 19103-2899. Accounting and Circulation Offices: Elsevier Inc., 3251 Riverport Lane, Maryland Heights, MO 63043. Periodicals postage paid at New York, NY and at additional mailing offices. Subscription prices are $228.00 per year (US individuals), $358.00 per year (US institutions), $100.00 per year (US students/residents), $283.00 per year (Canadian individuals), $383.00 per year (Canadian Institutions), $274.00 per year (foreign individuals), $383.00 per year (foreign institutions), and $120.00 per year (international students/residents), $100.00 per year (Canadian students/residents). Foreign air speed delivery is included in all *Clinics'* subscription prices. All prices are subject to change without notice. **POSTMASTER:** Send address changes to *Surgical Pathology Clinics*, Elsevier, 3251 Riverport Lane, Maryland Heights, MO 63043. **Customer Service: 1-800-654-2452 (US). From outside the United States, call 1-314-447-8871. Fax: 1-314-447-8029. E-mail: JournalsCustomerServiceusa@elsevier.com (for print support)** and **JournalsOnlineSupport-usa@elsevier.com (for online support)**.

Reprints. For copies of 100 or more, of articles in this publication, please contact the Commercial Reprints Department, Elsevier Inc., 360 Park Avenue South, New York, NY 10010-1710. Tel. 212-633-3874; Fax: 212-633-3820; E-mail: reprints@elsevier.com.

Surgical Pathology Clinics of North America is covered in *MEDLINE/PubMed (Index Medicus)*.

Printed in the United States of America.

Contributors

CONSULTING EDITOR

JASON L. HORNICK, MD, PhD
Director of Surgical Pathology and
Immunohistochemistry, Brigham and Women's
Hospital, Professor of Pathology, Harvard
Medical School, Boston, Massachusetts, USA

EDITOR

LAUREN L. RITTERHOUSE, MD, PhD
Associate Director, Center for Integrated
Diagnostics, Department of Pathology,
Massachusetts General Hospital, Assistant
Professor, Harvard Medical School, Boston,
Massachusetts, USA

AUTHORS

HIKMAT AL-AHMADIE, MD
Associate Member, Department of Pathology,
Memorial Sloan Kettering Cancer Center, New
York, New York, USA

CAMERON BEECH, MD
Gastrointestinal pathology fellow, Department
of Pathology, Yale New Haven Hospital, New
New Haven, Connecticut, USA

ALANNA J. CHURCH, MD
Department of Pathology, Boston Children's
Hospital, Harvard Medical School, Boston,
Massachusetts, USA

KATELYNN DAVIS, MD
Chief Resident Physician, Department of
Pathology, Johns Hopkins Medical Institutions,
Baltimore, Maryland, USA

FEI DONG, MD
Department of Pathology, Brigham and
Women's Hospital, Assistant Professor,
Harvard Medical School, Boston,
Massachusetts, USA

MARK D. EWALT, MD
Assistant Attending, Department of Pathology,
Memorial Sloan Kettering Cancer Center, New
York, New York, USA

KRISTYN GALBRAITH, MD
Clinical Fellow in Neuropathology, Department
of Pathology, NYU Langone Medical Center,
New York, New York, USA

MICHAEL C. HAFFNER, MD, PhD
Divisions of Human Biology and Clinical
Research, Fred Hutchinson Cancer Research
Center, Department of Pathology, University of
Washington, Seattle, Washington, USA;
Department of Pathology, Johns Hopkins
School of Medicine, Baltimore, Maryland, USA

JACLYN F. HECHTMAN, MD
Molecular and GI Pathologist, NeoGenomics
Laboratories, Fort Myers, Florida, USA

JUAN C. HERNANDEZ-PRERA, MD
Associate Member, Department of Pathology,
Moffitt Cancer Center, Tampa, Florida, USA

SUSAN J. HSIAO, MD, PhD
Assistant Professor, Department of Pathology
and Cell Biology, Columbia University Irving
Medical Center, New York, New York, USA

RAMON U. JIN, MD, PhD
Instructor, Section of Hematology/Oncology,
Department of Medicine, Baylor College of
Medicine, Houston, Texas, USA

ANNETTE S. KIM, MD, PhD
Associate Professor of Pathology, Department of Pathology, Brigham and Women's Hospital, Harvard Medical School, Boston, Massachusetts, USA

IBRAHIM KULAC, MD
Department of Pathology, Koç University School of Medicine, Istanbul, Turkey

GEORGE J. NETTO, MD
Professor and Chairperson, Department of Pathology, The University of Alabama at Birmingham, University of Alabama at Birmingham School of Medicine, Birmingham, Alabama, USA

ZEHRA ORDULU, MD
Department of Pathology, Brigham and Women's Hospital, Department of Pathology, Massachusetts General Hospital, Harvard Medical School, Boston, Massachusetts, USA

FRESIA PAREJA, MD, PhD
Assistant Attending, Department of Pathology, Memorial Sloan Kettering Cancer Center, New York, New York, USA

LAUREN L. RITTERHOUSE, MD, PhD
Associate Director, Center for Integrated Diagnostics, Department of Pathology, Massachusetts General Hospital, Assistant Professor, Harvard Medical School, Boston, Massachusetts, USA

DARA S. ROSS, MD
Associate Attending, Department of Pathology, Memorial Sloan Kettering Cancer Center, New York, New York, USA

MARTINE P. ROUDIER, MD, PhD
Department of Urology, University of Washington, Seattle, Washington, USA

SINCHITA ROY-CHOWDHURI, MD, PhD
Associate Professor, Department of Anatomic Pathology, Division of Pathology and Laboratory Medicine, The University of Texas MD Anderson Cancer Center, Houston, Texas, USA

SAM SADIGH, MD
Instructor of Pathology, Department of Pathology, Brigham and Women's Hospital, Harvard Medical School, Boston, Massachusetts, USA

JONATHAN C. SLACK, MD
Department of Pathology, Boston Children's Hospital, Harvard Medical School, Boston, Massachusetts, USA

MATIJA SNUDERL, MD
Director of Molecular Pathology and Diagnostics, Associate Professor, Department of Pathology, NYU Langone Medical Center, New York, New York, USA

MATTHEW D. STACHLER, MD, PhD
Assistant Professor, Department of Pathology, University of California, San Francisco, San Francisco, California, USA

ALISHA D. WARE, MD
Assistant Professor, Department of Pathology, Johns Hopkins Medical Institutions, Baltimore, Maryland, USA

JACLYN WATKINS, MD
Department of Pathology, Massachusetts General Hospital, Harvard Medical School, Boston, Massachusetts, USA

RENA R. XIAN, MD
Assistant Professor, Department of Pathology, Department of Oncology, Sidney Kimmel Comprehensive Cancer Center, Johns Hopkins Medical Institutions, Johns Hopkins School of Medicine, Baltimore, Maryland, USA

Contents

Pre-analytical factors in molecular oncology diagnostics are reviewed. Issues around sample collection, storage, and transport that might affect the stability of nucleic acids and the ability to perform molecular testing are addressed. In addition, molecular methods used commonly in clinical diagnostic laboratories, including newer technologies such as next-generation sequencing and digital droplet polymerase chain reaction, as well as their applications, are reviewed. Finally, we discuss considerations in designing a molecular test menu to deliver accurate and timely results in an efficient and cost-effective manner.

The identification of targetable genomic alterations in lung cancer is required as standard of care to guide optimal therapy selection. With a constantly evolving landscape of ancillary molecular and biomarker testing in lung cancer, pathologists need to be aware of what specimens to test, how the testing should be performed, and which targets to test for to provide the clinically relevant genomic information necessary to treat these patients. Several guideline statements on the topic are currently available to help pathologists and laboratory personnel best use the small specimens obtained from patients with lung cancer for ancillary molecular testing.

Gliomas are the most common adult and pediatric primary brain tumors. Molecular studies have identified features that can enhance diagnosis and provide biomarkers. IDH1/2 mutation with ATRX and TP53 mutations defines diffuse astrocytomas, whereas IDH1/2 mutations with 1p19q loss defines oligodendroglioma. Focal amplifications of receptor tyrosine kinase genes, TERT promoter mutation, and loss of chromosomes 10 and 13 with trisomy of chromosome 7 are characteristic features of glioblastoma and can be used for diagnosis. BRAF gene fusions and mutations in low-grade gliomas and histone H3 mutations in high-grade gliomas also can be used for diagnostics.

Molecular profiling studies have shed new light on the complex biology of prostate cancer. Genomic studies have highlighted that structural rearrangements are among the most common recurrent alterations. In addition, both germline and somatic mutations in DNA repair genes are enriched in patients with advanced disease. Primary prostate cancer has long been known to be multifocal, but recent studies demonstrate that a large fraction of prostate cancer shows evidence of multiclonality, suggesting that genetically distinct, independently arising tumor clones coexist. Metastatic prostate cancer shows a high level of morphologic and molecular diversity, which is associated with resistance to systemic therapies. The resulting high level of intratumoral heterogeneity has important implications for diagnosis and poses major challenges for the implementation of molecular studies. Here we provide a concise review of the molecular pathology of prostate cancer, highlight clinically relevant alterations, and discuss opportunities for molecular testing.

Urothelial carcinoma is characterized by the presence of a wide spectrum of histopathologic features and molecular alterations that contribute to its morphologic and genomic heterogeneity. It typically harbors high rates of somatic mutations with considerable genomic and transcriptional complexity and heterogeneity that is reflective of its varied histomorphologic and clinical features. This review provides an update on the recent advances in the molecular characterization and novel molecular taxonomy of urothelial carcinoma and variant histologies.

This review focuses on the diagnostic, prognostic, and predictive molecular biomarkers in ovarian epithelial neoplasms in the context of their morphologic classifications. Currently, most clinically actionable molecular findings are reported in high-grade serous carcinomas; however, the data on less common tumor types are rapidly accelerating. Overall, the advances in genomic knowledge over the last decade highlight the significance of integrating molecular findings with morphology in ovarian epithelial tumors for a wide-range of clinical applications, from assistance in diagnosis to predicting response to therapy.

Colorectal carcinoma is one of the most common cancer types in men and women, responsible for both the third highest incidence of new cancer cases and the third highest cause of cancer deaths. In the last several decades, the molecular mechanisms surrounding colorectal carcinoma's tumorigenesis have become clearer through research, providing new avenues for diagnostic testing and novel approaches to therapeutics. Laboratories are tasked with providing the most current information to help guide clinical decisions. In this review, we summarize the current knowledge surrounding colorectal carcinoma tumorigenesis and highlight clinically relevant molecular testing.

Upper gastroesophageal carcinomas consist of cancers arising from the esophagus and stomach. Squamous cell carcinomas and adenocarcinomas are seen in the esophagus and despite arising from the same organ have different biology. Gastric adenocarcinomas are categorized into 4 molecular subtypes: high Epstein-Barr virus load, microsatellite unstable cancers, chromosomal unstable (CIN) cancers, and genomically stable cancers. Genomically stable gastric cancers correlate highly with histologically defined diffuse-type cancers. Esophageal carcinomas and CIN gastric cancers often are driven by high-level amplifications of oncogenes and contain a high degree of intratumoral heterogeneity. Targeted therapeutics is an active area of research for gastroesophageal cancers.

pan-cancer biomarkers include sequence-altering mutations, copy number changes, gene rearrangements, and mutational signatures and have been demonstrated to predict response to targeted therapy. This article reviews issues surrounding current and emerging pan-cancer molecular biomarkers in clinical oncology: technological advances that enable the broad detection of cancer mutations across hundreds of genes, the spectrum of driver and passenger mutations derived from human cancer genomes, and implications for patient care now and in the near future.

Despite the apparent complexity of the molecular genetic underpinnings of myeloid neoplasms, most myeloid mutational profiles can be understood within a simple framework. Somatic mutations accumulate in hematopoietic stem cells with aging and toxic insults, termed clonal hematopoiesis. These "old stem cells" mutations, predominantly in the epigenetic and RNA spliceosome pathways, act as "founding" driver mutations leading to a clonal myeloid neoplasm when sufficient in number and clone size. Subsequent mutations can create the genetic flavor of the myeloid neoplasm ("backseat" drivers) due to their enrichment in certain entities or act as progression events ("aggressive" drivers) during clonal evolution.

Lymphoid malignancies are a broad and heterogeneous group of neoplasms. In the past decade, the genetic landscape of these tumors has been explored and cataloged in fine detail offering a glimpse into the mechanisms of lymphomagenesis and new opportunities to translate these findings into patient management. A myriad of studies have demonstrated both distinctive and overlapping molecular and chromosomal abnormalities that have influenced the diagnosis and classification of lymphoma, disease prognosis, and treatment selection.

SURGICAL PATHOLOGY CLINICS

SERIES OF RELATED INTEREST

Clinics in Laboratory Medicine
http://www.labmed.theclinics.com/
Medical Clinics
https://www.medical.theclinics.com/

THE CLINICS ARE AVAILABLE ONLINE!
Access your subscription at:
www.theclinics.com

Preface
The Evolving Role of Molecular Diagnostics in Pathology

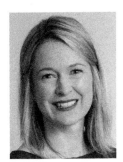

Lauren L. Ritterhouse, MD, PhD
Editor

The clinical implementation of molecular diagnostic technologies continues to expand across a wide variety of tumor types and has been shown to have utility for diagnostic, prognostic, and therapeutic implications. Genomic studies continue to expand our understanding of pathobiology with revelations that some differing tumor types are part of the same spectrum of disease; such is the case with esophageal adenocarcinoma and intestinal-type gastric adenocarcinomas of the proximal stomach (Stachler and Jin). Novel biomarkers are rapidly and continuously being identified, necessitating frequent workflow and best practice optimizations in both surgical pathology and the molecular diagnostic laboratory to facilitate the implementation of guideline recommended biomarker testing. In addition, there is an influx of new technologies and diagnostic assays available, such that curation of a molecular diagnostic pathology test menu for both in-house and send-out testing requires significant thought and collaboration with clinical colleagues (Hsaio and Ewalt). Depending on the tumor type and biomarkers to be evaluated, screening with immunohistochemistry may play an important role (Hernandez-Prera).

In addition, as many new biomarkers and targeted therapies have demonstrated evidence and efficacy across tumor types, the field of pan-tumor biomarkers continues to evolve (Dong). Prior to 2017, there were no Food and Drug Administration approvals for cancer therapies based exclusively on the presence of a biomarker and not tissue of origin. Since then, pembrolizumab has been approved for microsatellite-instability-high or mismatch repair deficient solid tumors in 2017, larotrectinib for solid tumors with NTRK gene fusions in 2018, and entrectinib for solid tumors with NTRK gene fusions in 2019. Although PARP inhibitors do not have a pan-tumor approval, several biomarkers, such as BRCA1/2 mutations and homologous recombination deficiency, may predict response to PARP inhibition across several tumor types, such as ovarian (Ordulu, Watkins, Ritterhouse) and prostate cancer (Kulac, Roudier, Haffner). Additional genes and signatures involved in DNA damage response and repair are also being evaluated as biomarkers predicting response to both chemo0-therapies and immunotherapies, exemplified in the case of urothelial carcinoma (Al-Ahmadie and Netto).

World Health Organization classifications for both central nervous system tumors and myeloid neoplasms have incorporated molecular and cytogenetic features into their classification criteria (Galbraith and Snuderl; Sadigh and Kim), and are expected to continue to evolve. New diagnostic entities are emerging in both sarcomas and pediatric solid tumors (Slack and Church) that are defined by their genetics, such as RET- and NTRK-rearranged mesenchymal tumors, which may be identical morphologically but respond to unique targeted therapies.

Surgical Pathology 14 (2021) xi–xii
https://doi.org/10.1016/j.path.2021.05.014
1875-9181/21/© 2021 Published by Elsevier Inc.

Frequent referencing of guideline statements, such as the National Comprehensive Cancer Network clinical practice guidelines in oncology, is highly recommended due to the constantly evolving nature of biomarkers. This is particularly true in tumor types such as non–small cell lung cancer in which genotyping is the standard of care to guide optimal therapy selection (Roy-Chowdhuri). In addition to genotyping at diagnosis, the role of molecular testing at recurrence or disease progression is growing as we learn more about resistance mechanisms to various therapies (Roy-Chowdhuri; Ross and Pareja). The utilization of so-called liquid biopsies (plasma-based circulating tumor DNA evaluation) continues to evolve, with potential applications in tumor heterogeneity, tissue inadequacy, and for emerging roles, such as predicting tumor recurrence in colorectal cancer (Beech and Hechtman). Finally, indications for measurable residual disease molecular testing are best established in hematopoietic neoplasms (Xian and Ware; Sadigh and Kim). As is evidenced in the following articles, molecular diagnostics is a promising, rapidly evolving, and integral part of the modern pathology practice.

Lauren L. Ritterhouse, MD, PhD
Center for Integrated Diagnostics
Department of Pathology
Massachusetts General Hospital
Harvard Medical School
Jackson Building
10th Floor, Suite 1015
55 Fruit Street
Boston, MA 02114, USA

E-mail address:
lritterhouse@mgh.harvard.edu

Molecular Methods
Clinical Utilization and Designing a Test Menu

Mark D. Ewalt, MD[a], Susan J. Hsiao, MD, PhD[b],*

KEYWORDS
- Molecular diagnostics • Pre-analytical • Methods • Next-generation sequencing
- Polymerase chain reaction

Key points

- Pre-analytical considerations, including sample collection, storage, and transport, as well as specimen assessment, are critical to ensure success of molecular diagnostic testing.
- Triaging tissue and maximizing material for molecular analyses are recommended for small specimens
- Molecular methodologies, such as sequencing-based, hybridization-based, or polymerase chain reaction–based have varying sensitivity and specificity and appropriate use depends on the application.
- Designing a molecular test menu requires consideration of the biomarker, prevalence, sample type, and limitations of the testing methodology.

ABSTRACT

Pre-analytical factors in molecular oncology diagnostics are reviewed. Issues around sample collection, storage, and transport that might affect the stability of nucleic acids and the ability to perform molecular testing are addressed. In addition, molecular methods used commonly in clinical diagnostic laboratories, including newer technologies such as next-generation sequencing and digital droplet polymerase chain reaction, as well as their applications, are reviewed. Finally, we discuss considerations in designing a molecular test menu to deliver accurate and timely results in an efficient and cost-effective manner.

BUILDING YOUR MOLECULAR TOOLBOX

Molecular diagnostics is focused on analyzing genetic changes in patient samples and encompasses a wide array of modalities to assess many types of target molecules. This article provides an overview of the most common test methods and applications in molecular oncology including analytical and pre-analytic considerations. The article also aims to discuss how to design and optimize a molecular diagnostics test menu based on the needs of your institution.

PRE-ANALYTICAL CONSIDERATIONS

Specimen collection, transport, and storage are all key factors in ensuring samples received for molecular oncology testing are analyzable and do not provide false negative results (**Table 1**). Typical samples that may be encountered in molecular oncology diagnostic laboratories include formalin-fixed paraffin-embedded (FFPE) tissue, cell blocks, smears, blood, bone marrow aspirates, and fresh or frozen tissue. Blood and bone marrow samples are typically collected in EDTA

[a] Department of Pathology, Memorial Sloan Kettering Cancer Center, 1275 York Avenue, S-618, New York, NY 10065, USA; [b] Department of Pathology & Cell Biology, Columbia University Medical Center, 630 West 168th Street, P&S11-453, New York, NY 10032, USA
* Corresponding author.
E-mail address: sjh2155@cumc.columbia.edu

Surgical Pathology 14 (2021) 359–368
https://doi.org/10.1016/j.path.2021.05.001
1875-9181/21/© 2021 Elsevier Inc. All rights reserved.

Table 1
Pre-analytical considerations for molecular testing

Pre-analytical Factors	Recommendations
Sample collection	• Use appropriate collection tubes (eg, EDTA; avoid heparin) • Minimize ischemic time for RNA analytes
Tissue fixation	• 10% Neutral buffered formalin • Alcohol-based fixatives • Frozen tissue
Decalcification	• Avoid unless using EDTA (acid-free)
Specimen storage and transport	• Minimize storage and transport times • Consider use of stabilizing reagents (for example for RNA or circulating tumor DNA (ctDNA) from blood specimens)
Specimen assessment	• Accurate assessment of tumor percentage important to prevent false negative results • Enrichment of tumor by macrodissection or microdissection is frequently necessary
Tissue triage for small specimens	• Embed cores into separate blocks • Avoid aggressive re-facing of blocks • Use all available material, including smears, cell blocks, ctDNA

or citrate tubes; other tubes, such as heparin-containing tubes, are generally not recommended for molecular analyses, as heparin may affect nucleic acid extraction and/or inhibit polymerase chain reaction (PCR) amplification.[1] Specialized tubes may be required for other applications. For example, for ribonucleic acid (RNA)-based assays, blood tubes with additives for RNA stabilization may be used; for circulating tumor deoxyribonucleic acid (ctDNA), blood tubes with agents that stabilize nucleated cells are often used.[2] FFPE tissue is another common specimen type, and multiple factors in the collection, fixation, and storage of FFPE tissue may affect the quantity and quality of DNA or RNA that may be extracted from this tissue.[3,4] Key pre-analytical considerations for molecular oncology specimens are summarized as follows.

SAMPLE COLLECTION

The time from when the specimen is collected until the time in which the specimen is preserved is referred to as ischemic time. Studies have found no significant difference in DNA quality/quantity based on ischemic time.[5,6] For RNA-based assays, however, ischemic time may have a profound effect, due to the lability of RNA. Long ischemic time has been reported to be associated with decreased RNA quantity and quality.[7] In particular, assays investigating gene expression are expected to be sensitive to such effects, and

thus ischemic time should be minimized when possible.

TISSUE FIXATION

10% Neutral Buffered Formalin is a standard fixative routinely used in anatomic pathology practices and preserves tissue by cross-linking DNA and protein. Other tissue fixatives, such as B5, Bouin, or Zenker fixatives, induce metal-protein complexes or depurination and are not recommended when subsequent molecular testing is desired.[8,9] Length of fixation may also affect nucleic acid quantity and yield. With 10% neutral buffered formalin, overfixation (longer than 72 hours of fixation) has been reported to affect DNA yields and quality.[10,11] Cytologic preparations, such as alcohol-fixed smears and cell blocks, also yield nucleic acids of high quality and may be used for molecular testing.[12,13]

DECALCIFICATION

Processing of tissues for decalcification may render samples unusable for molecular analyses and thus should be avoided when possible. Multiple decalcification solutions are available; however, many of these contain acid, which damages and depurinates DNA. Other decalcification solutions, such as EDTA, do not damage DNA and are compatible with molecular analyses.[3] Decalcification using EDTA is done using concentrations of 10% to 20% (typically 14%) and is pH dependent. The size of the biopsy

Table 2
Molecular methods

Methodology	Mutation	Fusion	Copy Number Variant	Advantages	Limitations
Sequencing methods				Detects known and novel variants	
Sanger	+	+/−		Fast Cheap Low input	Singleplex Not very sensitive (10%–20% LOD)
NGS	+	+	+	Multiplex Detects all types of variant Can be extremely sensitive (0.001%)	Slow Expensive Larger DNA input
Hybridization and other methods					
FISH		+	+	Fast Cheap Single-cell resolution	Only detects known/targeted variants Limited multiplexing
Array	+/−		+	Whole genome assessment High resolution	May not detect translocations
Karyotype		+	+	Whole genome assessment Single-cell resolution	Low resolution (10 MB) Slow Manual
IHC	+	+	+/−	• Fast • Single-cell resolution	Only a surrogate for fusion and copy number variants
PCR methods				Fast Cheap	Only detect known variants Limited multiplexing
qPCR	+	+	+	Sensitive 0.01%	
AS-PCR	+				
ddPCR	+	+	+	Sensitive 0.01%	

Abbreviations: AS-PCR, allele-specific PCR; ddPCR, digital droplet PCR; FISH, fluorescence in situ hybridization; IHC, immunohistochemistry; LOD, Limit of detection; NGS, next-generation sequencing; PCR, polymerase chain reaction; qPCR, quantitative PCR; +/-, In some specialized cases this assay modality may be used for the listed indication; however, it is not routinely used for this in most laboratories.

influences the rate of decalcification; small biopsies may take 16 to 24 hours, whereas larger biopsies may take several days. Other factors that influence the rate of decalcification include temperature, agitation, and sufficient decalcifier access (sufficient volume of EDTA solution is generally at a 20:1 ratio, and the EDTA solution should be changed regularly). Because it is difficult to predict when molecular testing may be necessary, it is not recommended to decalcify a specimen entirely with acid-based decalcification. Instead, one block of tissue should be reserved to undergo EDTA decalcification and noted in the report for use if molecular testing is required in the future.

SPECIMEN STORAGE AND TRANSPORT

Fresh tissues or fluids should be transported immediately to the laboratory and processed as soon as possible, particularly if RNA-based molecular testing is desired. Addition of stabilizing reagents, which lyse cells and inactivate nucleases, can preserve the sample for nucleic acid extraction at a later time. Another scenario in which specimen transport is critical is in circulating tumor DNA (ctDNA) testing. If a sample for ctDNA testing is collected in a tube without additives to stabilize nucleated cells, the sample should be processed within 6 hours of collection.[2] Samples should be stored under controlled conditions to minimize degradation. Long-term storage of samples in preservative may result in degradation of nucleic acids. Similarly, long-term storage of FFPE tissue has been found to be associated with DNA fragmentation and deamination of cytosine bases, and can result in poor DNA quality and failure of amplification and/or sequence artifacts.[14–19]

SPECIMEN ASSESSMENT

For somatic testing, the tumor cell content of the submitted specimen must be assessed. Sufficient tumor cell percentage is required to ensure that variants present in the tumor would be within the limit of detection established for the molecular testing requested on the specimen. Insufficient tumor cell percentage may result in false negative results. Assessment of tumor percentage is typically performed by manual review of hematoxylin-eosin–stained sections, although assessment using digital imaging is also used by some laboratories to reduce potential subjectivity in the tumor percentage assessment. Assays such as Sanger sequencing require tumor percentages of 20% to 40%, whereas other highly sensitive assays may require tumor percentages as low as a few percent. Enrichment of the tumor percentage beyond the minimum required to perform the assay is frequently performed nonetheless, due to the imprecise nature of estimating tumor percentage,[20] as well as to preserve the ability to detect variants in the presence of subclonal mutations or tumor heterogeneity. Macrodissection, a process in which areas of tumors are scraped using a scalpel or razor, or microdissection, a process in which a microscope is used to aid in targeting small areas of stained tissue sections for scraping, are frequently used for tumor enrichment.[21] Laser capture microdissection is another method that may be used for tumor enrichment, although the cost and time associated with this procedure have limited widespread adoption.[22]

MAXIMIZING TISSUE FOR MOLECULAR TESTING

Preservation of tissue to ensure sufficient amounts of material for diagnosis and subsequent molecular profiling may be challenging with small specimens obtained from minimally invasive approaches. In lung tumors, for example, biomarkers recommended to be evaluated include programmed death ligand 1 (PD-L1), *EGFR*, *ALK*, *ROS1*, *BRAF*, *KRAS*, *ERBB2*, *MET*, *RET*, and *NTRK*.[23] Testing for these biomarkers may be achieved by a combination of methodologies, such as immunohistochemistry (IHC), fluorescence in situ hybridization (FISH), targeted PCR, DNA sequencing, and/or RNA sequencing, each with their own minimal tissue requirements. If testing was ordered sequentially, and the block re-faced, the material may quickly become exhausted. Approaches to maximize material for testing include embedding cores into separate blocks, superficial facing of blocks, and utilization

of all available material, including cytology specimens such as smears, fine needle aspirates, cell blocks, and use of ctDNA.[13,24] Coordination of pathologists with oncologists, surgeons, interventional radiologists, and the histology, immunohistochemistry, cytogenetics, and molecular laboratories is important in the appropriate triaging of specimens.

MOLECULAR METHODS

Molecular methods focus on detecting changes in nucleic acids and can be grouped into classes based on the type of molecules they interrogate or the type of alterations they can detect (**Table 2**). The molecules tested include DNA, RNA, and protein, while these methods can detect sequence alterations, structural variation, copy number changes, and covalent modification of nucleic acids.

DEOXYRIBONUCLEIC ACID–BASED METHODS

There are a variety of methods used to test DNA molecules and these can be grouped into sequencing-based assays in which the full nucleotide sequence of target DNA molecules is assessed and non–sequencing-based methods.

The 2 primary methods of sequencing in clinical practice are Sanger sequencing and next-generation sequencing (NGS).[25]

Sanger sequencing, also called dideoxy sequencing, is a well-established method for generating DNA sequence information. It consists of extending a DNA fragment in the presence of a mixture of native deoxynucleoside triphosphate molecules (dNTPs) and dideoxynucleoside triphosphates (ddNTPs).[25] After a ddNTP is incorporated at a position in the growing DNA molecule, the extension reaction ends. The termination point occurs randomly along the length of the molecule and is repeated such that there are many fragments with the same termination point. These fragments are then separated by size, and the ddNTPs contain fluorescent tags corresponding to the base incorporated (A, T, G, or C), which can be detected by an instrument and correlated with the fragment size. In this way, the specific sequence can be "read" such that the first base in the strand is that which terminated the smallest fragment, and so on. Sanger sequencing has the benefits of being fast, allowing sequencing of longer reads than NGS, and the ability to detect single nucleotide variants and insertion/deletion variants (indels) in the region being tested.[25] However, Sanger suffers from limited analytical sensitivity and usually requires that at least 10% to 20% of the molecules in a mixture harbor a variant to be detected. As many variants in cancer are heterozygous, this requires 20% to 40% neoplastic cells in a sample to accurately detect an alteration by this method. In addition, the molecules sequenced by Sanger are read in a bulk fashion (all fragments of the same size are read simultaneously), which can make it difficult or impossible to determine if multiple variants in the same Sanger reaction are present on the same (in cis) strand of DNA or on alternate (in trans) strands of DNA.[26,27]

In the past 5 years, NGS, also called massively parallel sequencing, has become widely used in clinical oncology laboratories. Although different NGS platforms differ in the specifics of the chemistry used and detection methods (ionometric vs fluorometric), the basic principles of these technologies are shared.[25] The first steps of NGS are called library generation and target enrichment. For capture-based NGS, bulk genomic DNA molecules are fragmented and labeled with patient and sequencing platform specific DNA sequences ("tags" or "barcodes") added to the ends of the molecules to generate libraries. These are subsequently enriched for those molecules from the regions of clinical interest. In amplicon-based NGS, these steps may be combined by using PCR with primers that incorporate the patient and platform barcodes to generate target-enriched libraries. Each target-enriched patient-specific library is then pooled together for sequencing. The pooled libraries are then bound to a solid support such that single starting molecules are physically separated from one another on the support. Once bound, PCR is performed to increase the number of starting DNA molecules at each position on the solid support that will increase the assay signal. After this local amplification by PCR, sequencing is performed during which a signal is generated at (pH change for ionometric sequencing) or immediately following (fluorescence measurement in fluorometric sequencing) each base incorporation step. The instrument reads the series of signals at each position on the solid support and strings this together as individual sequences corresponding to each parent molecule at that location. These strings are called reads and are then processed by bioinformatics processes to generate human interpretable data.[25] Because NGS generates a distinct read from each separate molecule sequenced, it can be optimized to provide very high levels of sensitivity far below 1% through the use of unique molecular identifiers (UMIs). UMIs are short DNA sequences that are built into the adapters of each molecule during library generation and identify all reads that originated from a single original

molecule (with the same UMI). These reads can then be informatically combined based on consensus for all reads with the same UMI to suppress random errors.[28,29] In addition, when variants are located in close enough proximity to be on the same sequenced molecule, it is possible to assess the phase (cis/trans relationship) of these mutations. NGS also is able to interrogate many target regions simultaneously, whereas Sanger can only examine a single region. Unfortunately, NGS tends to require more input DNA, takes longer to process, and has a higher per reaction cost than Sanger sequencing.[30] It should be noted, however, that although a single Sanger sequencing reaction is faster and less expensive than an NGS reaction, the overall cost per base for NGS is orders of magnitude less expensive per base and therefore depending on the size of the target region, NGS may be far more cost-effective.[31]

Nonsequencing DNA methods of genetic testing include hybridization methods, karyotype analysis, and PCR-based methods.

In hybridization methods, fluorescently labeled short DNA sequences complementary to specific targets ("probes") are bound or hybridized to specific DNA targets.[32] In FISH, these probes can be used to perform several applications. They can enumerate copy number by comparing number of fluorescent signals to a control signal (ie, ERBB2 to CEN17).[33] They can demonstrate a breakapart within a gene where different colored probes are positioned at either end of a target region and the case is evaluated for a split signal pattern (ie, MYC breakapart) or they can be used to identify both partners in a fusion by labeling both sides of each partner with probes of the same color and then looking for an overlapping signal pattern (ie, BCR-ABL1 dual fusion).[34,35] FISH is rapid and highly sensitive for the specific alterations it targets; however, some variant alterations, particularly those smaller than the size of the FISH probe, or novel alterations may be missed by this method and only a few targets can be interrogated in each reaction.[36,37]

Chromosomal microarray (CMA) is typically now performed with probes for each of the possible alleles at thousands to millions of single nucleotide polymorphisms (SNPs) that are spread across the genome.[36] The fluorescent signal of each probe at each position determines the genotype for that SNP and reveals whether the patient is homozygous or heterozygous at each position. By looking across the genome, this can give information about copy number alterations at very high resolution (15 kb) and can provide specific genotype information at a single locus.[36,37] CMA provides whole genome assessment at high resolution but because it interrogates short probes, it usually cannot detect balanced translocation events that lead to no net change in the amount of DNA present.[36]

Karyotype is one of the most mature technologies used to evaluate genomic alterations and provides a full genome view in a single reaction.[32] In this technology, living cells are cultured, synchronized, and then halted at metaphase in the cell cycle. These cells are then gently lysed on the surface of a glass slide and stained (usually with Giemsa) to generate distinct banding patterns of the chromosomes. Each chromosome has specific banding patterns and expert technologists and geneticists can interpret these patterns to describe structural and copy number variants across the genome.[32] This method may take 3 to 7 days depending on the growth rate of the cells in culture and provides low resolution with chromosome bands generally corresponding to at least 10 Mb of DNA.[37]

PCR-based methods encompass a variety of techniques that use the specificity of the PCR reaction to detect alterations. At their most simple, allele-specific methods amplify (generate a PCR product) when a mutant sequence is present and fail to amplify in the absence of the target mutant allele.[38] Similar methods can be used to amplify translocations by using primers that would not amplify in the absence of a genetic rearrangement but bring the 2 primer regions in close proximity in the presence of the translocation so that PCR can generate a product; although this is more frequently performed from an RNA template, as discussed later in this article.[39] Another major PCR method used in clinical oncology is quantitative PCR (qPCR), which is sometimes referred to as a "real-time" PCR. In qPCR, a fluorescent signal is generated during each cycle of the PCR reaction and this signal is proportional to the amount of PCR product generated, which is also proportional to the amount of input target DNA in the reaction.[40] Using standard curves, one is able to quantitate the amount of starting material present. Another quantitative method for PCR is digital PCR (dPCR), whereby template DNA is diluted and partitioned to contain either 0 or 1 template molecule, hence the term digital.[41,42] One of the more common types of dPCR in use in clinical laboratories is digital droplet PCR (ddPCR). In this method, template DNA is diluted and emulsified to generate droplets that contain either 0 or 1 template DNA molecule.[43] Labeled PCR reactions are then performed for a particular genotype or genotypes, usually variant and normal. Quantification is reported either as the number of droplets of a particular genotype per unit volume or as the number of variant droplets divided by the total number of DNA-containing (variant + normal) droplets.[43] PCR-based methods are fast and relatively inexpensive with high sensitivity for the variants they interrogate. qPCR and ddPCR are able to detect 1 variant in 10,000 to 100,000 (1×10^{-4} to 10^{-5}) and are routinely used in minimal/measurable disease and ctDNA assessment.[44,45] Despite these advantages, PCR-based methods can only assess for known variants and have limited multiplexing capability such that only 4 to 8 variant targets can be interrogated in a single reaction.

Although the previously described DNA-based methods interrogate the specific DNA sequence, structure, or copy number, methylation-based methods can reveal the presence of the epigenetic covalent binding of a methyl group to the cytosine nucleotide. These methods either use specific restriction enzymes that cleave or fail to cleave at methylated sequence or use the bisulfite reaction to convert unmethylated cytosine residues to uracil residues and then perform a sequence-specific method (PCR or sequencing) to identify the methylation status of specific residues.[46]

RIBONUCLEIC ACID–BASED METHODS

Detection of RNA is performed by first using a reverse-transcriptase step during which RNA is converted into complementary DNA (cDNA). The cDNA is then interrogated through those methods described previously to analyze DNA.[47] RNA-based methods are particularly useful when interrogating fusion events and splice variants. In the case of fusion events, RNA-based methods remove the large intronic sequences leading to more efficient test methods.[48,49] In addition, assessing the RNA directly will allow determination if the resultant transcript is in-frame. For splice variants, DNA-based methods may predict a splice event; however, interrogating the RNA will definitively determine whether or not such an event has occurred.[50] RNA-based testing is also useful in assessing the relative expression levels of target genes.[51] This is frequently performed on array or NGS-based platforms.

PROTEIN-BASED METHODS

IHC is the predominant method used in clinical oncology to detect proteins and can be used as a marker of a range of underlying alterations. Qualitative IHC for a specific mutated protein such as *BRAF* p.V600E or *IDH1* p.R132H can rapidly detect the presence of an underlying DNA-level mutation event.[52,53] IHC can also be used quantitatively where high intensity of staining can be used as a surrogate for gene fusions (ie, *ALK* in lung cancer) or gene amplification (ie, *ERBB2* in breast cancer).[33,54–56] Depending on the clinical setting, these IHC surrogates may be used to triage to other testing modalities or be considered a final diagnostic assay in their own right.

CONSIDERATIONS IN DESIGNING A MOLECULAR TEST MENU

Molecular diagnostics provide critical information for the management of patients, and make possible the delivery of precision medicine. Selection of biomarkers to assess requires consideration of clinical utility, technical specifications, and cost-effectiveness. Clinically relevant biomarkers provide information on diagnoses, improve predictions of prognosis, and guide therapy choices or patient management. Consultation with ordering providers (eg, pathologists, oncologists, geneticists) and professional society guidelines can help guide the selection of biomarkers to test. Many biomarkers may be assessed by a variety of methods (reviewed previously in this article). For example, *IDH1* mutation status may be assessed by methods including IHC, real-time PCR, digital droplet PCR, Sanger sequencing, and NGS. To establish a diagnosis in glioma, IHC may be the preferred testing method, but to determine whether a targeted IDH1 inhibitor may be indicated in acute myeloid leukemia, a PCR or sequencing-based methodology may be optimal.

Turnaround time and cost-effectiveness are additional considerations that may influence test selection or necessitate utilization of a testing algorithm. As mentioned previously, in lung cancer, multiple biomarkers are recommended to be assessed.[21] Depending on the methodology, testing for single analytes or testing multiple analytes simultaneously may provide the best balance in terms of turnaround time and cost. An option some laboratories pursue is a sequential testing strategy. Alterations such as *KRAS* or *EGFR* mutations are more common than *ALK*, *RET*, or *ROS1* fusions, and these driver alterations are considered to be mutually exclusive. If separate assays are being run (and the clinical scenario permits), one could consider performing testing such a DNA-based sequencing assay for *KRAS* or *EGFR* mutations, and then an RNA-based assay to detect *ALK*, *RET*, or *ROS1* fusions only if the tumor is negative for *KRAS* or *EGFR* mutations. In other clinical scenarios in lung cancer, for example, with a patient with metastatic disease in whom immediate therapeutic options are needed, a rapid cartridge-based real-time PCR solution may be more appropriate.

Testing algorithms can become quite complex, especially when trying to detect a pan-tumor biomarker that can be detected with various methodologies and has varying prevalence. An example of this would be detection of NTRK gene fusions. NTRK gene fusions are targetable and range in prevalence from fewer than 5% to more than 75% of tumors, depending on the tumor type. From a practical standpoint, a single testing strategy will be difficult for many laboratories to achieve. One recommendation has been to combine several methodologies, including FISH, for tumors with high incidence of NTRK gene fusions, IHC for tumors that do not normally express TRK proteins and have a lower incidence of NTRK gene fusions, and broad NGS-based testing if tumors express TRK, or are negative by other testing.[57]

Following selection of biomarkers to detect and test methodology, a laboratory may choose to implement an FDA-approved or FDA-cleared assay or may choose a laboratory-developed procedure. FDA-approved or FDA-cleared assays are developed by In-vitro diagnostics (IVD) manufacturers and are approved or cleared by the FDA for clinical diagnostic use. Laboratory-developed procedures use test kits, research uses only reagents, analyte-specific reagents, and/or general purpose reagents to detect analytes. The performance of FDA-approved or FDA-cleared assays must be verified before use, whereas laboratory-developed procedures must undergo validation to establish the performance characteristics of the assay. Assay validation includes assessment of accuracy, precision, reportable range, reference range, analytical sensitivity, and analytical specificity. Obtaining appropriate calibrators, reference materials, and control samples is critical for this process.

Beyond developing biomarker testing in-house, algorithms also can be designed to work with reference laboratories such that common biomarkers in common diseases are tested in-house and rarer biomarkers are sent to a referral laboratory. This approach may allow a smaller laboratory to optimize its workflow and cost-effectiveness.

In summary, designing an effective molecular diagnostics menu can be a complex task; however, with careful planning and collaboration, it is possible to combine the methodologies described previously to develop comprehensive testing capabilities in many practice settings.

CLINICS CARE POINTS

- Use 10% neutral buffered formalin for fixation; avoid the use of acid-based decalcification solutions.

- Maximize tissue for molecular testing by embedding cores into separate blocks, using superficial facing of blocks, and utilizing cytology specimens.

- Consider features such as clinical utility, technical specifications of the molecular methodology, and cost-effectiveness when designing a test menu.

DISCLOSURE

S.J. Hsiao has received honoraria from Illumina, Loxo Oncology, Opentrons Labworks, and Medscape, and institutional research funding from Bristol Myers Squibb. M.D. Ewalt has received consulting revenue from Acceleron Pharma.

REFERENCES

1. Wilson IG. Inhibition and facilitation of nucleic acid amplification. Appl Environ Microbiol 1997;63:3741–51.
2. Merker JD, Oxnard GR, Compton C, et al. Circulating tumor DNA analysis in patients with cancer: American Society of Clinical Oncology and College of American Pathologists Joint Review. J Clin Oncol 2018;36:1631–41.
3. Bass BP, Engel KB, Greytak SR, et al. A review of preanalytical factors affecting molecular, protein, and morphological analysis of formalin-fixed, paraffin-embedded (FFPE) tissue: how well do you know your FFPE specimen? Arch Pathol Lab Med 2014;138:1520–30.
4. Srinivasan M, Sedmak D, Jewell S. Effect of fixatives and tissue processing on the content and integrity of nucleic acids. Am J Pathol 2002;161:1961–71.
5. Merkelbach S, Gehlen J, Handt S, et al. Novel enzyme immunoassay and optimized DNA extraction for the detection of polymerase-chain-reaction-amplified viral DNA from paraffin-embedded tissue. Am J Pathol 1997;150:1537–46.
6. Sepp R, Szabo I, Uda H, et al. Rapid techniques for DNA extraction from routinely processed archival tissue for use in PCR. J Clin Pathol 1994;47:318–23.
7. Guerrera F, Tabbo F, Bessone L, et al. The influence of tissue ischemia time on RNA integrity and patient-derived xenografts (PDX) engraftment rate in a non-small cell lung cancer (NSCLC) biobank. PLoS One 2016;11:e0145100.
8. Greer CE, Peterson SL, Kiviat NB, et al. PCR amplification from paraffin-embedded tissues. Effects of fixative and fixation time. Am J Clin Pathol 1991;95:117–24.
9. Howat WJ, Wilson BA. Tissue fixation and the effect of molecular fixatives on downstream staining procedures. Methods 2014;70:12–9.
10. Ferruelo A, El-Assar M, Lorente JA, et al. Transcriptional profiling and genotyping of degraded nucleic acids from autopsy tissue samples after prolonged formalin fixation times. Int J Clin Exp Pathol 2011;4:156–61.
11. Jackson DP, Lewis FA, Taylor GR, et al. Tissue extraction of DNA and RNA and analysis by the polymerase chain reaction. J Clin Pathol 1990;43:499–504.
12. Layfield LJ, Roy-Chowdhuri S, Baloch Z, et al. Utilization of ancillary studies in the cytologic diagnosis of respiratory lesions: the papanicolaou society of cytopathology consensus recommendations for respiratory cytology. Diagn Cytopathol 2016;44:1000–9.
13. Roy-Chowdhuri S, Aisner DL, Allen TC, et al. Biomarker testing in lung carcinoma cytology specimens: a perspective from members of the pulmonary pathology society. Arch Pathol Lab Med 2016; 140:1267–72.
14. Coombs NJ, Gough AC, Primrose JN. Optimisation of DNA and RNA extraction from archival formalin-fixed tissue. Nucleic Acids Res 1999;27:e12.
15. Do H, Dobrovic A. Dramatic reduction of sequence artefacts from DNA isolated from formalin-fixed cancer biopsies by treatment with uracil-DNA glycosylase. Oncotarget 2012;3:546–58.
16. Funabashi KS, Barcelos D, Visona I, et al. DNA extraction and molecular analysis of non-tumoral liver, spleen, and brain from autopsy samples: the effect of formalin fixation and paraffin embedding. Pathol Res Pract 2012;208:584–91.
17. Gall K, Pavelic J, Jadro-Santel D, et al. DNA amplification by polymerase chain reaction from brain tissues embedded in paraffin. Int J Exp Pathol 1993; 74:333–7.
18. Hewett PJ, Firgaira F, Morley A. The influence of age of template DNA derived from archival tissue on the outcome of the polymerase chain reaction. Aust N Z J Surg 1994;64:558–9.
19. Talaulikar D, Shadbolt B, McNiven M, et al. DNA amplification from formalin-fixed decalcified paraffin-embedded bone marrow trephine specimens: does the duration of storage matter? Pathology 2008;40:702–6.
20. Viray H, Li K, Long TA, et al. A prospective, multi-institutional diagnostic trial to determine pathologist accuracy in estimation of percentage of malignant cells. Arch Pathol Lab Med 2013;137:1545–9.
21. Aisner DL, Rumery MD, Merrick DT, et al. Do more with less: tips and techniques for maximizing small biopsy and cytology specimens for molecular and ancillary testing: the university of colorado experience. Arch Pathol Lab Med 2016;140:1206–20.

22. Fend F, Raffeld M. Laser capture microdissection in pathology. J Clin Pathol 2000;53:666–72.

23. Lindeman NI, Cagle PT, Aisner DL, et al. Updated molecular testing guideline for the selection of lung cancer patients for treatment with targeted tyrosine kinase inhibitors: guideline from the College of American Pathologists, the International Association for the Study of Lung Cancer, and the Association for Molecular Pathology. J Mol Diagn 2018;20: 129–59.

24. Rolfo C, Mack PC, Scagliotti GV, et al. Liquid biopsy for advanced non-small cell lung cancer (NSCLC): a statement paper from the IASLC. J Thorac Oncol 2018;13:1248–68.

25. Mardis ER. Next-generation sequencing platforms. Annu Rev Anal Chem (Palo Alto Calif 2013;6: 287–303.

26. Strom SP. Current practices and guidelines for clinical next-generation sequencing oncology testing. Cancer Biol Med 2016;13:3–11.

27. Tewhey R, Bansal V, Torkamani A, et al. The importance of phase information for human genomics. Nat Rev Genet 2011;12:215–23.

28. Schmitt MW, Kennedy SR, Salk JJ, et al. Detection of ultra-rare mutations by next-generation sequencing. Proc Natl Acad Sci U S A 2012;109:14508–13.

29. Young AL, Wong TN, Hughes AE, et al. Quantifying ultra-rare pre-leukemic clones via targeted error-corrected sequencing. Leukemia 2015;29:1608–11.

30. Horak P, Frohling S, Glimm H. Integrating next-generation sequencing into clinical oncology: strategies, promises and pitfalls. ESMO Open 2016;1: e000094.

31. Wetterstrand KA. DNA sequencing costs: data from the NHGRI Genome Sequencing Program (GSP). Available at: www.genome.gov/sequencingcosts-data. Accessed April 15, 2021.

32. Wan TS. Cancer cytogenetics: methodology revisited. Ann Lab Med 2014;34:413–25.

33. Wolff AC, Hammond MEH, Allison KH, et al. Human epidermal growth factor receptor 2 testing in breast cancer: American Society of Clinical Oncology/College of American Pathologists Clinical Practice Guideline Focused Update. Arch Pathol Lab Med 2018;142:1364–82.

34. Bentz M, Cabot G, Moos M, et al. Detection of chimeric BCR-ABL genes on bone marrow samples and blood smears in chronic myeloid and acute lymphoblastic leukemia by in situ hybridization. Blood 1994;83:1922–8.

35. Veronese ML, Ohta M, Finan J, et al. Detection of myc translocations in lymphoma cells by fluorescence in situ hybridization with yeast artificial chromosomes. Blood 1995;85:2132–8.

36. Gonzales PR, Carroll AJ, Korf BR. Overview of clinical cytogenetics. Curr Protoc Hum Genet 2016;89: 8 1 1–8 1 13.

37. Granada I, Palomo L, Ruiz-Xiville N, et al. Cytogenetics in the genomic era. Best Pract Res Clin Haematol 2020;33:101196.

38. Milbury CA, Li J, Makrigiorgos GM. PCR-based methods for the enrichment of minority alleles and mutations. Clin Chem 2009;55:632–40.

39. Westbrook CA. The role of molecular techniques in the clinical management of leukemia. Lessons from the Philadelphia chromosome. Cancer 1992;70:1695–700.

40. Netto GJ, Saad RD, Dysert PA 2nd. Diagnostic molecular pathology: current techniques and clinical applications, part I. Proc (Bayl Univ Med Cent) 2003;16:379–83.

41. Sykes PJ, Neoh SH, Brisco MJ, et al. Quantitation of targets for PCR by use of limiting dilution. Biotechniques 1992;13:444–9.

42. Vogelstein B, Kinzler KW. Digital PCR. Proc Natl Acad Sci U S A 1999;96:9236–41.

43. Pohl G, Shih Ie M. Principle and applications of digital PCR. Expert Rev Mol Diagn 2004;4:41–7.

44. Liang Z, Cheng Y, Chen Y, et al. EGFR T790M ctDNA testing platforms and their role as companion diagnostics: Correlation with clinical outcomes to EGFR-TKIs. Cancer Lett 2017;403:186–94.

45. Voso MT, Ottone T, Lavorgna S, et al. MRD in AML: the role of new techniques. Front Oncol 2019;9:655.

46. Kurdyukov S, Bullock M. DNA methylation analysis: choosing the right method. Biology (Basel) 2016;5:3.

47. Bachman J. Reverse-transcription PCR (RT-PCR). Methods Enzymol 2013;530:67–74.

48. Gabert J, Beillard E, van der Velden VH, et al. Standardization and quality control studies of 'real-time' quantitative reverse transcriptase polymerase chain reaction of fusion gene transcripts for residual disease detection in leukemia - a Europe Against Cancer program. Leukemia 2003; 17:2318–57.

49. Takeuchi K, Choi YL, Soda M, et al. Multiplex reverse transcription-PCR screening for EML4-ALK fusion transcripts. Clin Cancer Res 2008;14:6618–24.

50. Gow CH, Hsieh MS, Wu SG, et al. A comprehensive analysis of clinical outcomes in lung cancer patients harboring a MET exon 14 skipping mutation compared to other driver mutations in an East Asian population. Lung Cancer 2017;103:82–9.

51. Glaysher S, Gabriel FG, Cree IA. Measuring gene expression from cell cultures by quantitative reverse-transcriptase polymerase chain reaction. Methods Mol Biol 2011;731:381–93.

52. Kurt H, Bueso-Ramos CE, Khoury JD, et al. Characterization of IDH1 p.R132H mutant clones using mutation-specific antibody in myeloid neoplasms. Am J Surg Pathol 2018;42:569–77.

53. Ritterhouse LL, Barletta JA. BRAF V600E mutation-specific antibody: a review. Semin Diagn Pathol 2015;32:400–8.

54. Yi ES, Boland JM, Maleszewski JJ, et al. Correlation of IHC and FISH for ALK gene rearrangement in non-small cell lung carcinoma: IHC score algorithm for FISH. J Thorac Oncol 2011;6:459–65.

55. Wu YC, Chang IC, Wang CL, et al. Comparison of IHC, FISH and RT-PCR methods for detection of ALK rearrangements in 312 non-small cell lung cancer patients in Taiwan. PLoS One 2013;8: e70839.

56. Dowsett M, Bartlett J, Ellis IO, et al. Correlation between immunohistochemistry (HercepTest) and fluorescence in situ hybridization (FISH) for HER-2 in 426 breast carcinomas from 37 centres. J Pathol 2003;199:418–23.

57. Hsiao SJ, Zehir A, Sireci AN, et al. Detection of tumor NTRK gene fusions to identify patients who may benefit from tyrosine kinase (TRK) inhibitor therapy. J Mol Diagn 2019;21:553–71.

Molecular Pathology of Lung Cancer

Sinchita Roy-Chowdhuri, MD, PhD

KEYWORDS

- Non–small-cell lung cancer • Adenocarcinoma • Molecular testing • Next-generation sequencing
- Biomarkers • Lung cancer

Key points

- Molecular testing is standard of care in the clinical management of advanced-stage non–small-cell lung cancer.
- Molecular testing in lung cancer is a rapidly evolving field.
- Guideline recommendations from professional organizations have outlined the requirements for molecular testing.
- Guideline recommendations from professional organizations provide guidance for biomarkers to test and how to test them.
- Awareness of testing requirements is critical to judiciously triage small specimens and provide adequate testing results.

ABSTRACT

The identification of targetable genomic alterations in lung cancer is required as standard of care to guide optimal therapy selection. With a constantly evolving landscape of ancillary molecular and biomarker testing in lung cancer, pathologists need to be aware of what specimens to test, how the testing should be performed, and which targets to test for to provide the clinically relevant genomic information necessary to treat these patients. Several guideline statements on the topic are currently available to help pathologists and laboratory personnel best use the small specimens obtained from patients with lung cancer for ancillary molecular testing.

OVERVIEW

Lung cancer remains the leading cause of cancer death in the United States.[1] Over the past few decades, the management of patients with lung cancer, particularly non–small cell lung cancer (NSCLC), has increasingly relied on characterizing the oncogenic genomic alterations and biomarker phenotype that drive targeted therapies.[2] The rapid pace of identifying key biomarkers that drive oncogenesis in these tumors has led to an unprecedented number of new approvals by the US Food and Drug Administration (FDA) for NSCLC therapy in the past 1 year.[3] With a growing list of biomarkers currently recommended for testing in NSCLC and with emerging therapeutics targeting additional alterations, the list of biomarker-driven therapeutic options has expanded exponentially in recent years with targeted inhibitors, antibody conjugates, and combination therapies showing significantly improved patient outcomes.

Of the clinical practice guidelines available for managing patients with NSCLC, the National Comprehensive Cancer Network (NCCN) clinical practice guidelines in oncology for NSCLC are the most frequently updated, widely adopted, and reflect the current standard of care for managing these patients.[4] The NCCN guidelines are also

---

Department of Pathology, The University of Texas MD Anderson Cancer Center, 1515 Holcombe Boulevard Unit 83, Houston, TX 77030, USA
E-mail address: sroy2@mdanderson.org

Surgical Pathology 14 (2021) 369–377
https://doi.org/10.1016/j.path.2021.05.002
1875-9181/21/© 2021 Elsevier Inc. All rights reserved.

used by the health care payers in the United States, including the Centers for Medicare and Medicaid Services, to determine their coverage policies for NSCLC and therefore have financial implications for molecular laboratories and their NSCLC testing practices. The list of biomarkers that needs to be assessed for NSCLC has rapidly grown from just *EGFR, Anaplastic Lymphoma Kinase (ALK),* and *proto-oncogene tyrosine protein kinase ROS (ROS1),* to now include *BRAF* mutations, *MET* exon 14 skipping mutations, *RET* and *NTRK* gene rearrangements, and programmed death (PD)-ligand 1 (L1) expression. Currently, most drug approvals are for the management of patients with advanced-stage disease; however, the promise of precision oncology is likely to drive biomarker testing into the realm of early-stage disease in the near future.

SPECIMENS FOR TESTING

The biggest strides in oncogenic characterization of lung cancer has been primarily in NSCLC, particularly lung adenocarcinomas. Therefore, the pathologic diagnosis based on morphologic and immunohistochemical (IHC) profiling is critical for decisions regarding biomarker testing for oncologic management. In general, it is considered standard of care to test all patients with advanced stage nonsquamous NSCLC for targetable alterations, whereas PD-L1 assessment by IHC is recommended in both patients with squamous carcinoma and those with adenocarcinoma.[4] However, due to the inherent limitation of adequately evaluating tumor heterogeneity in limited volume samples, such as cytology or small biopsy specimens, physicians may perform biomarker testing even in tumors that do not necessarily demonstrate an adenocarcinoma histology, if clinical features suggest a high probability of an oncogenic driver.[5]

Molecular testing is performed primarily on formalin-fixed paraffin-embedded (FFPE) tissue blocks of histology or cytology specimens; however, the updated College of American Pathologists (CAP), the International Association for the Study of Lung Cancer (IASLC), and the Association for Molecular Pathology (AMP) lung molecular testing guidelines and the CAP thoracic small specimen collection and handling for ancillary studies guideline recommend the use of any cytology specimen preparation (ie, non-FFPE material), provided the substrate has been appropriately validated.[5]

TESTING METHODOLOGY

In the past, molecular testing was performed using a single gene testing model, with separate tests for

each target. However, with a limited amount of tumor in small biopsy and cytology specimens, a single-gene, single-test approach is not compatible with the multitarget biomarker testing needed for patients with NSCLC.[6] Hence, most molecular testing laboratories are rapidly moving toward a multiplexed sequencing approach as the preferred testing modality over separate single-gene tests. High-throughput multigene molecular profiling platforms, such as next-generation sequencing (NGS), have been gaining popularity because of their ability to provide the breadth of genomic information required for standard of care therapy, as well as identify additional therapeutic targets for enrollment in clinical trials.[7–9] Besides NGS and sequencing-based testing, some genomic targets, such as *ALK* and *ROS1* rearrangements, can be tested using alternative techniques, including fluorescence in situ hybridization (FISH) and IHC.[5] Evaluation of PD-L1 is currently performed by IHC alone.[10]

BIOMARKERS FOR TESTING

A comprehensive genomic profiling has become increasingly necessary in patients with NSCLC to make an optimal therapeutic selection. The currently approved targeted therapies in advanced stage NSCLC include actionable alterations in *EGFR, ALK, ROS1, BRAF, MET, RET,* and *NTRK.*[4] With a growing list of potential therapeutic targets, including *ERBB2* and *KRAS* mutations, high-level *MET* amplification, tumor mutational burden, and several other emerging genomic alterations, completion of successful clinical trial results followed by rapid FDA drug approvals will likely expand the armamentarium of effective therapeutic options for these patients.

In recent years, the field of immunotherapy has emerged as a major therapeutic choice for NSCLC tumors that do not harbor a targetable driver mutation. The FDA-approved immune checkpoint inhibitor drugs for NSCLC that target the PD-1/PD-L1 axis have demonstrated superior response rate and patient survival as compared with conventional chemotherapy.[11,12]

Clinically relevant biomarkers in NSCLC are briefly described in the following section and summarized in **Table 1.**

EPIDERMAL GROWTH FACTOR RECEPTOR

The discovery of a subset of patients with NSCLC harboring mutations in the epidermal growth factor receptor (*EGFR*) gene that sensitize them to tyrosine kinase inhibitor (TKI) therapy has led to a paradigm shift in the management of these

Table 1
Guideline recommended biomarkers required for clinical management of non–small-cell lung cancer

Biomarker	Evidence Level	Testing Methodology	Therapeutic Agent
EGFR Mutation	Required	PCR-based assays Sequencing (Sanger, NGS)	First-line therapy • Afatinib • Erlotinib • Dacomitinib • Gefitinib • Osimertinib • Erlotinib + ramucirumab • Erlotinib + bevacizumab (nonsquamous) Subsequent therapy • Osimertinib
ALK rearrangement	Required	FISH break-apart probe assay IHC NGS Real-time PCR	First-line therapy • Alectinib • Brigatinib • Crizotinib • Ceritinib Subsequent therapy • Alectinib • Brigatinib • Ceritinib • Lorlatinib
ROS1 rearrangement	Required	FISH break-apart probe assay IHC, with confirmation if positive NGS Real time PCR	First-line therapy • Crizotinib • Ceritinib • Entrectinib Subsequent therapy • Lorlatinib
BRAF V600E Mutation	Required	PCR-based assays Sequencing (Sanger, NGS) IHC (limited data)	First-line therapy • Dabrafenib/trametinib
MET exon 14 skipping mutation	Required	NGS, preferably RNA based	First-line therapy • Capmatinib • Crizotinib
RET rearrangement	Required	NGS RT-PCR FISH	First-line therapy • Selpercatinib • Pralsetinib • Cabozantinib • Vandetanib

(*continued on next page*)

Table 1
(continued)

Biomarker	Evidence Level	Testing Methodology	Therapeutic Agent
PD-L1 ≥1%	Required	IHC	First-line therapy • Carboplatin or cisplatin/ pemetrexed + pembrolizumab (non-squamous) • Carboplatin + paclitaxel+bevacizumab+atezolizumab (non-squamous) • Carboplatin + albumin-bound paclitaxel + atezolizumab (nonsquamous) • Nivolumab + ipilimumab + pemetrexed + carboplatin or cisplatin (nonsquamous) • Carboplatin + paclitaxel or albumin-bound paclitaxel + pembrolizumab (squamous) • Nivolumab + ipilimumab + paclitaxel + carboplatin (squamous) • Pembrolizumab • Nivolumab + ipilimumab
PD-L1 ≥50%	Required	IHC	First-line therapy • Pembrolizumab • Carboplatin or cisplatin/ pemetrexed + pembrolizumab • Atezolizumab • Carboplatin + paclitaxel+bevacizumab+atezolizumab (nonsquamous) • Carboplatin + albumin-bound paclitaxel + atezolizumab (nonsquamous) • Nivolumab + ipilimumab + pemetrexed + carboplatin or cisplatin • Nivolumab + ipilimumab
NTRK rearrangement	Required[a]	NGS, preferably RNA based FISH for *NTRK 1/2/3* IHC	First-line therapy • Larotrectinib • Entrectinib
ERBB2 (HER2) mutation	Emerging[a]	NGS (as part of broad molecular profiling))	• Trastuzumab • Afatinib
KRAS mutation	Emerging[a]	PCR-based assays NGS (as part of broad molecular profiling)	• Sotorasib
High level *MET* amplification	Emerging	NGS IHC FISH	• Crizotinib
Tumor mutational burden (TMB)	Emerging[a]	NGS	• Nivolumab + ipilimumab • Nivolumab

Based on National Comprehensive Cancer Network Guidelines for non–small-cell lung cancer version 2.2021.
   Abbreviations: FISH, fluorescence in situ hybridization; IHC, immunohistochemistry; NGS, next-generation sequencing; PCR, polymerase chain reaction; PD-L1, programmed death–ligand 1; RT, reverse transcriptase.
   [a] Recommended as part of a broad molecular profiling panel.

patients.[13–15] Oncogenic driver mutations in *EGFR* localize to the tyrosine kinase domain, with approximately 85% of activating mutations seen as deletions in exon 19 and a point mutation (L858R) in exon 21. TKI therapy, including erlotinib, gefitinib, and afatinib, has shown efficacy in treating patients harboring sensitizing *EGFR* mutations.[16] Disease progression is frequently seen, most often secondary to the acquisition of a resistance mutation (T790M) in exon 20 that is treated with osimertinib, a third-generation *EGFR* TKI.[17] Although osimertinib has shown documented efficacy in both first-line and second-line settings, patients inevitably develop resistance, encompassing *EGFR*-dependent as well as *EGFR*-independent mechanisms including *MET* and *ERBB2* amplification, activation of the RAS-mitogen-activated protein kinase (MAPK) or RAS-phosphatidylinositol 3-kinase (PI3K) pathways, novel fusion events, and histologic transformation to small cell carcinoma.[18] Mutation testing for *EGFR* is recommended by polymerase chain reaction (PCR)-based sequencing techniques using assays that are able to detect mutations in samples with as low as 20% tumor content.[19]

ALK

In approximately 4% to 5% patients with NSCLC, *ALK* can undergo gene fusion, most frequently with *EML4*, leading to a constitutively active EML4-ALK fusion protein driving oncogenesis. Several approved oral TKIs, including crizotinib, alectinib, and ceritinib, have shown efficacy in treating patients whose tumors harbor an *ALK* gene rearrangement.[20,21] Conventionally, biomarker testing for *ALK* gene rearrangements have used FISH break-apart probes for detecting *ALK* rearrangements; however, IHC assays using ALK 5A4 and D5F3 monoclonal antibodies have been FDA approved and can be used an equivalent alternative to *ALK* FISH.[19] As with *EGFR*-mutated tumors, resistance mechanisms, either due to *ALK* kinase secondary mutations or *ALK*-independent mechanisms eventually develop in these patients requiring switching to second-generation or third-generation *ALK* TKIs, such as lorlatinib.

ROS1

ROS1 gene rearrangements are seen in 1% to 2% of patients with NSCLC. Although gene partners for *ROS1* can vary (most commonly *CD74*, *SLC34A2*, *CCDC6*, and *FIG*), the resulting constitutively active kinase signaling of the ROS1 fusion protein drives oncogenesis in these tumors and responds dramatically to crizotinib, currently approved by the FDA as first-line treatment in these tumors.[22] Testing for *ROS1* fusions are performed either by FISH break-apart probes, reverse transcriptase (RT)-PCR for known fusion partners of *ROS1*, or ROS1 IHC using the D4D6 antibody clone. However, a positive ROS1 result by IHC requires confirmation by a molecular/cytogenetic method.[19] Resistance to crizotinib eventually develops in patients with *ROS1*-rearranged tumors, and subsequent sequencing-based testing may be used to identify secondary resistance mutations that can be treated with other TKIs, such as lorlatinib.

BRAF

BRAF mutations are seen in 1% to 2% patients with NSCLC, with the V600E point mutation being the most commonly encountered alteration seen in these patients. Patients who harbor a *BRAF* V600E mutation are eligible for the FDA-approved dual dabrafenib (*BRAF* inhibitor) and trametinib (*MEK* inhibitor) therapy.[4] Although the CAP/IASLC/AMP testing guidelines do not recommend *BRAF* molecular testing as a routine stand-alone assay outside of testing it as part of a larger testing panel, the American Society of Clinical Oncology (ASCO) endorsement of these guidelines and the NCCN guidelines include *BRAF* in the current recommendations for advanced stage NSCLC biomarker testing.[4,23] *BRAF* testing is usually performed using PCR/sequencing based methods. BRAF IHC using the VE1 clone may be an alternative testing option, although the published literature on the use of BRAF VE1 IHC in lung cancer is limited.

MET

Genomic alterations in NSCLC for *MET* include gene amplification, activating point mutations, or splice mutations such as the exon 14 skipping mutation.[24–26] The FDA recently approved capmatinib therapy for patients with *MET* exon 14 skipping mutations and is currently included in the NCCN guidelines as a recommended biomarker for patients with NSCLC.[4,27] *MET* exon 14 testing is usually performed as part of an expanded NGS panel, due to complexity of exon 14 splice sites. *MET* amplification can be tested via FISH or IHC.

RET

RET gene fusions in NSCLC can involve multiple gene targets leading to a constitutive activation of the *RET* signaling pathways. The FDA has approved selpercatinib and pralsetinib for patients with RET fusion positive advanced stage

NSCLC.[25,28] Testing for *RET* rearrangements may be performed by FISH or RT-PCR; however, NGS-based testing as part of an expanded fusion panel is gaining popularity.

NTRK

NTRK fusions are seen in fewer than 1% of patients with NSCLC and multiple fusion partners have been identified.[29–32] The FDA has approved larotrectinib and entrectinib as first-line therapy in any patients with solid tumor *NTRK* fusions, and the NCCN guidelines include a section recommending evaluating *NTRK* fusions in their testing algorithm.[4,33] Testing methodologies may include FISH, IHC, and/or NGS-based assays.

PROGRAMMED DEATH–LIGAND 1

Immune checkpoint inhibitor therapy has emerged as a major therapeutic choice for tumors that do not harbor a targetable driver mutation. PD-L1 biomarker testing relies on the assessment of PD-L1 expression by IHC on tumor cells using a tumor proportion score (TPS) to determine which patients are most likely to respond to immune checkpoint inhibitor therapy.[34–36] Currently, there are a number of immune checkpoint inhibitor drugs for NSCLC that are FDA approved or in clinical trials, with a paired assay comprising a different antibody clone and an associated staining platform, with different clinical cutoff definitions of positivity that qualify for immune checkpoint inhibitor therapy. The NCCN guidelines recommend testing advanced stage NSCLC using IHC evaluation.[4]

ERBB2

Emerging biomarkers for NSCLC include *ERBB2* (*HER2*) mutations that may be susceptible to targeted therapy that are currently being evaluated in clinical trials. Clinical trials are ongoing for treating NSCLC with *ERBB2* mutations with targeted agents including trastuzumab and afatinib.[4] Currently *ERBB2* mutation testing in NSCLC is largely PCR/sequencing based, and is focused on sequence alterations, specifically insertions and duplications in exon 20.

KRAS

Mutations in the *KRAS* gene are much more common in patients with NSCLC and seen in approximately 15% to 25% of patients. Although there are currently no specific FDA-approved targetable therapies for *KRAS*-mutated NSCLCs, emerging data from clinical trials have shown promising results using sotorasib in *KRAS* G12C-mutated lung tumors.[37] Testing for *KRAS* mutations is generally done via PCR/NGS-based methods but testing is currently not recommended by NCCN guidelines.

EMERGING TARGETS

With the use of expanded platforms interrogating NSCLC tumors, the list of rare genomic alterations continues to grow.[5] Although the clinical significance of these alterations may not be entirely clear at this time, ongoing preclinical and clinical trials will continue to identify potential actionable targeted therapeutics for these tumors with rare alterations.

The reality of lung cancer molecular testing is the rapid pace of discovery of novel therapeutic targets and the complexity of providing this genomic information in a timely fashion that aligns with the clinical management of these patients. The clinical practice guidelines, such as the NCCN, recommend the use of expanded multiplexed panels for molecular profiling, thus encouraging a shift from single-gene assays to larger NGS panels to provide the most effective and efficient way to identify clinically relevant biomarkers from limited volume specimens. The judicious use of the tissue specimen for diagnostic workup and subsequent biomarker testing is critical for patients with NSCLC, as oncologic management relies heavily on the adequacy of the tissue for all clinically relevant and guideline recommended biomarker testing.[38] However, even with the increasing use of multiplexed genomic profiling that offers a more tissue-conserving approach, 10% to 20% of small specimens remain inadequate for comprehensive testing.[39,40] Although most molecular laboratories perform biomarker testing on traditional FFPE tissue blocks, mounting evidence shows that non-FFPE specimens such as cytology direct smears, liquid-based cytology, and even specimen supernatants can be used for NGS testing, if properly validated.[6,41–44] Including additional specimen substrates can increase the molecular adequacy of small specimens used for biomarker testing. For patients in whom tissue is inadequate for lung cancer biomarker testing, options include repeat biopsy/sampling in an attempt to collect sufficient tumor tissue. However, not all patients may be amenable for repeat biopsy, and therefore, the use of liquid biopsies that use NGS to evaluate circulating tumor DNA from plasma as a surrogate for tumoral genomic profiling is gaining popularity.[45,46] Plasma-based biomarker testing has limited sensitivity and current clinical practice guidelines recommend using liquid biopsy as an alternative only when tissue-based testing is not feasible/available,[5] but with the clinical and technological advances in the field of biomarker testing, it is conceivable that the use of liquid biopsies will expand in the day-to-day clinical practice for NSCLC management.

SUMMARY

The identification of genomic alterations that play a role in lung cancer oncogenesis that can be treated with targeted therapeutics has been a paradigm shift in the management of these patients. Despite the clinical success of these targeted therapies in these patients, only a fraction of eligible patients with NSCLC worldwide currently have access to guideline-specified mandatory biomarker testing. Therefore, a multidisciplinary effort will be needed to optimize the adequate collection of tumor tissue for diagnosis and biomarker testing, to maximize the value of precision oncology for all patients who stand to benefit from these therapies.

CLINICS CARE POINTS

- The identification of genomic alterations in lung cancer targeted therapeutics has been a paradigm shift in the management of patients.

- While guideline recommendations have outlined the requirements for molecular testing, only a fraction of eligible patients with NSCLC worldwide currently have access to biomarker testing.

- A multidisciplinary effort to optimize the adequate collection of tumor tissue for diagnosis and biomarker testing is needed to treat all patients who stand to benefit from these therapies.

DISCLOSURE

The authors have nothing to disclose.

REFERENCES

1. National Cancer Institute (NIH), Surveillance, Epidemiology, and End Results Program (SEER). Cancer stat facts: lung and bronchus cancer, statistics at a glance. NIH SEER Web site. Available at: http://seer.cancer.gov/statfacts/html/lungb.html. Accessed April 6, 2020.

2. VanderLaan PA, Rangachari D, Costa DB. The rapidly evolving landscape of biomarker testing in non-small cell lung cancer. Cancer Cytopathol 2021;129(3):179–81.

3. Available at: https://www.fda.gov/drugs/resources-information-approved-drugs/hematologyoncology-cancer-approvals-safety-notifications. Accessed November 15, 2020.

4. National Comprehensive Cancer Network Clinical Practice Guidelines in Oncology (NCCN Guidelines). Non-small cell lung cancer, version 2.2021. Available at: https://www.nccn.org/professionals/physician_gls/pdf/nscl.pdf assessed 3/19/2021. Accessed March 19, 2021.

5. Lindeman NI, Cagle PT, Aisner DL, et al. Updated molecular testing guideline for the selection of lung cancer patients for treatment with targeted tyrosine kinase inhibitors: guideline from the College of American Pathologists, the International Association for the Study of Lung Cancer, and the Association for Molecular Pathology. Arch Pathol Lab Med 2018; 142(3):321–46.

6. Roy-Chowdhuri S, Pisapia P, Salto-Tellez M, et al. Invited review-next-generation sequencing: a modern tool in cytopathology. Virchows Arch 2019; 475(1):3–11.

7. Suh JH, Johnson A, Albacker A, et al. Comprehensive genomic profiling facilitates implementation of the national comprehensive cancer network guidelines for lung cancer biomarker testing and identifies patients who may benefit from enrollment in mechanism-driven clinical trials. Oncologist 2016; 21(6):684–91.

8. Jordan EJ, Kim HR, Arcila ME, et al. Prospective comprehensive molecular characterization of lung adenocarcinomas for efficient patient matching to approved and emerging therapies. Cancer Discov 2017;7(6):596–609.

9. Cancer Genome Atlas Research, Network. Comprehensive molecular profiling of lung adenocarcinoma. Nature 2014;511(7511):543–50.

10. Kerr KM, Tsao MS, Nicholson AG, et al. Programmed death-ligand 1 immunohistochemistry in lung cancer: in what state is this art? J Thorac Oncol 2015; 10(7):985–9.

11. Garon EB, Rizvi NA, Hui R, et al. Pembrolizumab for the treatment of non-small-cell lung cancer. N Engl J Med 2015;372(21):2018–28.

12. Rizvi NA, Hellmann MD, Snyder A, et al. Cancer immunology. Mutational landscape determines sensitivity to PD-1 blockade in non-small cell lung cancer. Science 2015;348(6230):124–8.

13. Lynch TJ, Bell DW, Sordella R, et al. Activating mutations in the epidermal growth factor receptor underlying responsiveness of non-small-cell lung cancer to gefitinib. N Engl J Med 2004;350(21): 2129–39.

14. Paez JG, Janne PA, Lee JC, et al. EGFR mutations in lung cancer: correlation with clinical response to gefitinib therapy. Science 2004;304(5676):1497–500.

15. Pao W, Miller V, Zakowski M, et al. EGF receptor gene mutations are common in lung cancers from "never smokers" and are associated with sensitivity of tumors to gefitinib and erlotinib. Proc Natl Acad Sci U S A 2004;101(36):13306–11.

16. Reck M, Rabe KF. Precision diagnosis and treatment for advanced non-small-cell lung cancer. N Engl J Med 2017;377(9):849–61.

17. Pao W, Miller VA, Politi KA, et al. Acquired resistance of lung adenocarcinomas to gefitinib or erlotinib is associated with a second mutation in the EGFR kinase domain. PLoS Med 2005;2(3):e73.

18. Leonetti A, Sharma S, Minari R, et al. Resistance mechanisms to osimertinib in EGFR-mutated non-small cell lung cancer. Br J Cancer 2019;121(9):725–37.

19. Lindeman NI, Cagle PT, Aisner DL, et al. Updated molecular testing guideline for the selection of lung cancer patients for treatment with targeted tyrosine kinase inhibitors: guideline from the College of American Pathologists, the International Association for the Study of Lung Cancer, and the Association for Molecular Pathology. J Thorac Oncol 2018;13(3):323–58.

20. de Mello RA, Neves NM, Tadokoro H, et al. New target therapies in advanced non-small cell lung cancer: a review of the literature and future perspectives. J Clin Med 2020;9(11):3543.

21. Arbour KC, Riely GJ. Systemic therapy for locally advanced and metastatic non-small cell lung cancer: a review. JAMA 2019;322(8):764–74.

22. Sequist LV. ROS1-targeted therapy in non-small cell lung cancer. Clin Adv Hematol Oncol 2012;10(12):827–8.

23. Kalemkerian GP, Narula N, Kennedy EB, et al. Molecular testing guideline for the selection of patients with lung cancer for treatment with targeted tyrosine kinase inhibitors: American Society of Clinical Oncology Endorsement of the College of American Pathologists/International Association for the Study of Lung Cancer/Association for molecular pathology clinical practice guideline update. J Clin Oncol 2018;36(9):911–9.

24. Kris MG, Arenberg DA, Herbst RS, et al. Emerging science and therapies in non-small-cell lung cancer: targeting the MET pathway. Clin Lung Cancer 2014;15(6):475.

25. Drilon A, Cappuzzo F, Ignatius Ou S-H, et al. Targeting MET in lung cancer: will expectations finally be MET? J Thorac Oncol 2017;12(1):15–26.

26. Yap TA, Popat S. Targeting MET Exon 14 skipping alterations: has lung cancer MET its match? J Thorac Oncol 2017;12(1):12–4.

27. Wolf J, Seto T, Han JY, et al. Capmatinib in MET Exon 14-mutated or MET-amplified non-small-cell lung cancer. N Engl J Med 2020;383(10):944–57.

28. Wright KM. FDA approves pralsetinib for treatment of adults with metastatic RET fusion-positive NSCLC. Oncology (Williston Park) 2020;34(10), 406-406;431.

29. Farago AF, Taylor MS, Doebele RC, et al. Clinicopathologic features of non-small-cell lung cancer harboring an NTRK gene fusion. JCO Precis Oncol 2018;2018:PO.18.00037.

30. Vaishnavi A, Le AT, Doebele RC. TRKing down an old oncogene in a new era of targeted therapy. Cancer Discov 2015;5(1):25–34.

31. Farago AF, Le LP, Zheng Z, et al. Durable clinical response to entrectinib in NTRK1-rearranged non-small cell lung cancer. J Thorac Oncol 2015;10(12):1670–4.

32. Vaishnavi A, Capeletti M, Le AT, et al. Oncogenic and drug-sensitive NTRK1 rearrangements in lung cancer. Nat Med 2013;19(11):1469–72.

33. Roth JA, Carlson JJ, Xia F, et al. The potential long-term comparative effectiveness of larotrectinib and entrectinib for second-line treatment of TRK fusion-positive metastatic lung cancer. J Manag Care Spec Pharm 2020;26(8):981–6.

34. Hirsch FR, McElhinny A, Stanforth D, et al. PD-L1 immunohistochemistry assays for lung cancer: results from phase 1 of the blueprint PD-L1 IHC assay comparison project. J Thorac Oncol 2017;12(2):208–22.

35. Lantuejoul S, Tsao MS, Cooper W, et al. PD-L1 testing for lung cancer in 2019: perspective from the IASLC pathology committee. J Thorac Oncol 2020;15(4):499–519.

36. Tsao MS, Kerr KM, Dacic S, et al. IASLC Atlas of PD-L1 IASLC Atlas of PD-L1 Immunohistochemistry Testing in Lung Cancer. 1st edition. International Association for the Study of Lung Cancer Denver, Colorado; 2017.

37. Hong DS, Fakih MG, Strickler JH, et al. KRAS(G12C) inhibition with sotorasib in advanced solid tumors. N Engl J Med 2020;383(13):1207–17.

38. Roy-Chowdhuri S, Dacic S, Ghofrani M, et al. Collection and handling of thoracic small biopsy and cytology specimens for ancillary studies: guideline from the College of American Pathologists in Collaboration with the American College of Chest Physicians, Association for Molecular Pathology, American Society of Cytopathology, American Thoracic Society, Pulmonary Pathology Society, Papanicolaou Society of Cytopathology, Society of Interventional Radiology, and Society of Thoracic Radiology. Arch Pathol Lab Med 2020;144(8):933–58.

39. Tam AL, Kim ES, Lee JJ, et al. Feasibility of image-guided transthoracic core-needle biopsy in the BATTLE lung trial. J Thorac Oncol 2013;8(4):436–42.

40. Sabir SH, Krishnamurthy S, Gupta S, et al. Characteristics of percutaneous core biopsies adequate for next generation genomic sequencing. PLoS One 2017;12(12):e0189651.

41. Rekhtman N, Roy-Chowdhuri S. Cytology specimens: a goldmine for molecular testing. Arch Pathol Lab Med 2016;140(11):1189–90.

42. Troncone G, Roy-Chowdhuri S. Key issues in molecular cytopathology. Arch Pathol Lab Med 2018; 142(3):289–90.

43. VanderLaan PA, Roy-Chowdhuri S. Current and future trends in non-small cell lung cancer biomarker testing: the American experience. Cancer Cytopathol 2020;128(9):629–36.

44. Roy-Chowdhuri S. Molecular testing of residual cytology samples: rethink, reclaim, repurpose. Cancer Cytopathol 2019;127(1):15–7.

45. Malapelle U, Pisapia P, Rocco D, et al. Next generation sequencing techniques in liquid biopsy: focus on non-small cell lung cancer patients. Transl Lung Cancer Res 2016;5(5):505–10.

46. Sholl LM, Aisner DL, Allen TC, et al. Liquid biopsy in lung cancer: a perspective from members of the pulmonary pathology society. Arch Pathol Lab Med 2016;140(8):825–9.

Molecular Pathology of Gliomas

Kristyn Galbraith, MD, Matija Snuderl, MD*

KEYWORDS

- IDH1/2 mutation • ATRX mutation • Histone H3 K27M mutation • 1p19q loss • BRAF fusion
- BRAF V600E mutation

Key points

- Isocitrate dehydrogenase 1/2 (IDH1/2) mutation status and 1p19q chromosomal arms status are critical for accurate classification of diffuse gliomas in adults.
- IDH1/2-mutated tumors have significantly better outcome than wild-type tumors.
- Diagnosis of glioblastoma can be based on characteristic molecular features alone in the absence of diagnostic histologic features.
- High-grade pediatric gliomas are characterized by histone H3 mutations with K27M or G34 mutations.
- Pediatric low-grade gliomas show MAPK pathway alterations most often via BRAF gene fusions or point mutations.

ABSTRACT

Gliomas are the most common adult and pediatric primary brain tumors. Molecular studies have identified features that can enhance diagnosis and provide biomarkers. *IDH1/2* mutation with *ATRX* and *TP53* mutations defines diffuse astrocytomas, whereas *IDH1/2* mutations with 1p19q loss defines oligodendroglioma. Focal amplifications of receptor tyrosine kinase genes, *TERT* promoter mutation, and loss of chromosomes 10 and 13 with trisomy of chromosome 7 are characteristic features of glioblastoma and can be used for diagnosis. *BRAF* gene fusions and mutations in low-grade gliomas and histone H3 mutations in high-grade gliomas also can be used for diagnostics.

OVERVIEW

Although primary central nervous system (CNS) tumors account for only 2% of all primary cancers, they cause 7% of deaths from cancer in those younger than 70 years old.[1] Median age of primary brain tumors is approximately 60 years and gliomas represent approximately 26% of all primary CNS tumors. Brain tumors are the second most common cancers in children 0 to 14 years old and a leading cause of cancer-related deaths in pediatric population. Gliomas biologically vary from relatively benign, slow growing, and well-demarcated to aggressive rapidly proliferating and diffusely infiltrative tumors. The category of glioma includes tumors originating from the glial cells of the CNS, including astrocytomas, oligodendrogliomas, in both molecular classification has changed the practice of pathology significantly.[2] Until recently, the classification of glioma has been based predominantly on histopathology, based on the resemblance of tumor cells to their presumed normal counterparts. The advance of molecular techniques has allowed for more precise classification of these tumors than before the 2016 World Health Organization (WHO) classification of CNS tumors.[3] Remarkable progress in

Department of Pathology, NYU Langone Medical Center, 240 East 38th Street, 22nd Floor, New York, NY 10016, USA
* Corresponding author.
E-mail address: Matija.Snuderl@nyulangone.org

Surgical Pathology 14 (2021) 379–386
https://doi.org/10.1016/j.path.2021.05.003
1875-9181/21/© 2021 Elsevier Inc. All rights reserved.

genome-wide genetic and epigenetic studies now enables more accurate classification of histologically similar-appearing tumors and disappearance of mixed and descriptive categories. In addition, mutation-specific antibodies enable diagnosis of the most critical mutations in situ.[4] The purpose of this review is to focus on the relevant molecular findings in gliomas and discuss how molecular classification has an impact on pathologic diagnosis and clinical management. In comparison with histopathology, molecular features also provide prognostic biomarkers predicting the natural progression of disease as well as predicting response to the therapy. A variety of molecular methods can be used for classification of gliomas. Although rapid development of large-scale molecular testing allows for extensive in-depth analysis using machine learning,[3] a basic but critical classification can be achieved by using immunohistochemical[4] and targeted molecular approaches.

DIFFERENTIAL DIAGNOSIS

Differential diagnosis of gliomas often can be achieved by combining clinical and imaging features before performing molecular studies. This is because, compared with other cancers, there is a striking correlation between age, location, and the molecular genetics of brain tumor, including gliomas.[5] Diffuse gliomas of small children tend to be located in the midline and carry histone H3 K27M mutation. On the contrary, more benign pediatric gliomas are driven by MAPK pathway alterations, most frequently *BRAF* gene fusion or point mutation, and are located either in the cerebellum or the optic pathway. Older children develop malignant hemispheric gliomas with histone H3 G34 mutation whereas slow-growing cortical tumors tend again to be driven by *BRAF* mutations and have well-demarcated growth. Young adults develop diffuse astrocytomas with a triple hit of *Isocitrate dehydrogenase 1/2 (IDH1/2)*, *TP53*, and *ATRX* mutations, which have to occur in an exact sequence.[6] Alternatively, *IDH1/2* mutation affects cells in a combination with a 1p19q chromosomal arm loss characteristic for oligodendroglioma. Oligodendrogliomas arise most frequently in the frontal lobe and are slow growing with calcifications. In older adults, greater than 60 years old, tumors are IDH–wild-type diffuse gliomas driven largely by copy number alterations and receptor tyrosine kinase (RTK), PI3K/PTEN/AKT and Rb pathway alterations. IDH-mutant and IDH–wild-type tumors also show striking differences in regards to clinical presentation, such as blood clotting and seizures. IDH-mutant tumors present more frequently with seizures and have lower risk of abnormal blood

clotting whereas IDH–wild-type diffuse gliomas have a high risk of thromboembolic complications.[7,8]

MOLECULAR PATHOLOGY FEATURES

DIFFUSE GLIOMA IDH-MUTANT

The discovery of *IDH1/2* mutations revolutionized understanding of glioma biology and upended a traditional grading system for diffuse gliomas.[9,10] *IDH1/2*-mutant astrocytomas are more likely to occur in younger adults and are associated with a better prognosis matching for grade than their IDH–wild-type counterparts. Studies have shown a significant association between *ATRX* and *TP53* mutations in *IDH1/2*-mutant gliomas. This close association suggests that the *ATRX* alterations are needed with *TP53* mutations in IDH-mutant astrocytomas to promote oncogenesis in adult gliomas.[6,11] In addition, studies have shown that MGMT promoter methylation is associated with IDH1 and TP53 mutations.[12] IDH-mutant and IDH–wild-type tumors represent distinct entities requiring a different grading system than the historically histologic grading.[13] The Consortium to Inform Molecular and Practical Approaches to CNS Tumor Taxonomy-Not Official WHO (working group has integrated the molecular features and proposed an integrated classification system, where IDH-mutant astrocytomas[14] are classified as

- Astrocytoma, IDH-mutant, WHO grade 2
  - Lacks anaplasia, has low mitotic activity, and does not have microvascular proliferation or necrosis
- Astrocytoma, IDH-mutant, WHO grade 3
  - Has anaplasia and significant mitotic activity but does not have microvascular proliferation or necrosis
- Astrocytoma, IDH-mutant, WHO grade 4
  - Microvascular proliferation or necrosis OR CDKN2A/B homozygous deletion

The *CDKN2A/B* homozygous deletion was incorporated into the grade 4 designation due to its strong association with shorter survival in patients with IDH-mutant astrocytomas. The recommendation was to not maintain the name glioblastoma (GBM) for IDH-mutated grade IV tumors.

Oligodendrogliomas are a subset of diffuse glioma, predominantly seen in the cerebral hemispheres of patients ages 50 years to 60 years old. They are classified by the WHO as grade 2 or grade 3 tumors. Studies have shown that one of the initial events in tumorigenesis of oligodendrogliomas is the acquisition of the mutation in IDH1/2, even before the loss of 1p/19q.[15] The mutation in *IDH1* or *IDH2* is followed by the codeletion of 1p/19q, required for the diagnosis of oligodendroglioma by the 2016 WHO classification. The codeletion of 1p/19q likely is associated with concurrent inactivating mutations of *FUBP1* and *CIC*, tumor suppressor genes on chromosomes 1p and 19q, respectively. A combination of *FUBP1* and *CIC* mutations is unique for oligodendrogliomas and these rarely are seen in other CNS tumors.[16] Additional mutations in oligodendrogliomas include *TERT* promoter mutations seen in approximately 80% of tumors and are mutually exclusive with *ATRX* mutations. The loss of 1p19q has been a defining feature of oligodendrogliomas.[17] Although a majority of tumors show a simple loss with 2 chromosomal arms of 1q, 1 arm of 1p, and 2 chromosomal arms of 19p and 1 arm of 19q, some tumors show a concurrent loss with a polysomy and variable ratio of 1p:1q and 19p:19q (2:4, 3:6, and so forth). This so-called relative loss, or superloss, has been associated with rapid progression.[18] The loss of 1p/19q with concurrent polysomy has been associated with adverse outcomes, younger age at disease onset, higher histologic tumor grade, and poor progression-free survival and overall survival. Recently a large multi-institutional study of 333 cases confirmed negative impact of polysomy on survival.[19] Loss of *CDKN2A/B* and *PIK3CA* alterations in oligodendroglioma also occasionally are present in high-grade tumors.

A strong association between *IDH1/2* with either *ATRX/TP53* in astrocytoma or with 1p19q loss in oligodendroglioma resulted in a diminished number of diffuse gliomas that could not be classified and would require a histologic diagnosis of oligoastrocytoma. A diagnosis of oligoastrocytoma is rarely supported molecularly[20] and in general is not recommended.[21]

Immunohistochemistry can be utilized readily for detection of the *IDH1* R132H mutation (**Figs. 1A** and **2A**), which is present in 80% to 90% of IDH-mutant gliomas using a mutation-specific antibody.[4] Other *IDH1/2* mutations are less common yet prognostically equally important and require detection by gene sequencing. Immunohistochemistry also can be used to aid in the detection of loss of *ATRX* expression (**Fig. 1B**) and strong p53 staining can suggest mutations in *TP53* (**Fig. 1C**); however, the commonly used antibodies are not mutation-specific and may require genetic confirmation. Assessment of 1p and 19q status is well-established across laboratories. Fluorescence in situ hybridization (FISH) (**Fig. 2B, C**), polymerase chain reaction loss of heterozygosity,

next-generation sequencing or genotyping, and methylation arrays (**Fig. 2D**) all can provide 1p19q status. In analysis of 1p19q arms, it is important to assess for loss of the entire arms of chromosomes 1p and 19q because isolated 19q loss is common in astrocytomas and focal loss of 1p frequently is seen in IDH–wild-type GBM.

DIFFUSE GLIOMA IDH–WILD-TYPE

Adult diffuse gliomas lacking *IDH1/2* mutation represent the most aggressive type of CNS gliomas. Although histology of GBM represents a majority of these tumors, studies have shown that there is a subset of histologically classified WHO grade II or grade III IDH–wild-type diffuse astrocytic gliomas that have poor survival similar to that seen in histologic GBM.[12] GBM is the most common primary malignant brain tumor of adults. *IDH1/2*–wild-type GBMs typically occur in older adults and carry a poor prognosis despite the most aggressive treatment. Most of the tumors are sporadic; however, GBMs are seen in variety of syndromes, such as Li-Fraumeni syndrome, Turcot syndrome, and neurofibromatosis type 1. GBMs are characterized by focal amplifications of RTK genes, including *PDGFRA*, *MET*, and *EGFR*, which is the most frequent driver, amplified in up to 40% of GBM.[22,23] EGFR amplification often is accompanied by EGFRvIII (EGFR variant III), a rearrangement with deletion of exons 2 to 7. Other molecular features include *TERT* promoter mutations, trisomy of chromosome 7, and loss of chromosome 10 with *PTEN* and chromosome 13 (*Rb*) whereas *TP53* mutations are less frequent. This allows for molecular diagnostics in tumors where histologic criteria are not definitive (**Fig. 1D**).

The cIMPACT-NOW update 3 proposed a class of a molecular GBM for tumors histologically classified as a lower grade but showing molecular features of a GBM. Studies have found that WHO grade II or grade III astrocytomas with *EGFR* amplification, *TERT* promoter mutation, or combined whole chromosome 7 gain and whole chromosome 10 loss (+7/−10) follow an aggressive course with shorter patient survival than other WHO grade II or grade III astrocytomas, similar to that of an IDH–wild-type GBM.[24] *CDKN2A/B* homozygous deletions frequently are seen with these so-called molecular GBMs.[24] A majority of IDH–wild-type infiltrating astrocytomas are primary GBMs, meaning they occur de novo without a precursor lesion.

Molecularly, tumors can be subclassified further either by RNA expression or DNA methylation[3] into several distinct groups, of which proneural,

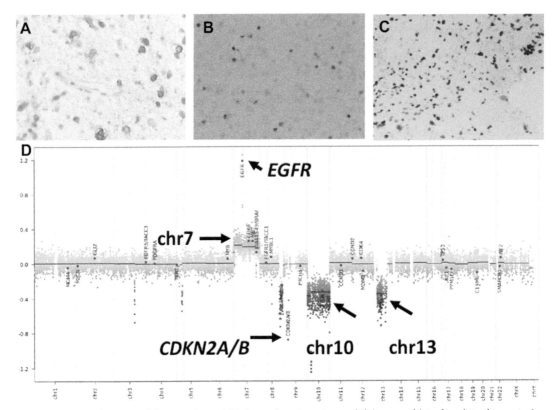

Fig. 1. Molecular features of low-grade and high-grade astrocytoma: (*A*) immunohistochemistry by mutation-specific antibodies for IDH1 R132H shows strong positivity in tumor cells, (Original magnification ×200) and (*B*) immunohistochemistry for ATRX loss shows loss in infiltrating glioma cells with preserved expression in the normal glial cells and neurons (Original magnification ×200). (*C*) Immunohistochemistry for p53 shows strong nuclear stain suggestive of a mutation. This triad is characteristic of an IDH-mutant glioma (Original magnification ×200). (*D*) Molecular features of IDH–wild-type astrocytoma, GBM include trisomy of chromosome 7 with focal amplification of EGFR, homozygous deletion of CDKN2A/B, and monosomy of chromosomes 10 and 13. The presence of these molecular features is diagnostic of GBM even in the absence of the high grade histologic features.

mesenchymal, and classic GBM are best characterized.[25] Although there may be some prognostic value, it is less striking than the effect of *IDH1/2* and 1p19q alterations. On the contrary, MGMT promoter methylation remains a powerful biomarker predicting response, albeit only short-lived, to adjuvant temozolomide and radiation therapy.[26,27]

PEDIATRIC MALIGNANT GLIOMA HISTONE H3–MUTATED

Diffuse intrinsic pontine glioma accounts for 75% of brainstem tumors in children and is known to be highly aggressive with a median survival of 11.2 months.[5,28] Previously this was thought to be a pediatric GBM, exclusively found in midline structures and diagnosed solely by imaging.[5,29] The discovery of the H3 K27M mutation showed that this tumor was distinct from GBMs and recognized in the 2016 WHO as a new entity.[30] This mutation in H3 resulting in the lysine to methionine

substitution at position 27 confers a worse prognosis than the wild-type cases.[31,32] The presence of the mutation on itself, however, is not sufficient for a diagnosis of GBM. The second cIMPACT-NOW update clarified that the diagnosis of H3 K27M diffuse midline glioma must be restricted to tumors that are diffusely infiltrative, present in midline structures, and not histologically compatible with a different tumor type as other tumors, such as pilocytic astrocytomas and gangliogliomas, which rarely can harbor this mutation[33,34] without the associated poor prognosis that would justify the WHO grade IV.[35] In addition, these tumors carry *TP53* mutations, *PDGFRA* amplification, and *FGFR1* mutations. Tumors with H3F3A or HIST1H3B/C carry activating mutations of *ACVR1* and are seen in the midline, often presenting histologically as lower-grade tumors before progressing to GBM. Biopsies of these tumors often are small and because histology may be low grade, the development of K27M mutation-

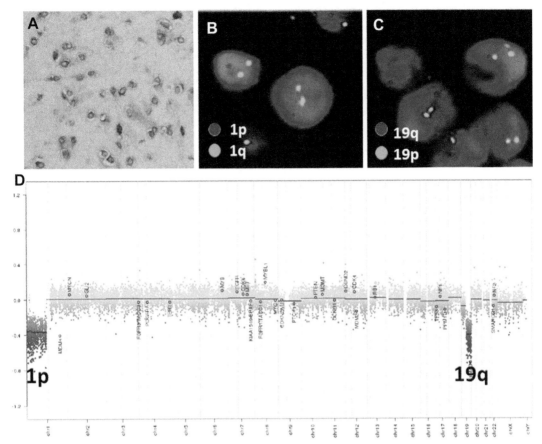

Fig. 2. Molecular features of an oligodendroglioma. (*A*) Oligodendroglioma is characterized by IDH1/2 mutation, which can be diagnosed using a mutation-specific antibody (Original magnification ×200). In addition, all oligodendrogliomas must show concurrent loss of chromosomal arms (*B*) 1p and (*C*) 19 q, either by FISH or by other methods, such as (*D*) whole-genome DNA methylation array analysis.

specific antibody provided a powerful tool for diagnosing these tumors properly.

In adolescents, histone H3–mutated tumors occur in the cortex and have a somewhat better prognosis although this may be attributed to a location that is more amenable to aggressive resection. The mutation is in G34 residue and is again accompanied with *TP53* and *ATRX* mutations.[32,36]

PEDIATRIC LOW-GRADE GLIOMAS

Low-grade gliomas are the most common type of brain tumor in children. Pilocytic astrocytomas, gangliogliomas, and pleomorphic xanthoastrocytomas (PXAs) are noninfiltrating tumors relatively well-demarcated tumors that are common in children and adolescents.[37–39] These tumors follow a benign clinical course and rarely show malignant progression. Pediatric low-grade gliomas do not carry *IDH1/2* or *ATRX* mutations, 1p19q loss, or RTK amplifications characteristic of adult tumors.

A large portion of these tumors is defined by *BRAF* alterations. Again, there is a strong correlation between molecular alteration and location with histology. Optic pathway, brainstem, cerebellar, and spinal cord pilocytic astrocytomas are driven by a fusion between *BRAF* and *KIAA1549*. On the contrary, cortical pilocytic astrocytoma, PXAs, and gangliogliomas are in most cases driven by *BRAF V600E* mutation.[40,41] Other alterations leading to activation of the RAF pathway include in-frame insertion in the *BRAF* gene, fusion of *BRAF* with *FAM131B*, and fusion of *SRGAP3* or *RAF1*.[42] Recognizing *BRAF* alterations is critical for diagnosis and clinical management. Although a complete surgical resection is desirable, it not always is possible, particularly in deep midline structures and optic pathways. MAPK pathway inhibitors represent an increasingly important therapeutic alternative for unresectable tumors.

Testing for *BRAF V600E* may be performed by mutation-specific antibody or sequencing and testing for BRAF fusions usually is performed by FISH or RNA next-generation sequencing.[43]

PXAs are WHO grade II and grade III gliomas of an astrocytic lineage that typically are relatively well demarcated and characterized by nuclear pleomorphism, eosinophilic granular bodies and xanthomatous cells. Microvascular proliferation and even necrosis can be present, and tumor may be difficult to distinguish from GBM. Many PXAs are driven by BRAF V600E mutation and occasionally RAF1 fusions.[44] Molecular features of anaplasia have not been defined clearly in PXA. Trisomy of chromosome 7 and homozygous deletion of CDKN2A/B as well as TERT mutations have been proposed but not firmly validated.[45]

In addition to BRAF-driven low-grade gliomas, pediatric diffuse gliomas represent a heterogenous group of glial tumors, which histologically often mimic oligodendrogliomas or astrocytomas. Proving the absence of IDH1/2 mutation, ATRX mutation, K27M, and G34 as well as RTK amplifications is paramount for clinical management. Studies have shown that the diffuse gliomas seen in children and adolescents are IDH–wild-type/H3–wild-type tumors with either a BRAF V600E mutation, FGFR alteration, or MYB or MYBL1 rearrangement and follow a more indolent clinical course with rare progression to a higher grade.[38] Diffuse gliomas with these molecular alterations are uncommon tumors and often present with seizures and slow growth in children. Histologically, these tumors can be graded as WHO grade II or grade III diffuse and must not be confused with diffuse astrocytoma or oligodendroglioma of adult type for management. According to the fourth cIMPACT NOW update, the defining genetic alterations are BRAF V600E mutation, MYB or MYBL1 structural variation including amplification, and FGFR1 alterations, either an internal tandem duplication of the tyrosine kinase domain or single-nucleotide variants.[38] Detection of these rare drivers often requires complex testing, including DNA and RNA next-generation sequencing or DNA methylation profiling.[3]

Due to the molecular and histologic heterogeneity of these tumors and the unknown impact on grading, the fourth cIMPACT NOW presented an integrated diagnostic classification with a tiered system, including integrated diagnosis, histologic classification, WHO grade, and molecular data.[38] It is paramount that these tumors are not managed as adult-type diffuse gliomas.

SUMMARY

Gliomas represent histologically and molecularly a diverse group of tumors. Although classification still is largely based on histology, molecular features are changing the practice of medicine. The discovery of IDH1/2 mutations and association with ATRX mutations and loss of 1p19q in astrocytoma and oligodendroglioma, respectively, and the definition of molecular IDH–wild-type GBM have dramatically changed the practice of neuropathology and WHO classification and markedly decreased the number of inconclusive diagnoses. Identifying BRAF gene fusions and mutations in low-grade gliomas and histone H3 mutations in high-grade gliomas can be used for diagnostics when histology is inconclusive. In addition, BRAF alterations represent a promising therapeutic target.

CLINICS CARE POINTS

- Diffuse gliomas are the most common primary brain tumors with strong correlation between age, tumor location, and molecular biology.

- In adults, IDH1/2 mutation status and 1p19q chromosomal arms status are critical for accurate classification.

- A combination of immunohistochemistry and molecular analysis can classify most adult diffuse gliomas.

- IDH1/2-mutated tumors show significantly better clinical outcomes.

- In pediatric gliomas, aggressive tumors are characterized by histone H3 mutations, whereas low-grade gliomas have MAPK pathway alterations most commonly are due to BRAF gene fusions or point mutations.

- In pediatric diffuse gliomas, mutations in IDH1/2 and other markers of adult gliomas must be excluded.

- BRAF alterations represent potential therapeutic targets.

ACKNOWLEDGEMENT

This work was in part supported by the Gray Family Foundation.

DISCLOSURE

The authors have nothing to disclose.

REFERENCES

1. Vigneswaran K, Neill S, Hadjipanayis CG. Beyond the World Health Organization grading of infiltrating

gliomas: advances in the molecular genetics of glioma classification. Ann Transl Med 2015;3(7):95.

2. Tabatabai G, Stupp R, van den Bent MJ, et al. Molecular diagnostics of gliomas: the clinical perspective. Acta Neuropathol 2010;120(5):585–92.

3. Capper D, Jones DTW, Sill M, et al. DNA methylation-based classification of central nervous system tumours. Nature 2018;555(7697):469–74.

4. Horbinski C, Kofler J, Kelly LM, et al. Diagnostic use of IDH1/2 mutation analysis in routine clinical testing of formalin-fixed, paraffin-embedded glioma tissues. J Neuropathol Exp Neurol 2009;68(12):1319–25.

5. Gajjar A, Bowers DC, Karajannis MA, et al. Pediatric brain tumors: innovative genomic information is transforming the diagnostic and clinical landscape. J Clin Oncol 2015;33(27):2986–98.

6. Modrek AS, Golub D, Khan T, et al. Low-grade astrocytoma mutations in IDH1, P53, and ATRX cooperate to block differentiation of human neural stem cells via repression of SOX2. Cell Rep 2017;21(5):1267–80.

7. Chen H, Judkins J, Thomas C, et al. Mutant IDH1 and seizures in patients with glioma. Neurology 2017;88(19):1805–13.

8. Unruh D, Schwarze SR, Khoury L, et al. Mutant IDH1 and thrombosis in gliomas. Acta Neuropathol 2016;132(6):917–30.

9. Yan H, Parsons DW, Jin G, et al. IDH1 and IDH2 mutations in gliomas. N Engl J Med 2009;360(8):765–73.

10. Cancer Genome Atlas Research Network, Brat DJ, Verhaak RG, Alfred Yung WK, et al. Comprehensive, integrative genomic analysis of diffuse lower-grade gliomas. N Engl J Med 2015;372(26):2481–98.

11. Kannan K, Inagaki A, Silber J, et al. Whole-exome sequencing identifies ATRX mutation as a key molecular determinant in lower-grade glioma. Oncotarget 2012;3(10):1194–203.

12. Appin CL, Brat DJ. Molecular pathways in gliomagenesis and their relevance to neuropathologic diagnosis. Adv Anat Pathol 2015;22(1):50–8.

13. Olar A, Wani KM, Alfaro-Munoz KD, et al. IDH mutation status and role of WHO grade and mitotic index in overall survival in grade II-III diffuse gliomas. Acta Neuropathol 2015;129(4):585–96.

14. Brat DJ, Aldape K, Colman H, et al. cIMPACT-NOW update 5: recommended grading criteria and terminologies for IDH-mutant astrocytomas. Acta Neuropathol 2020;139(3):603–8.

15. Watanabe T, Nobusawa S, Kleihues P, et al. IDH1 mutations are early events in the development of astrocytomas and oligodendrogliomas. Am J Pathol 2009;174(4):1149–53.

16. Bettegowda C, Agrawal N, Jiao Y, et al. Mutations in CIC and FUBP1 contribute to human oligodendroglioma. Science 2011;333(6048):1453–5.

17. Yip S, Butterfield YS, Morozova O, et al. Concurrent CIC mutations, IDH mutations, and 1p/19q loss distinguish oligodendrogliomas from other cancers. J Pathol 2012;226(1):7–16.

18. Snuderl M, Eichler AF, Ligon KL, et al. Polysomy for chromosomes 1 and 19 predicts earlier recurrence in anaplastic oligodendrogliomas with concurrent 1p/19q loss. Clin Cancer Res 2009;15(20):6430–7.

19. Chen H, Thomas C, Munoz FA, et al. Polysomy is associated with poor outcome in 1p19q co-deleted oligodendroglial tumors. Neuro Oncol 2019;21(9):1164–74.

20. Huse JT, Diamond EL, Wang L, et al. Mixed glioma with molecular features of composite oligodendroglioma and astrocytoma: a true "oligoastrocytoma"? Acta Neuropathol 2015;129(1):151–3.

21. Sahm F, Reuss D, Koelsche C, et al. Farewell to oligoastrocytoma: in situ molecular genetics favor classification as either oligodendroglioma or astrocytoma. Acta Neuropathol 2014;128(4):551–9.

22. Snuderl M, Fazlollahi L, Le LP, et al. Mosaic amplification of multiple receptor tyrosine kinase genes in glioblastoma. Cancer Cell 2011;20(6):810–7.

23. Joensuu H, Puputti M, Sihto H, et al. Amplification of genes encoding KIT, PDGFRalpha and VEGFR2 receptor tyrosine kinases is frequent in glioblastoma multiforme. J Pathol 2005;207(2):224–31.

24. Brat DJ, Aldape K, Colman H, et al. cIMPACT-NOW update 3: recommended diagnostic criteria for "Diffuse astrocytic glioma, IDH-wildtype, with molecular features of glioblastoma, WHO grade IV". Acta Neuropathol 2018;136(5):805–10.

25. Verhaak RG, Hoadley KA, Purdom E, et al. Integrated genomic analysis identifies clinically relevant subtypes of glioblastoma characterized by abnormalities in PDGFRA, IDH1, EGFR, and NF1. Cancer Cell 2010;17(1):98–110.

26. Cankovic M, Nikiforova MN, Snuderl M, et al. The role of MGMT testing in clinical practice: a report of the association for molecular pathology. J Mol Diagn 2013;15(5):539–55.

27. Hegi ME, Diserens AC, Gorlia T, et al. MGMT gene silencing and benefit from temozolomide in glioblastoma. N Engl J Med 2005;352(10):997–1003.

28. Jones C, Karajannis MA, Jones DTW, et al. Pediatric high-grade glioma: biologically and clinically in need of new thinking. Neuro Oncol 2017;19(2):153–61.

29. Spino M, Snuderl M. Genomic molecular classification of CNS malignancies. Adv Anat Pathol 2020;27(1):44–50.

30. Schwartzentruber J, Korshunov A, Liu XY, et al. Driver mutations in histone H3.3 and chromatin remodelling genes in paediatric glioblastoma. Nature 2012;482(7384):226–31.

31. Khuong-Quang DA, Buczkowicz P, Rakopoulos P, et al. K27M mutation in histone H3.3 defines clinically and biologically distinct subgroups of pediatric diffuse intrinsic pontine gliomas. Acta Neuropathol 2012;124(3):439–47.

32. Sturm D, Witt H, Hovestadt V, et al. Hotspot mutations in H3F3A and IDH1 define distinct epigenetic and biological subgroups of glioblastoma. Cancer Cell 2012;22(4):425–37.

33. Orillac C, Thomas C, Dastagirzada Y, et al. Pilocytic astrocytoma and glioneuronal tumor with histone H3 K27M mutation. Acta Neuropathol Commun 2016; 4(1):84.

34. Pages M, Beccaria K, Boddaert N, et al. Co-occurrence of histone H3 K27M and BRAF V600E mutations in paediatric midline grade I ganglioglioma. Brain Pathol 2018;28(1):103–11.

35. Louis DN, Giannini C, Capper D, et al. cIMPACT-NOW update 2: diagnostic clarifications for diffuse midline glioma, H3 K27M-mutant and diffuse astrocytoma/anaplastic astrocytoma, IDH-mutant. Acta Neuropathol 2018;135(4):639–42.

36. Korshunov A, Capper D, Reuss D, et al. Histologically distinct neuroepithelial tumors with histone 3 G34 mutation are molecularly similar and comprise a single nosologic entity. Acta Neuropathol 2016;131(1): 137–46.

37. Collins VP, Jones DT, Giannini C. Pilocytic astrocytoma: pathology, molecular mechanisms and markers. Acta Neuropathol 2015;129(6):775–88.

38. Ellison DW, Hawkins C, Jones DTW, et al. cIMPACT-NOW update 4: diffuse gliomas characterized by MYB, MYBL1, or FGFR1 alterations or BRAF(V600E) mutation. Acta Neuropathol 2019;137(4):683–7.

39. Ida CM, Rodriguez FJ, Burger PC, et al. Pleomorphic xanthoastrocytoma: natural history and long-term follow-up. Brain Pathol 2015;25(5):575–86.

40. Horbinski C. To BRAF or not to BRAF: is that even a question anymore? J Neuropathol Exp Neurol 2013; 72(1):2–7.

41. Lassaletta A, Zapotocky M, Mistry M, et al. Therapeutic and prognostic implications of BRAF V600E in pediatric low-grade gliomas. J Clin Oncol 2017; 35(25):2934–41.

42. Cin H, Meyer C, Herr R, et al. Oncogenic FAM131B-BRAF fusion resulting from 7q34 deletion comprises an alternative mechanism of MAPK pathway activation in pilocytic astrocytoma. Acta Neuropathol 2011;121(6):763–74.

43. Horbinski C, Miller CR, Perry A. Gone FISHing: clinical lessons learned in brain tumor molecular diagnostics over the last decade. Brain Pathol 2011; 21(1):57–73.

44. Phillips JJ, Gong H, Chen K, et al. The genetic landscape of anaplastic pleomorphic xanthoastrocytoma. Brain Pathol 2019;29(1):85–96.

45. Tang K, Kurland D, Vasudevaraja V, et al. Exploring DNA methylation for prognosis and analyzing the tumor microenvironment in pleomorphic xanthoastrocytoma. J Neuropathol Exp Neurol 2020;79(8): 880–90.

Molecular Pathology of Prostate Cancer

Ibrahim Kulac, MD[a], Martine P. Roudier, MD, PhD[b], Michael C. Haffner, MD, PhD[c,d,e,f,*]

KEYWORDS

• Prostate cancer • AR • ERG • PTEN • Intratumoral heterogeneity • Metastasis • Morphology

---

Key points

- Numerous profiling studies have delineated the molecular blue print of prostate cancer in the past years.
- Pertinent genomic alterations include recurrent rearrangements (in particular gene fusions involving erythroblast transformation-specific transcription factors) and copy number alterations (eg, copy number loss of *PTEN*, copy number gain of *AR*).
- DNA repair gene alterations are common and can be present as germline and somatic variants. These mutations have important prognostic and predictive implications.
- Primary prostate cancers are often multifocal and composed of independently arising tumor cell clones, which has major implications for diagnosis and treatment.
- Metastatic prostate cancer is a highly heterogeneous disease. Lineage plasticity characterized by the loss of prostatic lineage markers is a common feature of therapy-resistant prostate cancer.

ABSTRACT

Molecular profiling studies have shed new light on the complex biology of prostate cancer. Genomic studies have highlighted that structural rearrangements are among the most common recurrent alterations. In addition, both germline and somatic mutations in DNA repair genes are enriched in patients with advanced disease. Primary prostate cancer has long been known to be multifocal, but recent studies demonstrate that a large fraction of prostate cancer shows evidence of multiclonality, suggesting that genetically distinct, independently arising tumor clones coexist. Metastatic prostate cancer shows a high level of morphologic and molecular diversity, which is associated with resistance to systemic therapies. The resulting high level of intratumoral heterogeneity has important implications for diagnosis and poses major challenges for the implementation of molecular studies. Here we provide a concise review of the molecular pathology of prostate cancer, highlight clinically relevant alterations, and discuss opportunities for molecular testing.

OVERVIEW

Prostate cancer (PC) is the most common noncutaneous malignancy in men in the United States and makes up almost 20% of all newly diagnosed cancer cases.[1] The initial presentation and clinical course of PC can vary greatly between patients.

---

[a] Department of Pathology, Koç University School of Medicine, Davutpasa Caddesi No:4, Istanbul 34010, Turkey; [b] Department of Urology, University of Washington, Northeast Pacific Street, Seattle, WA 98195, USA; [c] Division of Human Biology, Fred Hutchinson Cancer Research Center, 1100 Fairview Avenue, Seattle, WA 98109, USA; [d] Division of Clinical Research, Fred Hutchinson Cancer Research Center, 1100 Fairview Avenue, Seattle, WA 98109, USA; [e] Department of Pathology, University of Washington, Seattle, WA, USA; [f] Department of Pathology, Johns Hopkins University School of Medicine, Baltimore, MD, USA

* Corresponding author. Division of Human Biology, Fred Hutchinson Cancer Research Center, 1100 Fairview Avenue, Seattle, WA 98109.
E-mail address: mhaffner@fredhutch.org

Surgical Pathology 14 (2021) 387–401
https://doi.org/10.1016/j.path.2021.05.004
1875-9181/21/© 2021 Elsevier Inc. All rights reserved.

The clinical spectrum ranges from indolent disease with an exceedingly low risk of progression to highly aggressive disease variants with early recurrence and high rates of cancer-related death.[2-4] Given this disease heterogeneity, understanding factors that predict the future clinical behavior of PC in an individual patient has been of the highest interest in the field. For decades, the assessment of histopathologic features such as Gleason grade and grade group tumor grade, tumor volume, and tumor stage have been the most pertinent prognostic parameters on which clinical decision-making is based. This factor strongly emphasizes the important relevance of the pathologist in the care of PC patients. Over the past years, molecular diagnostic applications have been penetrating more and more into the daily practice of genitourinary pathology. Many of these novel molecular tools have the potential to improve diagnostic accuracy and predictive values and ultimately lead to better clinical outcomes. In the multidisciplinary care for patients with PC, pathologists will play an essential role in bridging molecular studies and clinical decision-making.

In this review, we aim to provide a concise overview of relevant molecular alterations in PC and highlight opportunities for precision pathology in clinical practice, as well as delineate the challenges posed by the complex biology of PC.

PROSTATE CANCER ETIOLOGY AND GERMLINE ALTERATIONS

Although the etiologic factors that contribute to PC initiation remain a matter of intensive research, recent studies have highlighted the role of chronic unresolved inflammation, infection, and persistent epithelial cell injury as well as the exposure to dietary carcinogens, in particular heterocyclic amines in the pathogenesis of PC.[5-8] These exposure risk factors (which are to some extent modifiable) need to be evaluated in the context of germline genetic risk predisposition. Inherited genetic risk factors are an important determinant for PC development. Indeed, genome-wide association studies have revealed numerous genetic risk variants linked to PC.[9,10] Interestingly, some variants involve genes that regulate inflammation and pathogen response (eg, RNASEL, MSR1) highlighting the interplay between environment and host factors.[2] Although the individual contribution of these low penetrant risk alleles might be limited, models combining multiple risk loci can identify individuals with more than 5-fold increased risk for developing PC.[11] Importantly, a recent study demonstrated that certain germline risk alleles determine somatic

epigenome alterations in PC suggesting that germline alterations can influence a plethora of somatic changes.[12] In addition, several highly penetrant germline variants, in particular in HOXB13 (G48E) and BRCA2 were identified.[13,14] Although these alterations are relatively uncommon, they are associated with a substantial (5- to 7-fold) increased risk for developing PC.[14,15] For current clinical practice, it is relevant to highlight the association of germline mutations as they relate to familial tumor syndromes. In particular, germline alterations in BRCA1 and BRCA2 in addition to genes associated with Lynch Syndrome can be found in PC patients which warrants germline genetic testing and genetic counseling of family members in a subset of PC patients (discussed elsewhere in this article).[13]

PRECURSORS LESIONS

Although the definition of the cell of origin of PC is a matter of ongoing debate in the literature, almost all primary PCs show features of prostatic luminal epithelial cell differentiation, which is characterized by the expression of the androgen receptor (AR) and AR target genes such as prostate-specific antigen (PSA). Collectively, these findings suggest that a luminal cell phenotype is the dominant cellular differentiation in primary PC.[16-18] Precursor lesions of PC have been studied extensively over that past decades.[19-21] Currently, the most widely accepted PC precursor lesion is high-grade prostatic intraepithelial neoplasia (HG-PIN), which is characterized by cytologically atypical cells confined to preexisting ducts and acini by intact basal cells.[19,20] HG-PIN often shares molecular alterations with adjacent invasive carcinoma, which was originally used to define HG-PIN as a precursor lesion.[21-23] However, more recent in-depth genomic studies of this putative precursor lesion have suggested that at least a subset of lesions with morphologic features of HG-PIN are in fact invasive carcinoma cells, retrogradely colonizing preexisting ductal and acinar spaces.[21,24-26] These lesions appear morphologically as HG-PIN, but are on the molecular level consistent with invasive carcinoma.[24] This observation has important implications for screening and provides some explanation for the association between the extent of HG-PIN and the risk for subsequent cancer detection on repeat biopsies.[21,27]

THE MULTIFOCAL AND MULTICLONAL NATURE OF PROSTATE CANCER

It is well-established that primary PCs often show several distinct tumor nodules.[28-30] Indeed, multifocal tumor lesions can be found in up to 80% of radical prostatectomy specimens.[31-34] Individual

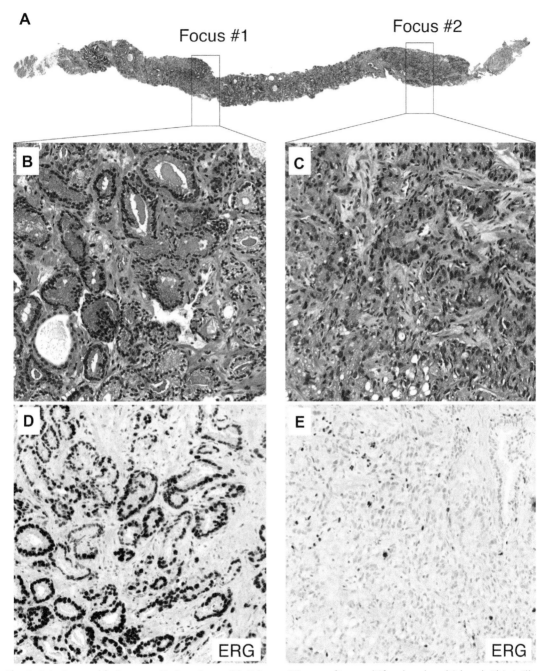

Fig. 1. Intratumoral heterogeneity in primary PC. Primary PCs are often multifocal and multiclonal. This is illustrated by a needle core biopsy [original magnification 20x] (*A*), which shows 2 noncontiguous tumor foci. Notably, the 2 tumor foci differ in tumor grade (focus 1, Gleason score 3 + 3 = 6 [original magnification 20x] [*B*]; focus 2, Gleason score 4 + 4 = 8 (original magnification 20x) [*C*]) and ERG rearrangement status assessed by ERG IHC (focus 1, ERG positive [original magnification 20x] [*D*], focus 2, negative (original magnification 20x) [*E*]), strongly suggesting that these 2 lesions are of independent clonal origin.

tumor foci can be separated spatially and show distinct morphologic features.[32] More recent genomic studies have shown that up to 70% of cases of multifocal PC consists of genomically distinct tumors with nonoverlapping mutation profiles.[29,35–38] This finding suggests, that a prostate gland can harbor multiple separate tumors that likely arise independently and show distinct molecular alterations and biological behavior.[29,35,38,39] The observation that primary PCs can be composed of distinct tumor clones sets PC apart from most other solid tumors. The resulting high level of spatiogenomic heterogeneity represents a major challenge for primary PC diagnosis. As shown in **Fig. 1**, a given prostate core biopsy can sample 2 tumor foci, with distinct morphologies (see **Fig. 1**). In situ assays, such as immunohistochemical staining for ERG, which can be used to infer the clonal relationship demonstrate that in this biopsy core 2 genomically distinct tumors were represented. This scenario is not uncommon. In fact, a recent study showed that around 25% of biopsies with noncontiguous core involvement tumors sample 2 separate tumor clones.[40] This finding illustrates the complexity of multifocality and multiclonality in PC core biopsies. It is therefore important to consider this high level of intratumoral heterogeneity when selecting biopsy samples for molecular analysis. Using a targeted sequencing approach, the heterogeneity of genomic alterations in biopsy samples and matched radical prostatectomy samples was studied recently.[41] Of a total of 22 genomically distinct tumor lesions, only 10 were represented on diagnostic biopsy samples.[41] More broadly, this finding also implies that systematic needle biopsies are probably insufficient to detect all relevant tumor clones and subclones.[39,42] This finding is particularly relevant for clinical practice, where the primary tumor sample information is often used to make decisions about actionable alterations in distant metastases.[43]

In addition, these observations challenge the assumptions of both standard template biopsy, as well as image-guided targeted biopsies and call into question the concept of a "dominant lesion," which is defined solely by size or histologic criteria, being largely responsible for a patient's clinical course. This finding is supported by studies showing that certain genomic and molecular features, rather than size or histology alone, can identify tumor foci that are more likely to contribute to disease progression.[35,38,39,44] For instance, we reported a case several years ago, in which we were able to demonstrate that the lethal metastatic cell clone in a patient who died of PC originated from a small well differentiated (Gleason pattern 3) lesion in the primary tumor. Importantly, this small low-grade lesion that showed evidence for molecular alterations that are tightly linked to aggressive disease, such as genomic alterations in *PTEN* and *TP53*, was associated with a bulky clonally distinct and higher grade tumor that did not contribute to the lethal tumor burden.[38] The study of intratumor heterogeneity in PC can be technically challenging

and although the literature on intratumor heterogeneity in PC has expanded dramatically over the past years, future studies are needed to more directly address the clinical challenges that arise from the multiclonal nature of PC.

CLINICALLY RELEVANT MOLECULAR ALTERATIONS

Recent large-scale profiling studies have laid out a blueprint of the genomic and transcriptomic landscape of PC.[45–50] Although the overall point mutation rate in PC is relatively low, copy number alterations and structural rearrangements are very common and often involve driver gene changes. We have summarized several key pathways that are frequently altered in PC and contribute to tumor progression and therapy resistance.

GENOMIC ALTERATIONS

Androgen Receptor

The vast majority of PCs crucially depend on AR signaling.[51] The AR is a nuclear hormone receptor that is required for maintaining prostatic differentiation, but is subverted in PC to fuel cancer growth.[52] Although initial and often profound responses to therapies that lower testosterone levels or interfere with AR signaling are common, most PCs become refractory to these interventions and progress to castration-resistant PC (CRPC). Importantly, despite AR pathway inhibition, tumor cells maintain aberrant AR activity through a number of genomic and nongenomic mechanisms. These include high-level copy number gains of the *AR* gene itself or its distant enhancer and gain-of-function mutations in AR.[48,52,53] Collectively, more than 60% of metastatic CRPC (mCRPC) cases show evidence for genomic *AR* alterations.[48,52,53] In addition, the *AR* gene locus can give rise to constitutively active *AR* splice variants.[54] Importantly, *AR* genomic alterations and splice variants can be detected in blood-based assays from cell free DNA and circulating tumor cells.[54–58] Their presence has been associated with resistance to first- and second-line hormonal therapies and is currently explored as a predictive biomarker for advanced PC.[54,55] In addition to alterations in the *AR* gene itself, several other genes involved in AR signaling including *FOXA1*, *MED12*, *ZBTB16*, *NCOR1*, and *NCOR2* harbor genomic alterations in PC.[48] Because these AR alterations are almost exclusively present in treatment-refractory metastatic disease, there is currently limited experience with tissue-based assessment.[59] However, with increasing frequency of biopsies from mCRPC, investigation of the AR signaling axis will likely become important for clinical management in the future (discussed elsewhere in this article).

Erythroblast Transformation-Specific Transcription Factors

The most common recurrent genomic alterations in PC are rearrangements involving erythroblast transformation-specific transcription factors, which include ERG, ETV1, ETV4, ETV5, and FLI1. In up to 80% of cases erythroblast transformation-specific genes become juxtaposed to androgen-regulated genes through genomic rearrangements resulting in their overexpression in PC.[60,61] By far the most common rearrangement comprises the 5′ end of the androgen regulated of TMPRSS2 fused to ERG. TMPRSS2-ERG rearrangements seem to be an early event in PC development and functionally contribute to cell invasion and transcriptional reprogramming.[62,63] This scenario suggests that structural alterations likely represent key driver events in PC. Importantly, a large fraction of these structural alterations shows a complex chain architecture involving numerous genome fragments often encompassing multiple driver genes. Such complex chained rearrangements (also termed "chromoplexy") are unlikely to arise from sequential independent events but rather suggest a coordinated underlying mechanism. This finding supports a model of punctate evolution in which a large number of driver alterations are generated in a small number of events rather than gradual accumulation over time.[64] There is a growing body of literature suggesting that transcriptional processes rather than DNA replication may represent important events resulting in genomic instability in PC.[65,66] For instance, it was noted that androgen signaling can induce DNA double-strand breaks, in a process that involves class 2 topoisomerase activity.[67] Such androgen-induced breaks can seed rearrangements (eg, recurrent rearrangement between TMPRSS2 and ERG) and are likely also involved in general genomic instability in PC.[65,66] Indeed, several studies have highlighted that sites of genomic rearrangements in PC are enriched for AR-binding site and numerous complex rearrangements involve at least one androgen-regulated gene.[64,68,69]

The prognostic relevance of ERG rearrangements has been analyzed in numerous studies, but ERG as single marker did not show any robust association with disease outcomes or aggressive PC phenotypes.[70–72] ERG expression, however, can serve in certain settings as a helpful marker to determine the presence of PC and as shown elsewhere in this article (see **Fig. 1**) is extremely valuable for assessing clonality.

DNA Repair

As noted elsewhere in this article, despite the relatively low mutation rate, copy number and structural variants are very common in PC, suggesting potential alterations in pathways involved in DNA repair.[46,48,64,73] Genes encoding for proteins involved in both single- and double-strand break sensing and repair have been found to harbor both somatic and germline alterations in men with PC. Sequencing studies over the past years have demonstrated that key DNA repair genes including BRCA2, ATM, CHEK2, BRCA1, and ATR show somatic inactivating mutations, which are enriched in advanced metastatic PC.[13,15,74,75] Collectively, around 20% of all metastatic PC cases show alterations in DNA damage-response (DDR) genes. Of particular interest is that a large fraction of these alterations is present already in the germline DNA with cumulatively around 10% of men with advanced PC harboring germline mutation in BRCA2, ATM, and BRCA1.[13] Importantly, men with germline alterations in these genes are more likely to show disease progression and adverse outcomes.[13,15,75–77] Given the importance for patient management as well as the implications for cancer risk in other family members, genetic testing for germline DDR gene alterations followed by appropriate genetic counseling should be considered in men with localized disease with a Gleason score of 8 or greater (grade group ≥4) and/or a PSA of 20 or greater and any patient with metastatic disease.[59] Testing for DNA repair gene alterations also provides important predictive information. Tumors with certain DDR gene defects show a high sensitivity to poly (ADP-ribose) polymerase inhibitors and platinum compounds (such as cisplatin).[78] Several clinical trials have shown high response rates in men with DDR defects to the poly (ADP-ribose) polymerase inhibitors olaparib and rucaparib, which prompted the recent US Food and Drug Administration approval of these drugs for mCRPC.[79,80] Although responses seem to be robust in cases with BRCA2 mutations, it is unclear if this finding can be extrapolated to other DDR gene alterations.[81–83] More broadly, targeting DNA repair defects will likely become an important therapy option for advanced PC. With an increasing number of highly specific inhibitors to key DNA repair proteins, appropriate patient selection and the development of robust companion diagnostic tests will be extremely important.[84] In addition to homologous DNA repair defects, alterations in mismatch repair (MMR) genes (including MSH2, MSH6, MLH1 and PMS2), which results in microsatellite instability have been observed in primary PC (<3%) and mCRPC (approximately 10%). In localized PC, MMR alterations are associated with higher Gleason grade and are enriched for cases with ductal morphology.[85,86] Germline alterations of MMR genes are less common than other homologous repair gene alterations but should be considered owing to their association with the Lynch syndrome. The rationale that MMR generates hundreds to thousands of somatic mutations that encode potential neoantigens led the US Food and Drug Administration to approve pembrolizumab for all tumor types with MMR alterations.[87] Although MMR-deficient PC cases might be rare, their identification is therapeutically meaningful because they can show durable responses to anti-programmed cell death and programmed cell death ligand 1 therapies.[88]

Cell Cycle

P53 is a stress-induced transcription factor that regulates cell cycle arrest, senescence, and apoptosis among many other cellular pathway.[89] TP53 is mutated in approximately 10% of primary PCs, but shows a strong enrichment in mCRPC, with up to 50% of metastatic PCs harboring TP53 alterations. TP53 mutations seem to be early truncal events in PC and are associated with high-grade disease and adverse clinical outcomes.[38,44,90] However, it is important to note that not all TP53 mutations lead to a loss of tumor suppressive function. Rather, some TP53 mutations can result in a specific functional gain that contributes to tumor progression.[91] In PC, there is a near even split between classical loss-of-function mutations (homozygous deletions, truncating mutations) and missense mutations, which can potentially result in context-dependent gain- or loss-of-function and dominant negative phenotypes.[48,91,92] Although the clinical relevance of different TP53 alterations is unclear, ongoing preclinical studies and early clinical trials are currently testing novel approaches to restore p53 function or specifically target TP53 mutant cancers.[93]

RB1 is an important tumor suppressor gene involved in cell cycle regulation, but also controls independent protumorigenic transcriptional programs.[94,95] Although RB1 alterations are relatively rare in primary PC (1%), RB1 loss (most commonly through copy number alterations) is enriched in advanced CRPC (9%).[96,97] In fact, a recent large-scale genomics study showed that RB1 alterations have the strongest association with poor outcomes

in metastatic PC.[88] Notably, concomitant RB1 and TP53 loss is a common feature of small cell neuroendocrine PC (NEPC). Whereas in murine PC models deletion of Rb1 and Tp53 results in high-grade carcinoma with neuroendocrine differentiation,[98] these two genomic alterations by themselves seem to be insufficient to induce a small cell phenotype in human PC.[99,100]

PI3K/PTEN

Alterations in the tumor suppressor gene PTEN occur in up to 20% of localized prostate and 40% of mCRPC. Most cases with PTEN loss harbor copy number changes, resulting in a complete absence of PTEN protein expression.[101–104] Therefore, PTEN status can be interrogated robustly using genetically validated immunohistochemical approaches.[102–104] Several studies have highlighted the prognostic potential of PTEN immunohistochemistry in large retrospective studies, demonstrating that PTEN loss is associated with increased rates of biochemical recurrence and shorter survival in contemporary biopsy and radical prostatectomy cohorts.[103,105,106] Furthermore, there is evidence that PTEN loss in lower grade tumors is associated with the presence of adjacent higher grade lesions.[107] In addition to its role as a prognostic marker, PTEN loss can potentially also serve as a predictive biomarker for therapies targeting the PI3K-AKT axis.[108]

Wnt

Wnt comprises a group of signaling pathways involved in cell proliferation, cellular homeostasis, stem cell renewal and cell migration.[109,110] Wnt signaling pathways have been shown to harbor genomic alterations in 10% to 20% of cases with advanced PC, with an enrichment in activating mutations in CTNNB1 and RSPO2 and inactivating mutations in APC, RNF43, and ZNRF3.[48] These alterations are associated with adverse histopathologic findings and earlier clinical progression. Importantly, the wnt pathway has been mechanistically implicated in regulating AR signaling and tumors with wnt pathway activating mutations show decreased responsiveness to second-generation hormonal therapies abiraterone and enzalutamide.[111,112] In addition, nongenomic alterations of wnt signaling, in particular increased expression of wnt signaling intermediates such as WNT5A and DKK1 are present in a large fraction of mCRPC.[113,114] These findings open up new opportunities for cotargeting of wnt together with other signaling pathways in PC.

EPIGENETIC ALTERATIONS

In addition to genomic changes, epigenetic alterations are increasingly recognized as important driver alterations in PC.[115,116] The spectrum of epigenome modifications is broad and encompasses all potentially heritable changes that alter gene expression.[115,116] Likely owing to the availability of robust analytical tools, DNA methylation changes have been extensively explored in PC over the past decade.[115–118] The methylation of cytosine in the context of CpG dinucleotides is an important regulator of gene transcription and defines cellular identity. Alterations in DNA methylation patterns are universal in PC and occur early during PC initiation.[115] Although DNA methylation changes are potentially reversible, several studies have documented that cancer specific DNA methylation marks are highly recurrent (eg, hypermethylation of GSTP1 can be found in up to 90% of PCs) and remarkably stable and maintained throughout disease progression.[116,119] These findings suggest that DNA methylation changes could serve as valuable biomarkers in PC. Indeed, numerous studies have evaluated methylation-based biomarkers for PC detection in the blood and urine,[119–122] and a commercial test (ConfirmMDx, MDxHealth, Irvine, CA) is available for assessing the risk of cancer detection on repeat biopsies.[123] Because PC is characterized by a paucity of recurrent genomic alterations, DNA methylation changes could be used as attractive cancer-specific analytes for the early detection of PC, as well as disease monitoring in the metastatic setting.[55,124,125] Although most of these assays are currently in early stages of clinical development and validation, there will likely be a wave of innovative DNA methylation-based biomarkers with diverse clinical applications in the near future.

TRANSCRIPTOMIC ALTERATIONS

Extensive expression profiling efforts in PC have highlighted transcriptional alterations that can provide relevant prognostic information. Several expression signatures have been turned into commercial "genomic classifiers" (ie, Polaris, OncotypeDx, Decipher) that provide prognostic value in addition to existing clinicopathologic data (reviewed in[126,127]). Although these assays have been validated extensively in retrospective cohorts, prospective studies are currently missing and the clinical settings in which these assays are most impactful has yet to be defined.[126,128] In addition, other expression signatures, such as the PAM50 classifier, which was originally developed to subtype breast cancers into luminal and basal types, has been suggested to provide prognostic as well as predictive information for response to hormonal therapy in PC.[129] This intriguing finding suggests that certain transcriptional changes seem to be associated with more aggressive disease phenotypes, irrespective of the tissue of origin.[130] Although most expression analyses focus on annotated protein coding genes, more recent studies have investigated long noncoding RNAs, which do not contain protein coding sequences, but can have important structural functions.[131] In PC, several long noncoding RNAs with potentially useful biomarker properties have been identified (NEAT1, PCA3, PCAT-1, and SChLAP1).[132–137] The detection of PCA3 in the urine can, for instance, improve the performance of cancer detection in PSA screening cohorts.[136] SCHLAP1 expression, in contrast, hand has been described as a robust prognostic marker and high SChLAP1 levels are associated with increased rates of recurrence and mortality.[132,133] Interestingly, SCHLAP1 expression has been associated with more aggressive morphologic variants of PC including intraductal and cribriform morphologies.[138]

ASSESSING METASTATIC PROSTATE CANCER

HISTOMORPHOLOGIC FEATURES OF METASTATIC PROSTATE CANCER

Over the past decades, the vast majority of PC pathology was limited to the assessment of prostate biopsies and prostatectomy specimens. However, with improved methodologies for obtaining metastatic PC biopsies from both soft tissue and bone and the increasing importance of the assessment of molecular alterations in metastases for patient management, it is likely that the number of metastatic PC specimens seen by surgical pathologists will greatly increase in the coming years. With the evolution of novel therapies for PC, the spectrum of morphologies of metastatic PC has greatly changed. Our group has recently studied the morphologic features of metastatic PC obtained in a large rapid autopsy cohort and found a broad spectrum of variant histologies (**Fig. 2**). This encompasses common PC morphologies such as acinar and cribriform architectures, but also poorly differentiated and anaplastic carcinomas. In addition, squamous features and neuroendocrine differentiation (carcinoid-like pattern and small cell carcinoma) are present in a large number of mCRPC (see **Fig. 2**). These diverse patterns found in mCRPC, which often show minimal to no resemblance to primary PC, highlight the difficulties in assessing PC in the metastatic setting.

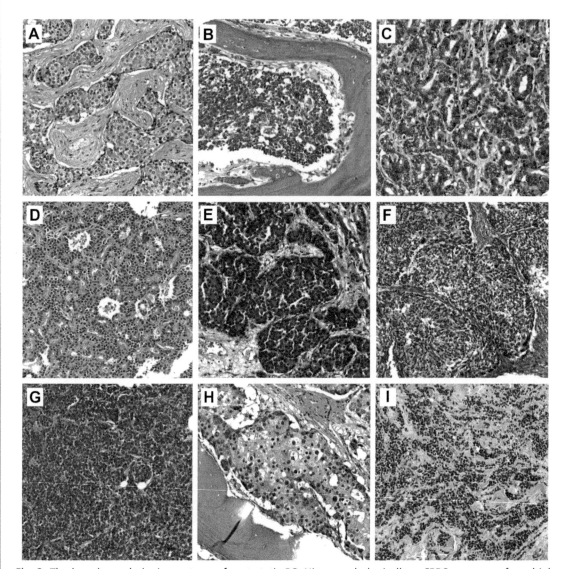

Fig. 2. The broad morphologic spectrum of metastatic PC. Histomorphologically, mCRPC can range from high grade carcinoma with squamous features [original magnification 20x] (*A*), high-grade carcinoma with pleomorphic giant cells [original magnification 20x] (*B*), adenocarcinoma [original magnification 20x] (*C*), adenocarcinoma with cribriform architecture [original magnification 20x] (*D*), carcinoid-like tumors [original magnification 20x] (*E*), high-grade neuroendocrine tumors with spindle cell morphology [original magnification 20x] (*F*), poorly differentiated carcinoma not otherwise specified [original magnification 20x] (*G*, *H*), and small cell neuroendocrine carcinoma [original magnification 20x] (*I*).

Although in the majority of cases AR expression will still be maintained and AR-regulated lineage markers such as PSA, PSAP, and NKX3.1 are positive, recent studies have shown that a substantial number of PCs loose AR expression and are subsequently negative for PSA and NKX3.1 (discussed elsewhere in this article).[139] HOXB13 has been suggested as a robust marker for prostatic differentiation in the metastatic setting[140]; however, similar to other prostate lineage markers,

HOXB13 expression can be lost in tumors with neuroendocrine differentiation.

LINEAGE PLASTICITY

The widespread clinical use of highly potent AR-targeting therapies, including enzalutamide and abiraterone, has greatly shaped the phenotypic landscape of metastatic PC.[125,139,141,142] Increasingly recognized in clinical practice is a subset of

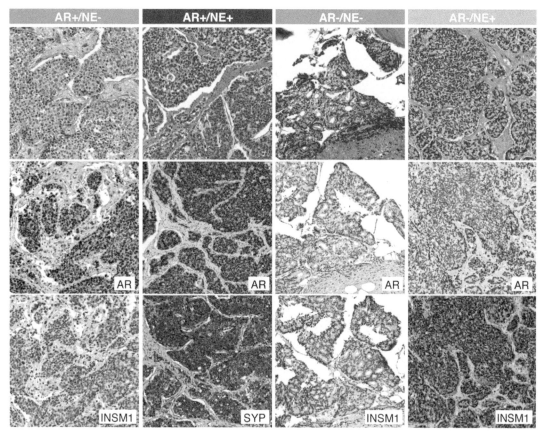

Fig. 3. Molecular subtypes of metastatic PC. Based on the expression of AR and AR target genes as well as neuro-endocrine markers (NE; eg, INSM1; SYP, synaptophysin) metastatic treatment refractory PCs can be subdivided into 4 molecular subtypes characterized by AR expression in the absence of NE marker expression, expression of AR and NE markers (in particular SYP), absence of AR and NE markers (double-negative PC [DNPC]) and neuro-endocrine PC (NEPC) characterized by absence of AR but strong NE marker expression.

patients with advanced CRPC who show evolution to a rapidly progressing disease that is refractory to hormone therapy and exhibits a visceral dissemination pattern.[143,144] Such tumors often show loss of AR and gain of neuroendocrine marker expression. Morphologically, this clinically aggressive variant of PC can show features of poorly differentiated carcinoma or even small cell morphology[143] (**Fig. 3**). Although de novo small cell carcinoma of the prostate is exceedingly rare,[145] therapy-related NEPCs are present in up to 20% of patients undergoing contemporary AR targeted therapies.[144,146,147] Recent preclinical and clinical evidence suggest that these tumors likely arise through trans-differentiation of a preexisting adenocarcinoma as an adaptive resistance mechanism to AR targeted therapies.[143,145,147–149] The accurate distinction between high-grade adenocarcinoma and NEPC is of clinical importance since the management for these entities differs; whereas NEPC is mostly resistant to

conventional androgen deprivation therapies, these tumors show sensitivity to platinum-based chemotherapies or other targeted therapies.[143,150] While there is currently no well-established panel of immunohistochemical markers, the use of prostate lineage markers AR, PSA and NKX3.1 together with neuroendocrine markers, in particular INSM1, synaptophysin and FOXA2 have shown value in assessing neuroendocrine differentiation in both de novo and treatment associated NEPC.[151,152] In addition to tumors that loose AR and gain neuroendocrine marker expression, a third molecular subtype of metastatic PC was recently described. These double negative PC (DNPC) are characterized by the absence of both AR and neuroendocrine marker and make up around 20% of all mCRPC (see **Fig. 3**).[139,149] Although the biology of these tumors is currently under investigation, they show a dependence on MAPK and FGF signaling and likely represent a distinct subgroup with unique therapeutic vulnerabilities. Lastly, a group of mCRPC termed amphicrine PC shows co-expression of AR and a subset of neuroendocrine markers (in particular synaptophysin, see **Fig. 3**).[149] It is presently unclear if these tumors represent a distinct subgroup or an intermediate in the transdifferentiating from a conventional adenocarcinoma to a NEPC. Assessment of AR and neuroendocrine markers on metastatic biopsies will be likely become very important in the diagnostic workup for patients with mCRPC. Although currently used mostly in the setting of clinical trials, the important information gained from such tissue-based studies will be extremely relevant for the optimal diagnostic management in the future. However, before widespread clinical use, markers and assays used in this setting will need to be carefully validated in multi-institutional studies.

SUMMARY

There is no doubt that the use of molecular testing in PC will improve patient outcomes; however, their clinical implementation will likely be challenging. Challenges will arise from the complex biology of PC, in particular the high level of intertumoral and intratumoral heterogeneity, but also from the necessity of a coordinated multidisciplinary approach to the care of PC patients. The plethora of prognostic tests available for localized PC will require an active interface between urologists and pathologists in determining the clinical significance of different assay platforms and most importantly the accessibility of tissue. The complex presentation of metastatic PC and the increased appreciation of resistance mechanisms that involve loss of classical lineage features will necessitate an even more focused interaction between pathologists and oncologists. In addition, an increasing interaction between pathology and radiology will likely be at the center of PC clinical diagnostics in the future. The major improvements in multiparametric MRI imaging have allowed to visualize tumors more robustly and will enable a more focused sampling. It will be important in future studies to correlate these histomorphologic and molecular findings with imaging studies. Similarly, advanced functional imaging will open a real-time window to studying tumor heterogeneity in the setting of metastatic disease. However, these powerful new technologies will be most clinically useful when combined with advanced tissue based and liquid biopsy approaches. This process will require novel computational frameworks to analyze the complex multidimensional data

generated as part of such diagnostic workup studies.[153] Therefore, in the paradigm of multidisciplinary care, the role of the pathologist as a steward who bridges molecular diagnostic and clinical care will be ever more important.

CONFLICTS OF INTEREST AND SOURCES OF FUNDING

The authors have no significant relationships with, or financial interest in, any commercial companies pertaining to this article. Research reported in this publication was supported in part by the NIH/NCI (P50CA097186), the U.S. Department of Defense Prostate Cancer Research Program (W81XWH-20-1-0111), and the Safeway Foundation.

REFERENCES

1. Siegel RL, Miller KD, Jemal A. Cancer statistics, 2020. CA Cancer J Clin 2020;70:7–30.
2. Nelson WG, De Marzo AM, Isaacs WB. Prostate cancer. N Engl J Med 2003;349:366–81.
3. Attard G, Parker C, Eeles RA, et al., Prostate cancer. Lancet 2016;387:79-82.
4. Litwin MS, Tan H-J. The diagnosis and treatment of prostate cancer: a review. JAMA 2017;317: 2532–42.
5. Puhr M, De Marzo A, Isaacs W, et al. Inflammation, microbiota, and prostate cancer. Eur Urol Focus 2016;2:374–82.
6. Sfanos KS, Yegnasubramanian S, Nelson WG, et al. The inflammatory microenvironment and microbiome in prostate cancer development. Nat Rev Urol 2018;15:11–24.
7. de Bono JS, Guo C, Gurel B, et al. Prostate carcinogenesis: inflammatory storms. Nat Rev Cancer 2020;20:455–69.
8. Nelson WG, DeMarzo AM, Yegnasubramanian S. The diet as a cause of human prostate cancer. Cancer Treat Res 2014;159:51–68.
9. Kote-Jarai Z, Easton DF, Stanford JL, et al. Multiple novel prostate cancer predisposition loci confirmed by an international study: the PRACTICAL Consortium. Cancer Epidemiol Biomarkers Prev 2008; 17:2052–61.
10. Eeles RA, Olama AAA, Benlloch S, et al. Identification of 23 new prostate cancer susceptibility loci using the iCOGS custom genotyping array. Nat Genet 2013;45:385–91, 391.e1-2.
11. Zheng SL, Sun J, Wiklund F, et al. Cumulative association of five genetic variants with prostate cancer. N Engl J Med 2008;358:910–9.
12. Houlahan KE, Shiah Y-J, Gusev A, et al. Genome-wide germline correlates of the epigenetic

landscape of prostate cancer. Nat Med 2019;25: 1615–26.

13. Pritchard CC, Mateo J, Walsh MF, et al. Inherited DNA-repair gene mutations in men with metastatic prostate cancer. N Engl J Med 2016;375:443–53.

14. Ewing CM, Ray AM, Lange EM, et al. Germline mutations in HOXB13 and prostate-cancer risk. N Engl J Med 2012;366:141–9.

15. Castro E, Goh C, Olmos D, et al. Germline BRCA mutations are associated with higher risk of nodal involvement, distant metastasis, and poor survival outcomes in prostate cancer. J Clin Oncol 2013; 31:1748–57.

16. De Marzo AM, Nelson WG, Bieberich CJ, et al. Prostate cancer: new answers prompt new questions regarding cell of origin. Nat Rev Urol 2010; 7:650–2.

17. Strand DW, Goldstein AS. The many ways to make a luminal cell and a prostate cancer cell. Endocr Relat Cancer 2015;22:T187–97.

18. Guo W, Li L, He J, et al. Single-cell transcriptomics identifies a distinct luminal progenitor cell type in distal prostate invagination tips. Nat Genet 2020; 52:908–18.

19. Epstein JI. Precursor lesions to prostatic adenocarcinoma. Virchows Arch 2009;454:1–16.

20. Bostwick DG. Prospective origins of prostate carcinoma. Prostatic intraepithelial neoplasia and atypical adenomatous hyperplasia. Cancer 1996;78: 330–6.

21. De Marzo AM, Haffner MC, Lotan TL, et al. Premalignancy in prostate cancer: rethinking what we know. Cancer Prev Res (Phila) 2016;9:648–56.

22. Furusato B, Gao C-L, Ravindranath L, et al. Mapping of TMPRSS2-ERG fusions in the context of multifocal prostate cancer. Mod Pathol 2008;21:67–75.

23. Bostwick DG, Qian J. High-grade prostatic intraepithelial neoplasia. Mod Pathol 2004;17:360–79.

24. Haffner MC, Weier C, Xu MM, et al. Molecular evidence that invasive adenocarcinoma can mimic prostatic intraepithelial neoplasia (PIN) and intraductal carcinoma through retrograde glandular colonization. J Pathol 2016;238:31–41.

25. Haffner MC, Barbieri CE. Shifting paradigms for high-grade prostatic intraepithelial neoplasia. Eur Urol 2016;69:831–3.

26. Trabzonlu L, Kulac I, Zheng Q, et al. Molecular pathology of high-grade prostatic intraepithelial neoplasia: challenges and opportunities. Cold Spring Harb Perspect Med 2019;9:a030403.

27. Netto GJ, Epstein JI. Widespread high-grade prostatic intraepithelial neoplasia on prostatic needle biopsy: a significant likelihood of subsequently diagnosed adenocarcinoma. Am J Surg Pathol 2006;30:1184–8.

28. Mitchell T, Neal DE. The genomic evolution of human prostate cancer. Br J Cancer 2015;1–6. https://doi.org/10.1038/bjc.2015.234.

29. Løvf M, Zhao S, Axcrona U, et al. Multifocal primary prostate cancer exhibits high degree of genomic heterogeneity. Eur Urol 2018. https://doi.org/10.1016/j.eururo.2018.08.009.

30. Fraser M, Berlin A, Bristow RG, et al. Genomic, pathological, and clinical heterogeneity as drivers of personalized medicine in prostate cancer. Urol Oncol 2015;33:85–94.

31. Andreoiu M, Cheng L. Multifocal prostate cancer: biologic, prognostic, and therapeutic implications. Hum Pathol 2010;41:781–93.

32. Arora R, Koch MO, Eble JN, et al. Heterogeneity of Gleason grade in multifocal adenocarcinoma of the prostate. Cancer 2004;100:2362–6.

33. Cheng L, Song SY, Pretlow TG, et al. Evidence of independent origin of multiple tumors from patients with prostate cancer. J Natl Cancer Inst 1998;90: 233–7.

34. Miller GJ, Cygan JM. Morphology of prostate cancer: the effects of multifocality on histological grade, tumor volume and capsule penetration. J Urol 1994;152:1709–13.

35. Boutros PC, Fraser M, Harding NJ, et al. Spatial genomic heterogeneity within localized, multifocal prostate cancer. Nat Genet 2015;47:736–45.

36. Lindberg J, Klevebring D, Liu W, et al. Exome sequencing of prostate cancer supports the hypothesis of independent tumour origins. Eur Urol 2013;63:347–53.

37. Van Etten JL, Dehm SM. Clonal origin and spread of metastatic prostate cancer. Endocr Relat Cancer 2016;23:R207–17.

38. Haffner MC, Mosbruger T, Esopi DM, et al. Tracking the clonal origin of lethal prostate cancer. J Clin Invest 2013;123:4918–22.

39. Haffner MC, De Marzo AM, Yegnasubramanian S, et al. Diagnostic challenges of clonal heterogeneity in prostate cancer. J Clin Oncol 2015;33: e38–40.

40. Fontugne J, Davis K, Palanisamy N, et al. Clonal evaluation of prostate cancer foci in biopsies with discontinuous tumor involvement by dual ERG/SPINK1 immunohistochemistry. Mod Pathol 2016; 29:157–65.

41. Kristiansen A, Bergström R, Delahunt B, et al. Somatic alterations detected in diagnostic prostate biopsies provide an inadequate representation of multifocal prostate cancer. Prostate 2019;79:920–8.

42. Salami SS, Hovelson DH, Kaplan JB, et al. Transcriptomic heterogeneity in multifocal prostate cancer. JCI Insight 2018;3:3.

43. Brastianos PK, Carter SL, Santagata S, et al. Genomic characterization of brain metastases

reveals branched evolution and potential therapeutic targets. Cancer Discov 2015;5:1164–77.

44. Hong MKH, Macintyre G, Wedge DC, et al. Tracking the origins and drivers of subclonal metastatic expansion in prostate cancer. Nat Commun 2015;6:6605–12.

45. Lawrence MS, Stojanov P, Mermel CH, et al. Discovery and saturation analysis of cancer genes across 21 tumour types. Nature 2015;505:495–501.

46. Frank S, Nelson P, Vasioukhin V. Recent advances in prostate cancer research: large-scale genomic analyses reveal novel driver mutations and DNA repair defects. F1000Res 2018;7:1173.

47. Fraser M, Sabelnykova VY, Yamaguchi TN, et al. Genomic hallmarks of localized, non-indolent prostate cancer. Nature 2017;541:359–64.

48. Robinson D, Van Allen EM, Wu Y-M, et al. Integrative clinical genomics of advanced prostate cancer. Cell 2015;161:1215–28.

49. Wedge DC, Gundem G, Mitchell T, et al. Sequencing of prostate cancers identifies new cancer genes, routes of progression and drug targets. Nat Genet 2018;50:682–92.

50. Quigley DA, Dang HX, Zhao SG, et al. Genomic hallmarks and structural variation in metastatic prostate cancer. Cell 2018;174:758–69.e9.

51. Mitsiades N. A road map to comprehensive androgen receptor axis targeting for castration-resistant prostate cancer. Cancer Res 2013;73:4599–605.

52. Watson PA, Arora VK, Sawyers CL. Emerging mechanisms of resistance to androgen receptor inhibitors in prostate cancer. Nat Rev Cancer 2015;15:701–11.

53. Viswanathan SR, Ha G, Hoff AM, et al. Structural alterations driving castration-resistant prostate cancer revealed by linked-read genome sequencing. Cell 2018;174:433–47.e19.

54. Maughan BL, Antonarakis ES. Clinical relevance of androgen receptor splice variants in castration-resistant prostate cancer. Curr Treat Options Oncol 2015;16:57.

55. Wu A, Attard G. Plasma DNA analysis in prostate cancer: opportunities for improving clinical management. Clin Chem 2019;65:100–7.

56. Romanel A, Gasi Tandefelt D, Conteduca V, et al. Plasma AR and abiraterone-resistant prostate cancer. Sci Transl Med 2015;7:312re10.

57. Antonarakis ES, Lu C, Wang H, et al. AR-V7 and resistance to enzalutamide and abiraterone in prostate cancer. N Engl J Med 2014;371:1028–38.

58. Guedes LB, Morais CL, Almutairi F, et al. Analytic validation of RNA In Situ Hybridization (RISH) for AR and AR-V7 expression in human prostate cancer. Clin Cancer Res 2016;22:4651–63.

59. Lotan TL, Tomlins SA, Bismar TA, et al. Report from the International Society of Urological Pathology (ISUP) Consultation Conference on Molecular Pathology of Urogenital Cancers. I. Molecular biomarkers in prostate cancer. Am J Surg Pathol 2020;44:e15–29.

60. Tomlins SA, Rhodes DR, Perner S, et al. Recurrent fusion of TMPRSS2 and ETS transcription factor genes in prostate cancer. Science 2005;310:644–8.

61. Kumar-Sinha C, Tomlins SA, Chinnaiyan AM. Recurrent gene fusions in prostate cancer. Nat Rev Cancer 2008;8:497–511.

62. Tomlins SA, Laxman B, Varambally S, et al. Role of the TMPRSS2-ERG gene fusion in prostate cancer. Neoplasia 2008;10:177–88.

63. Perner S, Mosquera J-M, Demichelis F, et al. TMPRSS2-ERG fusion prostate cancer: an early molecular event associated with invasion. Am J Surg Pathol 2007;31:882–8.

64. Baca SC, Prandi D, Lawrence MS, et al. Punctuated evolution of prostate cancer genomes. Cell 2013;153:666–77.

65. Ashour ME, Atteya R, El-Khamisy SF. Topoisomerase-mediated chromosomal break repair: an emerging player in many games. Nat Rev Cancer 2015;15:137–51.

66. Haffner MC, De Marzo AM, Meeker AK, et al. Transcription-induced DNA double strand breaks: both oncogenic force and potential therapeutic target? Clin Cancer Res 2011;17:3858–64.

67. Haffner MC, Aryee MJ, Toubaji A, et al. Androgen-induced TOP2B-mediated double-strand breaks and prostate cancer gene rearrangements. Nat Genet 2010;42:668–75.

68. Weischenfeldt J, Simon R, Feuerbach L, et al. Integrative genomic analyses reveal an androgen-driven somatic alteration landscape in early-onset prostate cancer. Cancer Cell 2013;23:159–70.

69. Berger MF, Lawrence MS, Demichelis F, et al. The genomic complexity of primary human prostate cancer. Nature 2011;470:214–20.

70. Toubaji A, Albadine R, Meeker AK, et al. Increased gene copy number of ERG on chromosome 21 but not TMPRSS2-ERG fusion predicts outcome in prostatic adenocarcinomas. Mod Pathol 2011;24:1511–20.

71. Albadine R, Latour M, Toubaji A, et al. TMPRSS2-ERG gene fusion status in minute (minimal) prostatic adenocarcinoma. Mod Pathol 2009;22:1415–22.

72. Ahearn TU, Pettersson A, Ebot EM, et al. A prospective investigation of PTEN loss and ERG expression in lethal prostate cancer. J Natl Cancer Inst 2016;108:djv346.

73. Mateo J, Boysen G, Barbieri CE, et al. DNA repair in prostate cancer: biology and clinical implications. Eur Urol 2017;71:417–25.

74. Mohler JL, Antonarakis ES, Armstrong AJ, et al. Prostate cancer, version 2.2019, NCCN clinical practice guidelines in oncology. J Natl Compr Canc Netw 2019;17:479–505.

75. Na R, Zheng SL, Han M, et al. Germline mutations in ATM and BRCA1/2 distinguish risk for lethal and indolent prostate cancer and are associated with early age at death. Eur Urol 2017;71:740–7.

76. Carter HB, Helfand B, Mamawala M, et al. Germline mutations in ATM and BRCA1/2 are associated with grade reclassification in men on active surveillance for prostate cancer. Eur Urol 2019; 75:743–9.

77. Marshall CH, Fu W, Wang H, et al. Prevalence of DNA repair gene mutations in localized prostate cancer according to clinical and pathologic features: association of Gleason score and tumor stage. Prostate Cancer Prostatic Dis 2019;22: 59–65.

78. Marshall CH, Antonarakis ES. Therapeutic targeting of the DNA damage response in prostate cancer. Curr Opin Oncol 2020;32:216–22.

79. de Bono J, Mateo J, Fizazi K, et al. Olaparib for metastatic castration-resistant prostate cancer. N Engl J Med 2020;382:2091–102.

80. Abida W, Patnaik A, Campbell D, et al. Rucaparib in men with metastatic castration-resistant prostate cancer harboring a BRCA1 or BRCA2 gene alteration. J Clin Oncol 2020. https://doi.org/10.1200/JCO.20.01035. JCO2001035.

81. Marshall CH, Sokolova AO, McNatty AL, et al. Differential response to olaparib treatment among men with metastatic castration-resistant prostate cancer harboring BRCA1 or BRCA2 versus ATM mutations. Eur Urol 2019;76:452–8.

82. Abida W, Campbell D, Patnaik A, et al. Non-BRCA DNA damage repair gene alterations and response to the PARP inhibitor rucaparib in metastatic castration-resistant prostate cancer: analysis from the phase II TRITON2 study. Clin Cancer Res 2020;26:2487–96.

83. Schweizer MT, Cheng HH, Nelson PS, et al. Two steps forward and one step back for precision in prostate cancer treatment. J Clin Oncol 2020;38: 3740–2.

84. Brown JS, O'Carrigan B, Jackson SP, et al. Targeting DNA repair in cancer: beyond PARP inhibitors. Cancer Discov 2017;7:20–37.

85. Schweizer MT, Antonarakis ES, Bismar TA, et al. Genomic characterization of prostatic ductal adenocarcinoma identifies a high prevalence of DNA repair gene mutations. JCO Precis Oncol 2019;3:1–9.

86. Guedes LB, Antonarakis ES, Schweizer MT, et al. MSH2 loss in primary prostate cancer. Clin Cancer Res 2017;23:6863–74.

87. Marabelle A, Le DT, Ascierto PA, et al. Efficacy of pembrolizumab in patients with noncolorectal high microsatellite instability/mismatch repair-deficient cancer: results from the phase II KEYNOTE-158 study. J Clin Oncol 2020;38:1–10.

88. Abida W, Cheng ML, Armenia J, et al. Analysis of the prevalence of microsatellite instability in prostate cancer and response to immune checkpoint blockade. JAMA Oncol 2019;5:471–8.

89. Levine AJ, Oren M. The first 30 years of p53: growing ever more complex. Nat Rev Cancer 2009;9:749–58.

90. Navone NM, Troncoso P, Pisters LL, et al. p53 protein accumulation and gene mutation in the progression of human prostate carcinoma. J Natl Cancer Inst 1993;85:1657–69.

91. Brosh R, Rotter V. When mutants gain new powers: news from the mutant p53 field. Nat Rev Cancer 2009;9:701–13.

92. Guedes LB, Almutairi F, Haffner MC, et al. Analytic, preanalytic, and clinical validation of p53 IHC for detection of TP53 missense mutation in prostate cancer. Clin Cancer Res 2017;23:4693–703.

93. Bykov VJN, Eriksson SE, Bianchi J, et al. Targeting mutant p53 for efficient cancer therapy. Nat Rev Cancer 2018;18:89–102.

94. Burkhart DL, Morel KL, Sheahan AV, et al. The role of RB in prostate cancer progression. Adv Exp Med Biol 2019;1210:301–18.

95. McNair C, Xu K, Mandigo AC, et al. Differential impact of RB status on E2F1 reprogramming in human cancer. J Clin Invest 2018;128:341–58.

96. Abida W, Cyrta J, Heller G, et al. Genomic correlates of clinical outcome in advanced prostate cancer. Proc Natl Acad Sci U S A 2019;116:11428–36.

97. Cancer Genome Atlas Research Network. The molecular taxonomy of primary prostate cancer. Cell 2015;163:1011–25.

98. Ku S-Y, Rosario S, Wang Y, et al. Rb1 and Trp53 cooperate to suppress prostate cancer lineage plasticity, metastasis, and antiandrogen resistance. Science 2017;355:78–83.

99. Nyquist MD, Corella A, Coleman I, et al. Combined TP53 and RB1 loss promotes prostate cancer resistance to a spectrum of therapeutics and confers vulnerability to replication stress. CellReports 2020;31:107669.

100. Tan H-L, Sood A, Rahimi HA, et al. Rb loss is characteristic of prostatic small cell neuroendocrine carcinoma. Clin Cancer Res 2014;20:890–903.

101. Yoshimoto M, Cutz J-C, Nuin PAS, et al. Interphase FISH analysis of PTEN in histologic sections shows genomic deletions in 68% of primary prostate cancer and 23% of high-grade prostatic intra-epithelial neoplasias. Cancer Genet Cytogenet 2006;169: 128–37.

102. Lotan TL, Gurel B, Sutcliffe S, et al. PTEN protein loss by immunostaining: analytic validation and prognostic indicator for a high risk surgical cohort of prostate cancer patients. Clin Cancer Res 2011;17:6563–73.

103. Lotan TL, Wei W, Morais CL, et al. PTEN loss as determined by clinical-grade immunohistochemistry assay is associated with worse recurrence-free survival in prostate cancer. Eur Urol Focus 2016;2:180–8.

104. Chaux A, Peskoe SB, Gonzalez-Roibon N, et al. Loss of PTEN expression is associated with increased risk of recurrence after prostatectomy for clinically localized prostate cancer. Mod Pathol 2012;25:1543–9.

105. Lotan TL, Carvalho FL, Peskoe SB, et al. PTEN loss is associated with upgrading of prostate cancer from biopsy to radical prostatectomy. Mod Pathol 2014. https://doi.org/10.1038/modpathol.2014.85.

106. Jamaspishvili T, Berman DM, Ross AE, et al. Clinical implications of PTEN loss in prostate cancer. Nat Rev Urol 2018;15:222–34.

107. Trock BJ, Fedor H, Gurel B, et al. PTEN loss and chromosome 8 alterations in Gleason grade 3 prostate cancer cores predicts the presence of un-sampled grade 4 tumor: implications for active surveillance. Mod Pathol 2016;29:764–71.

108. de Bono JS, De Giorgi U, Rodrigues DN, et al. Randomized phase II study evaluating akt blockade with ipatasertib, in combination with abiraterone, in patients with metastatic prostate cancer with and without PTEN loss. Clin Cancer Res 2019;25:928–36.

109. Murillo-Garzón V, Kypta R. WNT signalling in prostate cancer. Nat Rev Urol 2017;14:683–96.

110. Nusse R, Clevers H. Wnt/β-catenin signaling, disease, and emerging therapeutic modalities. Cell 2017;169:985–99.

111. Isaacsson Velho P, Fu W, Wang H, et al. Wnt-pathway activating mutations are associated with resistance to first-line abiraterone and enzalutamide in castration-resistant prostate cancer. Eur Urol 2020;77:14–21.

112. Lee E, Ha S, Logan SK. Divergent androgen receptor and beta-catenin signaling in prostate cancer cells. PLoS One 2015;10:e0141589. Culig Z, ed.

113. Miyamoto DT, Zheng Y, Wittner BS, et al. RNA-Seq of single prostate CTCs implicates noncanonical Wnt signaling in antiandrogen resistance. Science 2015;349:1351–6.

114. Wise DR, Schneider JA, Armenia J, et al. Dickkopf-1 can lead to immune evasion in metastatic castration-resistant prostate cancer. JCO Precis Oncol 2020;4:1167–79.

115. Nelson WG, De Marzo AM, Yegnasubramanian S. Epigenetic alterations in human prostate cancers. Endocrinology 2009;150:3991–4002.

116. Yegnasubramanian S, De Marzo AM, Nelson WG. Prostate cancer epigenetics: from basic mechanisms to clinical implications. Cold Spring Harb Perspect Med 2019;9:a030445.

117. Baylin SB, Jones PA. A decade of exploring the cancer epigenome - biological and translational implications. Nat Rev Cancer 2011;11:726–34.

118. Jones PA, Baylin SB. The epigenomics of cancer. Cell 2007;128:683–92.

119. Aryee MJ, Liu W, Engelmann JC, et al. DNA methylation alterations exhibit intraindividual stability and interindividual heterogeneity in prostate cancer metastases. Sci Transl Med 2013;5:169ra10.

120. Yegnasubramanian S, Kowalski J, Gonzalgo ML, et al. Hypermethylation of CpG islands in primary and metastatic human prostate cancer. Cancer Res 2004;64:1975–86.

121. O'Reilly E, Tuzova AV, Walsh AL, et al. epiCaPture: a urine DNA methylation test for early detection of aggressive prostate cancer. JCO Precis Oncol 2019;2019:1–18.

122. Yegnasubramanian S, Haffner MC, Zhang Y, et al. DNA hypomethylation arises later in prostate cancer progression than CpG island hypermethylation and contributes to metastatic tumor heterogeneity. Cancer Res 2008;68:8954–67.

123. Partin AW, van Criekinge W, Trock BJ, et al. Clinical evaluation of an epigenetic assay to predict missed cancer in prostate biopsy specimens. Trans Am Clin Climatol Assoc 2016;127:313–27.

124. Wu A, Cremaschi P, Wetterskog D, et al. Genome-wide plasma DNA methylation features of metastatic prostate cancer. J Clin Invest 2020;130:1991–2000.

125. Beltran H, Romanel A, Conteduca V, et al. Circulating tumor DNA profile recognizes transformation to castration-resistant neuroendocrine prostate cancer. J Clin Invest 2020;130:1653–68.

126. Vince RA, Tosoian JJ, Jackson WC, et al. Tissue-based genomics: which test and when. Curr Opin Urol 2019;29:598–604.

127. Loeb S, Ross AE. Genomic testing for localized prostate cancer: where do we go from here? Curr Opin Urol 2017;27:495–9.

128. Abdollah F, Dalela D, Haffner MC, et al. The role of biomarkers and genetics in the diagnosis of prostate cancer. Eur Urol Focus 2015;1:99–108.

129. Zhao SG, Chang SL, Erho N, et al. Associations of luminal and basal subtyping of prostate cancer with prognosis and response to androgen deprivation therapy. JAMA Oncol 2017;3:1663–72.

130. Zhao SG, Chen WS, Das R, et al. Clinical and genomic implications of luminal and basal

subtypes across carcinomas. Clin Cancer Res 2019;25:2450–7.

131. Slack FJ, Chinnaiyan AM. The role of non-coding RNAs in oncology. Cell 2019;179:1033–55.

132. Prensner JR, Iyer MK, Sahu A, et al. The long noncoding RNA SChLAP1 promotes aggressive prostate cancer and antagonizes the SWI/SNF complex. Nat Genet 2013;45:1392–8.

133. Prensner JR, Zhao S, Erho N, et al. RNA biomarkers associated with metastatic progression in prostate cancer: a multi-institutional high-throughput analysis of SChLAP1. Lancet Oncol 2014;15:1469–80.

134. Mehra R, Udager AM, Ahearn TU, et al. Overexpression of the long non-coding RNA SChLAP1 independently predicts lethal prostate cancer. Eur Urol 2016;70:549–52.

135. Prensner JR, Iyer MK, Balbin OA, et al. Transcriptome sequencing across a prostate cancer cohort identifies PCAT-1, an unannotated lincRNA implicated in disease progression. Nat Biotechnol 2011;29:742–9.

136. Hessels D, Gunnewiek JMTK, van Oort I, et al. DD3(PCA3)-based molecular urine analysis for the diagnosis of prostate cancer. Eur Urol 2003; 44:8–15, [discussion: 15–6].

137. Chakravarty D, Sboner A, Nair SS, et al. The oestrogen receptor alpha-regulated lncRNA NEAT1 is a critical modulator of prostate cancer. Nat Commun 2014;5:5383.

138. Chua MLK, Lo W, Pintilie M, et al. A prostate cancer "nimbosus": genomic instability and SChLAP1 dysregulation underpin aggression of intraductal and cribriform subpathologies. Eur Urol 2017;72: 665–74.

139. Bluemn EG, Coleman IM, Lucas JM, et al. Androgen receptor pathway-independent prostate cancer is sustained through FGF signaling. Cancer Cell 2017;32:474–89.e6.

140. Varinot J, Furudoï A, Drouin S, et al. HOXB13 protein expression in metastatic lesions is a promising marker for prostate origin. Virchows Arch 2016; 468:619–22.

141. Beltran H, Hruszkewycz A, Scher HI, et al. The role of lineage plasticity in prostate cancer therapy resistance. Clin Cancer Res 2019;25: 6916–24.

142. Davies AH, Beltran H, Zoubeidi A. Cellular plasticity and the neuroendocrine phenotype in prostate cancer. Nat Rev Urol 2018;5:9.

143. Beltran H, Tomlins S, Aparicio A, et al. Aggressive variants of castration-resistant prostate cancer. Clin Cancer Res 2014;20:2846–50.

144. Aparicio AM, Shen L, Tapia ELN, et al. Combined tumor suppressor defects characterize clinically defined aggressive variant prostate cancers. Clin Cancer Res 2016;22:1520–30.

145. Epstein JI, Amin MB, Beltran H, et al. Proposed morphologic classification of prostate cancer with neuroendocrine differentiation. Am J Surg Pathol 2014;38:756–67.

146. Aggarwal R, Huang J, Alumkal JJ, et al. Clinical and genomic characterization of treatment-emergent small-cell neuroendocrine prostate cancer: a multi-institutional prospective study. J Clin Oncol 2018;36:2492–503.

147. Beltran H, Prandi D, Mosquera J-M, et al. Divergent clonal evolution of castration-resistant neuroendocrine prostate cancer. Nat Med 2016;22: 298–305.

148. Palmgren JS, Karavadia SS, Wakefield MR. Unusual and underappreciated: small cell carcinoma of the prostate. Semin Oncol 2007;34:22–9.

149. Labrecque MP, Coleman IM, Brown LG, et al. Molecular profiling stratifies diverse phenotypes of treatment-refractory metastatic castration-resistant prostate cancer. J Clin Invest 2019;130: 4492–505.

150. Conteduca V, Oromendia C, Eng KW, et al. Clinical features of neuroendocrine prostate cancer. Eur J Cancer 2019;121:7–18.

151. Park JW, Lee JK, Witte ON, et al. FOXA2 is a sensitive and specific marker for small cell neuroendocrine carcinoma of the prostate. Mod Pathol 2017;30:1262–72.

152. Xin Z, Zhang Y, Jiang Z, et al. Insulinoma-associated protein 1 is a novel sensitive and specific marker for small cell carcinoma of the prostate. Hum Pathol 2018;79:151–9.

153. Harmon SA, Tuncer S, Sanford T, et al. Artificial intelligence at the intersection of pathology and radiology in prostate cancer. Diagn Interv Radiol 2019;25:183–8.

Molecular Pathology of Urothelial Carcinoma

Hikmat Al-Ahmadie, MD[a],*, George J. Netto, MD[b],*

KEYWORDS

• Urothelial carcinoma • Molecular pathology • Molecular classification

Key points

- Urothelial carcinoma is a morphologically, clinically and genomically heterogeneous disease.
- Urothelial carcinoma harbors a high rate of somatic mutations that are dominated by APOBEC mutagenesis.
- Expression profiling identifies many molecular subtypes with important insights into the biology of urothelial neoplasia.
- Divergent differentiation and variant histologies are common in urothelial carcinoma, some of which may harbor specific genetic alterations, but the majority harbor mutations similar to those seen in classic urothelial carcinoma.

ABSTRACT

Urothelial carcinoma is characterized by the presence of a wide spectrum of histopathologic features and molecular alterations that contribute to its morphologic and genomic heterogeneity. It typically harbors high rates of somatic mutations with considerable genomic and transcriptional complexity and heterogeneity that is reflective of its varied histomorphologic and clinical features. This review provides an update on the recent advances in the molecular characterization and novel molecular taxonomy of urothelial carcinoma and variant histologies.

(UC) and provided insights into the molecular biology and pathogenesis of UC and some of its variants.[1] One of the main challenges in UC is the presence of considerable intratumoral and intertumoral heterogeneity that can be appreciated at the clinical, morphologic, genomic, and transcriptomic levels.[2] Many UC variant histologies are recognized and can be pure or, more frequently, mixed with UC–not otherwise specified. These variants historically have been based on defined morphologic features and more recently new molecular studies provided valuable insights into them.[1,3] The aim of this review is to provide an update on recent advances in molecular features of UC and a subset of its variants and potential clinical applications.

OVERVIEW

Recent advances in molecular biology and next-generation sequencing technologies have greatly enhanced our knowledge and understanding of the genomic landscape of urothelial carcinoma

MOLECULAR CHARACTERIZATION OF INVASIVE UROTHELIAL CARCINOMA

Multiple somatic mutation clones can be detected in the normal-appearing urothelial lining of the

Funding resources: This article was supported in part by Sloan Kettering Institute for Cancer Research Cancer Center Support Grant (P30CA008748), SPORE in Bladder Cancer (P50CA221745), and NCI (P01CA221757).

[a] Department of Pathology, Memorial Sloan Kettering Cancer Center, 1275 York Avenue, New York, NW 10065, USA; [b] Department of Pathology, University of Alabama at Birmingham, University of Alabama at Birmingham School of Medicine, WP Building, Suite P230, 619 19th Street South, Birmingham, AL 35249-7331, USA

* Corresponding authors.

E-mail addresses: alahmadh@mskcc.org (H.A.-A.); gnetto@uab.edu (G.J.N.)

Surgical Pathology 14 (2021) 403–414
https://doi.org/10.1016/j.path.2021.05.005
1875-9181/21/© 2021 Elsevier Inc. All rights reserved.

bladder in both healthy and diseased bladders.[4,5] This mutational background provides a permissive environment field effect for the development of UC through a process of clonal expansion such that the ultimate invasive disease is composed of multiple clones sharing ancestral mutations but also harboring many novel and unique mutations, which was revealed by multiregions sequencing from the same bladder.[4,6,7]

Recent studies with focus on the genomic landscape of UC consistently identified high rates of somatic mutations (>7 mutations per megabase), surpassed only by lung carcinomas and melanoma, which is characteristic of a carcinogen-induced malignancy.[8–10] By mutation signature analysis from whole-exome sequencing, APOBEC mutagenesis was the main mutational signature, which is attributed to a family of cytidine deaminase enzymes responsible for innate immunity that restricts the propagation of retroviruses and retrotransposons.[8] In muscle-invasive bladder cancer (MIBC) cohort reported by The Cancer Genome Atlas (TCGA), 2 APOBEC-mediated mutation signatures were associated with 66% of the single-nucleotide variants (SNVs), and the presence of APOBEC3-associated mutation signature was associated with better prognosis and improved 5-year overall survival.[10–12] Another mutational signature associated with ERCC2 mutation corresponded to approximately 20% of all SNVs in MIBC. This mutational signature additionally was shown to be associated with smoking independent of ERCC2 mutation status.[13] ERCC2 encodes a DNA helicase with a central role in a highly conserved DNA repair pathway through nucleotide-excision repair mechanism. Mutations in ERCC2, as well as other genes involved in DNA damage response and repair (DDR), recently were shown to be associated with improved response to cisplatin based chemotherapy as well as immune checkpoint blockade and radiation therapy for advanced UC.[14–18] Moreover, the presence of putative deleterious DDR gene alterations in pretreatment tumor tissue was strongly predictive of chemosensitivity, durable response, and superior long-term survival in MIBC patients treated with neoadjuvant dose-dense gemcitabine and cisplatin (ddGC).[19] Based on these results, there now are clinical trials designed to prospectively profile transurethral resection tumor samples by NGS for the presence of alterations in DDR genes and correlation with response to neoadjuvant ddGC, with the possibility of bladder preservation in patients demonstrating response to this treatment (clinical trial NCT03609216).

Besides the genes involved in DDR, many other genes are significantly mutated in UC that are involved in important cellular signaling pathways and canonical functions (**Fig. 1**). Most alterations were identified in genes involved in regulating the cell cycle, chromatin modification, receptor tyrosine kinase signaling, gene transcription, and other functions.[9,10,20] For example, one of the most commonly mutated genes is the cell cycle regulator TP53 (mutated in approximately half of MIBCs), which generally is mutually exclusive with MDM2 amplifications (present in approximately 7% of MIBCs). Other relatively common inactivating alterations occur in RB1 (mutation and deletion) and CDKN2A (deletion). Oncogenic alterations in several genes involved in cell signaling also are present, including activating hotspot mutations in receptor tyrosine kinases FGFR3 (and less frequently FGFR3 fusion and amplification), ERBB2 (including ERBB2 amplification), and ERBB3 and PIK3CA. Such alterations are important therapeutic targets in many cancer types but have not shown similar efficacy in bladder cancer, which could be related to mutation heterogeneity and clonality within the tumor or comutation pattern, as was reported by the neratinib basket trial for tumors with oncogenic ERBB2 and ERBB3 mutations.[21] One exception that is showing promise in the application of targeted therapy in UC is the presence of oncogenic alterations in FGFR3 (mutation, amplification, and fusion). Recent reports showed that FGFR3-targeted agents erdafitinib and BGJ398 (infigratinib) demonstrated efficacy in patients with advanced and metastatic UC that harbored FGFR3 mutations and overexpression.[22,23] Supported by these results, erdafitinib now is approved by the Food and Drug Administration for the treatment of patients with locally advanced or metastatic UC with FGFR3 or FGFR2 alterations who have disease progression following chemotherapy.[24]

The most frequent mutation in UC that was not reported in large-scale exome-based sequencing studies is the recurrent point mutations in TERT promoter region. In many studies, TERT promoter mutations were identified in UC in different grades and stages and spectrum of morphologic variants but not in benign proliferative conditions, such as cystitis cystica et glandularis and florid von Brunn nests,[25–28] or benign urothelial neoplasms, such as urothelial papilloma and inverted papilloma.[29–32] These findings have important clinical implications in facilitating the distinction between UC with deceptively bland morphologic features, such as nested variant of UC (NVUC), from its benign mimics (namely, cystitis cystica, florid von Brunn nests, and inverted urothelial papilloma). The detection of TERT promoter mutation in early-

Fig. 1. The genomic landscape of MIBC as reported by the TCGA cohort[10] with co-occurring alterations in canonical cellular functions and signaling pathways.[89,90] This oncoprint is generated from cBio-Portal (https://www.cbio-portal.org). *Data from* Cerami, E., et al., The cBio cancer genomics portal: an open platform for exploring multidimensional cancer genomics data. Cancer Discov, 2012. 2(5): p. 401-4, Gao, J., et al., Integrative analysis of complex cancer genomics and clinical profiles using the cBio-Portal. Sci Signal, 2013. 6(269): p. pl1.

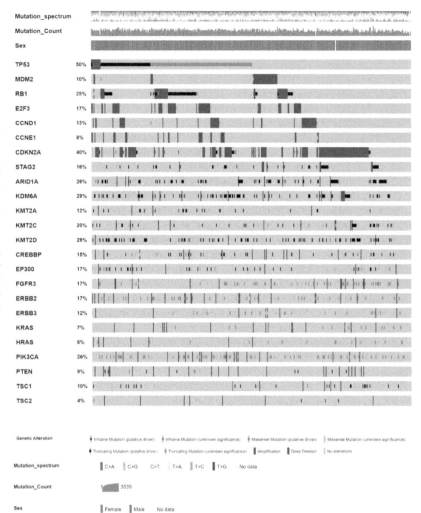

stage and low-grade disease suggests that it is an early genetic event in the development of UC.[29] More importantly, this alteration also can be detected from urine samples, making it a potential biomarker for urothelial neoplasia that can be detected by noninvasive procedures.[33,34]

The genetic landscape of early-stage UC overall is similar to that reported in MIBC but differs in the frequency of certain mutations. For example, mutations in *FGFR3* and chromatin modifier *KDM6A* are significantly more frequent in early-stage and low-grade UC compared with MIBC, whereas mutations in *TP53*, *RB1*, and chromatin modifier *ARID1A* show the reverse pattern.[35]

MOLECULAR TAXONOMY OF UROTHELIAL CARCINOMA

Expression profiling of UC by RNA and/or immunohistochemistry revealed several molecular subtypes and several classification schemes, some of which were linked to prognosis or response to a variety of therapies. Different classifications used different names for different subtypes, but there is significant overlap among them.[10,36–39] The most comprehensive and widely used classifications are those proposed by the Lund University group and that of the TCGA.[10,39,40] To further provide uniformity to the terminology applied to RNA-based classification, a recent international effort led by the Bladder Cancer Molecular Taxonomy Group provided a consensus molecular classification of MIBC that was based on reanalyzing 1750 MIBC transcriptomic profiles from 18 data sets, 16 of which already were published (**Figs. 2** and **3**).[41,42] Central to these various classification systems is the presence of 2 major categories, luminal and basal, with additional subtypes of these 2 major categories. This basal-luminal division of MIBC initially was

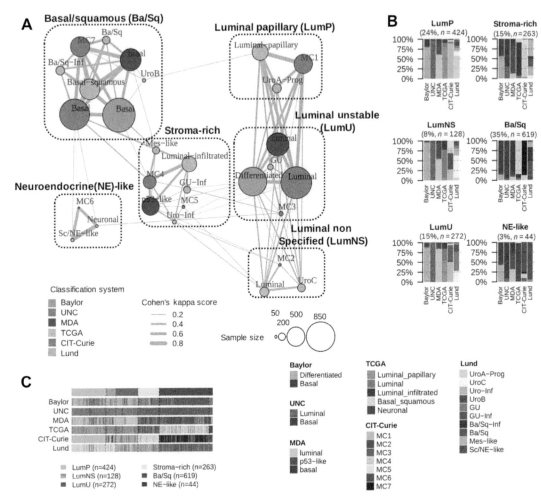

Fig. 2. Consensus molecular classification of muscle invasive UC. (*A*) Clustered network of consensus classification based on 1750 transcriptomes originally classified according to 6 different input molecular subtypes. The circles inside each clique represent subtype contribution from each input subtype matched by color. Circle size is proportional to the number of samples assigned to the subtype. (*B*) Input subtypes repartitioned among each consensus class. (*C*) Relationship between subtyping results from the 6 input classification schemes. Samples are ordered by predicted consensus classes. MDA, MD Anderson Cancer Center; UNC, University of North Carolina.[41] (*From* Kamoun, A., et al., A Consensus Molecular Classification of Muscle-invasive Bladder Cancer. Eur Urol, 2020. 77(4): p. 420-433.)

adopted following perceived similarities to the expression profiles of breast cancer. As such, basal bladder tumors typically express basal type keratins (eg, KRT5, KRT6, and KRT14), whereas luminal tumors typically have high expression levels of FGFR3, transcription factors PPARG, GATA3, FOXA1, and ELF3, uroplakin genes found in umbrella cells, and KRT20.[36,37,43] The TCGA analysis further expanded and refined this classification and identified 3 subgroups within the luminal subtype along with a basal-squamous subtype as well a distinct neuronal cluster (total of 5 subtypes) (**Fig. 4**). The identified subgroups within the luminal subtype—luminal-

papillary, luminal-infiltrated, and luminal—correspond approximately to the luminal subtypes by consensus molecular classification, namely luminal papillary (LumP), luminal nonspecified (LumNS), luminal unstable (LumU), and stroma-rich subtypes. The TCGA luminal-papillary subtype is enriched with papillary tumors, lower stage, and FGFR3 overexpression as a result of FGFR3 mutations, amplification, and FGFR3-TACC3 fusions. The TCGA luminal-infiltrated subtype is characterized by the presence of myofibroblast and smooth muscle gene signatures, lymphocytic infiltrate, and increased expression of immune markers, such as CD274 (PD-L1) and PDCD1

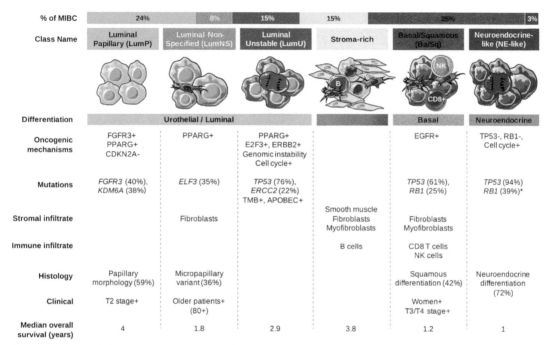

% of MIBC	24%	8%	15%	15%	35%	3%
Class Name	Luminal Papillary (LumP)	Luminal Non-Specified (LumNS)	Luminal Unstable (LumU)	Stroma-rich	Basal/Squamous (Ba/Sq)	Neuroendocrine-like (NE-like)
Differentiation	Urothelial / Luminal				Basal	Neuroendocrine
Oncogenic mechanisms	FGFR3+ PPARG+ CDKN2A-	PPARG+	PPARG+ E2F3+, ERBB2+ Genomic instability Cell cycle+		EGFR+	TP53-, RB1-, Cell cycle+
Mutations	FGFR3 (40%), KDM6A (38%)	ELF3 (35%)	TP53 (76%), ERCC2 (22%) TMB+, APOBEC+		TP53 (61%), RB1 (25%)	TP53 (94%) RB1 (39%)*
Stromal infiltrate		Fibroblasts		Smooth muscle Fibroblasts Myofibroblasts	Fibroblasts Myofibroblasts	
Immune infiltrate				B cells	CD8 T cells NK cells	
Histology	Papillary morphology (59%)	Micropapillary variant (36%)			Squamous differentiation (42%)	Neuroendocrine differentiation (72%)
Clinical	T2 stage+	Older patients+ (80+)			Women+ T3/T4 stage+	
Median overall survival (years)	4	1.8	2.9	3.8	1.2	1

Fig. 3. Summary of the main characteristics of the consensus molecular classes. (*Top to bottom*) Proportion of consensus classes in the 1750 tumor samples; consensus class names; schematic graphical representation of tumor cells and their microenvironments (immune cells, fibroblasts, and smooth muscle cells); and a table listing the main characteristics, such as oncogenic mechanisms, mutations, stromal infiltrate, immune infiltrate, histology, clinical characteristics, and median overall survival. NK, natural killer.[41] (*From* Kamoun, A., et al., A Consensus Molecular Classification of Muscle-invasive Bladder Cancer. Eur Urol, 2020. 77(4): p. 420-433.)

(PD-1). Similar expression patterns were linked to a wild-type p53 signature and chemoresistance in 1 study[36] but were reported to derive most benefit from anti–PD-L1 treatment in another study.[44] The basal subtype is enriched with tumors exhibiting squamous morphology by histopathologic review and thus was called basal-squamous but also included tumors that were devoid of unequivocal squamous differentiation (SqD).[10,41] This subtype is associated with high expression of basal and stemlike markers, such as CD44, KRT5, KRT6A, and KRT14 (**Fig. 5**), and SqD markers, such as desmocollins (DSC1-3) and desmogleins (DSG1–4), TGM1 (transglutaminase 1), and PI3 (elafin). The basal-squamous subtype also is enriched in TP53 mutations, more common in women, and shows increased lymphocytic infiltrates and a strong immune gene signature expression. The TCGA neuronal subtype corresponded to the neuroendocrine-like consensus subtype (and small cell/neuroendocrine-like carcinoma subtype [SmCC] by Lund University classification) and is enriched with tumors with neuroendocrine morphology and consistently showed relatively high expression levels of genes involved in neuronal differentiation and development as well as typical neuroendocrine and neural differentiation markers, such as chromogranin, PEG10, PLEKHG4, and TUBB2B.[10,40,41] Although a majority of tumors in this cluster (85%) had alterations in genes in the p53/cell cycle pathway, only a subset was associated with mutations in both TP53 and RB1, which is the hallmark alteration in SmCC.[45] Nonetheless, this subtype was associated with the worst clinical outcome.[10,46]

RNA-based molecular classification has been applied in many studies as a means for patient risk stratification and association with outcome[10,41,46] and reported correlation with responses to chemotherapy or immunotherapy in advanced disease.[36,44,47] Although these molecular classifications provide important biologic insights of MIBC, molecular subtyping continues to evolve and, as such, may not be ready yet for routine clinical applications because several questions remain unanswered and prospective validation still is lacking. Further work and investigation are needed to delineate the exact roles of these different classification schema and the effect of intratumoral heterogeneity and therapeutic intervention on the stability of such molecular subtypes. This is highlighted by studies showing intratumoral heterogeneity of molecular subtype

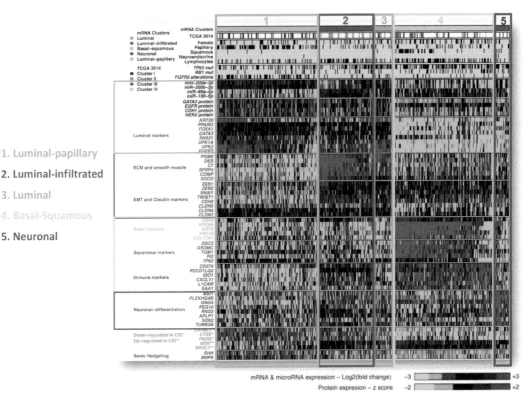

Fig. 4. TCGA molecular subtypes of muscle invasive UC by RNA expression profiling. (*Top to bottom*) Five mRNA expression subtypes (luminal-papillary, luminal-infiltrated, luminal, basal-squamous, and neuronal); 4 previously reported TCGA subtypes; selected clinical covariates and key genetic alterations; and normalized expression for miRNAs and proteins for selected genes. Samples within the 3 luminal subtypes, the basal-squamous subtype, and the neuronal subtype are ordered by luminal, basal, and neuroendocrine signature scores, respectively.[10] (*From* Robertson, A.G., et al., Comprehensive Molecular Characterization of Muscle-Invasive Bladder Cancer. Cell, 2017. 171(3): p. 540-556 e25.)

assignment to different parts of the same tumor,[48,49] to primary versus metastatic tumors from the same patient,[50] or to initial versus recurrent or progressed tumors from the same patient.[51]

There also is preclinical evidence of switch between luminal and basal subtypes in organoid generated from luminal bladder cancers,[52] further underscoring the need for more investigations into the biology and stability of these molecular subtypes.

MOLECULAR UPDATES ON HISTOLOGIC VARIANTS OF UROTHELIAL CARCINOMA

SqD is the most common divergent differentiation in UC, identified in up to 30% of high-grade and/or high-stage disease.[3,53] Expression profiling studies that included UC with SqD consistently reported that this tumor type nearly always clustered with the basal/squamous subtypes in virtually all classification schema.[10,36–38,54] These tumors

characteristically show overexpression of high molecular weight keratins (CK5, CK6, and CK14) and epidermal growth factor receptor as well as down-regulation of markers of urothelial differentiation, such as uroplakins, GATA3, FOXA1, PPARG, and thrombomodulin. Because these studies were based on bulk samples with mixed squamous and urothelial components, they were unable to provide insights into the exact mechanisms involved in the development of squamous morphology in this setting.

Two studies investigated intratumoral heterogeneity within UC with SqD by analyzing separate areas of urothelial and squamous morphology from the same tumor.[48,49] They reported that in a subset of cases the expression profiles of the urothelial area were classified as luminal whereas the squamous areas were mostly classified as basal/squamous.

Glandular differentiation is reported in variable incidences in different studies, ranging from 8% to 18%.[53,55–57] There is limited literature on the molecular characteristics of glandular differentiation

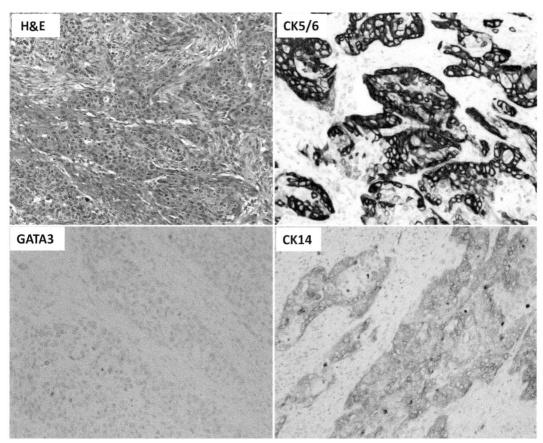

Fig. 5. Basal UC. In this example of invasive UC without morphologic evidence of SqD, there is near absence of luminal marker GATA3 expression and overexpression of basal markers CK5/6 and CK14, consistent with basal subtype (original magnification x100).

in UC but the available evidence suggests that there is overlap with those of UC, particularly the presence of high rates of mutations in *TERT* promoter region and in chromatin remodeling genes.[27,58]

Plasmacytoid UC (PUC) is a rare and aggressive variant of UC with a diffuse and infiltrating pattern of discohesive, individual, or small clusters of tumor cells, generally with minimal stromal reaction. Tumor cell nuclei typically are eccentrically located, giving a superficial resemblance to plasma cells and, in most cases, tumor cells contain intracytoplasmic vacuoles that push and compress the nucleus resulting in signet ring cell morphology.[59–61] PUC usually presents at advanced stage and is associated with high mortality rate, high propensity for relapse and frequent peritoneal carcinomatosis despite sometimes the apparent initial response to chemotherapy.[59–63] Next-generation sequencing and functional studies identified the presence of *CDH1* truncating mutations, and less frequently CDH1 promoter hypermethylation, as the defining features of

PUC that were specific to this histologic variant.[59] These mutations results in loss of E-cadherin expression in a majority of cases (**Fig. 6**). Beyond CDH1 alterations, the overall genomic landscape of PUC generally is similar to that of UC-NOS, with frequent mutations in chromatin modifiers, cell cycle regulators, and *TERT* promoter.[59,64]

In contrast to the presence of germline *CDH1* mutations in patients with hereditary diffuse gastric cancers and a subset of mammary lobular carcinoma, no germline *CDH1* mutations were identified in PUC, including in a patient with 2 primary tumors driven by *CDH1* loss, a primary breast lobular carcinoma, and a primary bladder PUC.[59,65]

Micropapillary UC (MPUC) is a rare variant of UC with reported aggressive clinical behavior. By molecular analysis, MPUC consistently harbors higher rates of *ERBB2* amplification than classic UC, which in some reports was associated with worse outcome following radical cystectomy.[66–68] The distribution of *ERBB2* amplification within MPUC tumors is variable, but it is preferentially

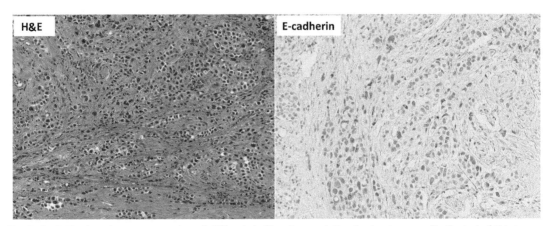

Fig. 6. PUC. The invasive tumor consists of diffusely infiltrating and discohesive tumor cells. Typical of this tumor, there is complete loss of E-cadherin expression in tumor cells. Next-generation sequencing identified a *CDH1* (X337_splice) mutation (original magnification x100).

present in the micropapillary component in tumors containing both MP and UC areas[69] (**Fig. 7**), despite the higher rate of *ERBB2* amplification in the UC areas in these mixed MPUC-UC tumors than the reported rates in pure UC or those not mixed with MP components.[10,20,70] Recurrent hotspots *ERBB2* mutations have been reported in bladder MPUC,[71] but it is likely that their frequency is similar to that reported in classic UC. By expression profiling, MPUC generally is luminal and displays enrichment of *PPARG* and suppression of p63 target genes.[41,72]

SmCC is rare and is morphologically similar to that of the lung and other organs and can be admixed with a urothelial or other divergent differentiation component.[53] By molecular analysis, SmCC is characterized by the presence of *TP53* and *RB1* comutations, which, in 1 study, was identified in 90% and 87% of cases, respectively (80% of tumors displayed co-alterations of both genes).[45] Furthermore, even in tumors without *RB1* deletion or loss of function mutations, there was loss of RB expression by immunohistochemistry, suggesting an alternative mechanism for retinoblastoma (RB) protein loss of expression, such as epigenetic silencing. Moreover, genes that were commonly mutated in UC also were found to be mutated in bladder SmCC, including *TERT*

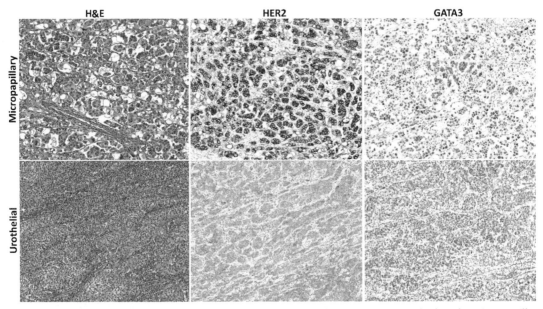

Fig. 7. Micropapillary UC. In this mixed MPUC-UC tumor, there is HER2 overexpression (+3) in the micropapillary component only, which was associated with 8-fold *ERBB2* amplification by next-generation sequencing. Consistent with a luminal phenotype, this tumor expresses luminal marker GATA3 in both components (original magnification x100).

promoter mutations (95%) and truncating alterations in genes involved in chromatin modification, such as *CREBBP*, *EP300*, *ARID1A*, and *KMT2D*, in approximately 75% of samples.[45,73] This mutation pattern can be helpful in determining a urothelial origin of a SmCC tumor from a metastatic location or when the site of origin is not obvious (for example, urothelial vs prostatic vs pulmonary).

SmCC is associated with a high level of chromosomal instability that is characterized by the presence of whole genome duplication in 72% of tumors, in particular those with *TP53* missense mutations that resulted in biallelic silencing. Compared with that of the lung, bladder SmCC is enriched for APOBEC mutation signature in contrast to the dominant smoking signature that is associated with lung SmCC.[45,54] These findings support the precursor urothelial origin of bladder SmCC. A recent study confirmed these observations and reported a urothelial-to-neural phenotypic switch with a dysregulated epithelial-to-mesenchymal transition network in bladder SmCC.[74]

Sarcomatoid UC is a rare form of bladder cancer in which a component of the tumor exhibits mesenchymal phenotype that can in some tumors be true heterologous elements in the form of cartilaginous, osseous, rhabdomyoblastic, or other elements.[75–77] Like other variants of UC, it has been reported that the sarcomatous and urothelial components within the same tumor share common clonal origin and that sarcomatoid UC is enriched with mutations in *TP53*, *RB1*, and *PIK3CA* and is associated with dysregulation of epithelial-mesenchymal transition (EMT) network and overexpression of EMT markers.[76–79] By expression profiling, they share features of the basal molecular subtype of UC, characterized by down-regulation of luminal markers, such as FOXA1 and GATA3, and up-regulation of basal markers in a subset of tumors, such as keratins 5, 6, and 14.[41,78]

NVUC is another rare variant of UC characterized by deceptively bland morphologic features that can be associated with aggressive clinical course.[80,81] A large nested variant of UC recognized where the invading tumor nests are noticeably large and irregular.[82,83] Identifying this variant can be diagnostically challenging because it shares overlapping features with benign entities, such as proliferative cystitis, von Brunn nest hyperplasia, nephrogenic adenoma, or inverted papilloma.[82,84,85] So far, a few molecular findings have been reported in this tumor type, the most common of which is the high rate of *TERT* promoter mutations that was not found in benign mimickers,[25,26,86] as well as occasional mutations in

TP53, *JAK3*, and *CTNNB1*, suggesting that this tumor likely harbors molecular alterations similar to those of UC. A recent study on large nested UC reported FGFR3 mutations in a vast majority of cases.[87] Nested UC typically exhibits luminal expression pattern by studies that were based on IHC expression of luminal markers, in particular FOXA1, GATA3, and CK20.[86–88]

SUMMARY AND FUTURE DIRECTIONS

Recent advances in the molecular biology and genomics of UC provided great insights into the molecular mechanisms underlying the development, progression, and heterogeneity of this disease. The recently proposed molecular classifications provide additional important insights into the biology of MIBC and a consensus on a molecular classification scheme that is applicable to routine clinical use urgently is needed. Ideally such classification will help to address several unanswered questions including how stable these molecular subtypes are within a given tumor (questions of intratumoral heterogeneity within the primary tumor, or primary vs metastasis) and following therapy. It also would be helpful to determine whether molecular subtyping should be incorporated into clinical decision making and, if so, in which disease states and/or treatment settings. Addressing these questions should hopefully enhance our ability to provide novel and precise biomarker-directed therapies.

REFERENCES

1. Al-Ahmadie H, Netto GJ. Updates on the genomics of bladder cancer and novel molecular taxonomy. Adv Anat Pathol 2020;27(1):36–43.

2. Meeks JJ, Al-Ahmadie H, Faltas BM, et al. Genomic heterogeneity in bladder cancer: challenges and possible solutions to improve outcomes. Nat Rev Urol 2020;17(5):259–70.

3. Moch H, Cubilla AL, Humphrey PA, et al. WHO Classification of tumours of the urinary system and male genital organs. In: Bosman FT, et al, editors. World Health Organization classification of tumours. 4th edition. Lyon (France): International Agency for Research on Cancer; 2016.

4. Lawson ARJ, Abascal F, Coorens THH, et al. Extensive heterogeneity in somatic mutation and selection in the human bladder. Science 2020;370(6512):75–82.

5. Li R, Du Y, Chen Z, et al. Macroscopic somatic clonal expansion in morphologically normal human urothelium. Science 2020;370(6512):82–9.

6. Thomsen MB, Nordentoft I, Lamy P, et al. Spatial and temporal clonal evolution during development of

metastatic urothelial carcinoma. Mol Oncol 2016; 10(9):1450–60.

7. Heide T, Maurer A, Eipel M, et al. Multiregion human bladder cancer sequencing reveals tumour evolution, bladder cancer phenotypes and implications for targeted therapy. J Pathol 2019;248(2):230–42.

8. Lawrence MS, Stojanov P, Polak P, et al. Mutational heterogeneity in cancer and the search for new cancer-associated genes. Nature 2013;499(7457): 214–8.

9. Gui Y, Guo G, Huang Y, et al. Frequent mutations of chromatin remodeling genes in transitional cell carcinoma of the bladder. Nat Genet 2011;43(9):875–8.

10. Robertson AG, Kim J, Al-Ahmadie H, et al. Comprehensive molecular characterization of muscle-invasive bladder cancer. Cell 2017;171(3):540–56.e25.

11. Glaser AP, Fantini D, Shilatifard A, et al. The evolving genomic landscape of urothelial carcinoma. Nat Rev Urol 2017;14(4):215–29.

12. Vlachostergios PJ, Faltas BM. Treatment resistance in urothelial carcinoma: an evolutionary perspective. Nat Rev Clin Oncol 2018;15(8).

13. Kim J, Mouw KW, Polak P, et al. Somatic ERCC2 mutations are associated with a distinct genomic signature in urothelial tumors. Nat Genet 2016;48(6): 600–6.

14. Teo MY, Bambury RM, Zabor EC, et al. DNA damage response and repair gene alterations are associated with improved survival in patients with platinum-treated advanced urothelial carcinoma. Clin Cancer Res 2017;23(14):3610–8.

15. Teo MY, Bambury RM, Zabor EC, et al. Alterations in DNA damage response and repair genes as potential marker of clinical benefit from PD-1/PD-L1 blockade in advanced urothelial cancers. J Clin Oncol 2018;36(17):1685–94.

16. Desai NB, Scott SN, Zabor EC, et al. Genomic characterization of response to chemoradiation in urothelial bladder cancer. Cancer 2016;122(23):3715–23.

17. Van Allen EM, Mouw KW, Kim P, et al. Somatic ERCC2 mutations correlate with cisplatin sensitivity in muscle-invasive urothelial carcinoma. Cancer Discov 2014;4(10):1140–53.

18. Mouw KW, D'Andrea AD. DNA repair deficiency and immunotherapy response. J Clin Oncol 2018;36(17): 1710–3.

19. Iyer G, Balar AV, Milowsky MI, et al. Multicenter prospective phase II trial of neoadjuvant dose-dense gemcitabine plus cisplatin in patients with muscle-invasive bladder cancer. J Clin Oncol 2018;36(19):1949–56.

20. Iyer G, Al-Ahmadie H, Schultz N, et al. Prevalence and co-occurrence of actionable genomic alterations in high-grade bladder cancer. J Clin Oncol 2013;31(25):3133–40.

21. Hyman DM, Piha-Paul SA, Won H, et al. HER kinase inhibition in patients with HER2- and HER3-mutant cancers. Nature 2018;554(7691):189–94.

22. Pal SK, Rosenberg JE, Hoffman-Censits JH, et al. Efficacy of BGJ398, a fibroblast growth factor receptor 1-3 inhibitor, in patients with previously treated advanced urothelial carcinoma with FGFR3 alterations. Cancer Discov 2018;8(7):812–21.

23. Loriot Y, Necchi A, Park SH, et al. Erdafitinib in locally advanced or metastatic urothelial carcinoma. N Engl J Med 2019;381(4):338–48.

24. FDA grants accelerated approval to erdafitinib for metastatic urothelial carcinoma. Available at: https://www.fda.gov/drugs/resources-information-approved-drugs/fda-grants-accelerated-approval-erdafitinib-metastatic-urothelial-carcinoma.

25. Taylor AS, McKenney JK, Osunkoya AO, et al. PAX8 expression and TERT promoter mutations in the nested variant of urothelial carcinoma: a clinicopathologic study with immunohistochemical and molecular correlates. Mod Pathol 2020;33(6):1165–71.

26. Zhong M, Tian W, Zhuge J, et al. Distinguishing nested variants of urothelial carcinoma from benign mimickers by TERT promoter mutation. Am J Surg Pathol 2015;39(1):127–31.

27. Vail E, Zheng X, Zhou M, et al. Telomerase reverse transcriptase promoter mutations in glandular lesions of the urinary bladder. Ann Diagn Pathol 2015;19(5):301–5.

28. Brown NA, Lew M, Weigelin HC, et al. Comparative study of TERT promoter mutation status within spatially, temporally and morphologically distinct components of urothelial carcinoma. Histopathology 2018;72(2):354–6.

29. Kinde I, Munari E, Faraj SF, et al. TERT promoter mutations occur early in urothelial neoplasia and are biomarkers of early disease and disease recurrence in urine. Cancer Res 2013;73(24):7162–7.

30. Isharwal S, Hu W, Sarungbam J, et al. Genomic landscape of inverted urothelial papilloma and urothelial papilloma of the bladder. J Pathol 2019; 248(3):260–5.

31. Wang CC, Huang CY, Jhuang YL, et al. Biological significance of TERT promoter mutation in papillary urothelial neoplasm of low malignant potential. Histopathology 2018;72(5):795–803.

32. Isharwal S, Audenet F, Drill E, et al. Prognostic value of TERT alterations, mutational and copy number alterations burden in urothelial carcinoma. Eur Urol Focus 2017;5(2):201–4.

33. Springer SU, Chen CH, Rodriguez Pena MDC, et al. Non-invasive detection of urothelial cancer through the analysis of driver gene mutations and aneuploidy. Elife 2018;7:e32143.

34. Eich ML, Rodriguez Pena MDC, Springer SU, et al. Incidence and distribution of UroSEEK gene panel in a multi-institutional cohort of bladder urothelial carcinoma. Mod Pathol 2019;32(10):1544–50.

35. Pietzak EJ, Bagrodia A, Cha EK, et al. Next-generation sequencing of nonmuscle invasive bladder

cancer reveals potential biomarkers and rational therapeutic targets. Eur Urol 2017;72(6):952–9.

36. Choi W, Porten S, Kim S, et al. Identification of distinct basal and luminal subtypes of muscle-invasive bladder cancer with different sensitivities to frontline chemotherapy. Cancer Cell 2014;25(2):152–65.

37. Damrauer JS, Hoadley KA, Chism DD, et al. Intrinsic subtypes of high-grade bladder cancer reflect the hallmarks of breast cancer biology. Proc Natl Acad Sci U S A 2014;111(8):3110–5.

38. Sjodahl G, Lauss M, Lövgren K, et al. A molecular taxonomy for urothelial carcinoma. Clin Cancer Res 2012;18(12):3377–86.

39. Sjodahl G, Lövgren K, Lauss M, et al. Toward a molecular pathologic classification of urothelial carcinoma. Am J Pathol 2013;183(3):681–91.

40. Sjodahl G, Eriksson P, Liedberg F, et al. Molecular classification of urothelial carcinoma: global mRNA classification versus tumour-cell phenotype classification. J Pathol 2017;242(1):113–25.

41. Kamoun A, de Reyniès A, Allory Y, et al. A consensus molecular classification of muscle-invasive bladder cancer. Eur Urol 2020;77(4):420–33.

42. Lerner SP, McConkey DJ, Hoadley KA, et al. Bladder cancer molecular taxonomy: summary from a consensus meeting. Bladder Cancer 2016;2(1):37–47.

43. Kim J, Robertson G, Akbani R, et al. Genomic assessment of muscle-invasive bladder cancer: insights from the cancer genome atlas (TCGA) project. In: Hansel DE, Lerner SP, editors. Precision molecular pathology of bladder cancer. Cham (Switzerland): Springer International Publishing; 2018. p. 43–64.

44. Rosenberg JE, Hoffman-Censits J, Powles T, et al. Atezolizumab in patients with locally advanced and metastatic urothelial carcinoma who have progressed following treatment with platinum-based chemotherapy: a single-arm, multicentre, phase 2 trial. Lancet 2016;387(10031):1909–20.

45. Chang MT, Penson A, Desai NB, et al. Small cell carcinomas of the bladder and lung are characterized by a convergent but distinct pathogenesis. Clin Cancer Res 2017;24(8):1965–73.

46. Marzouka NA, Eriksson P, Rovira C, et al. A validation and extended description of the Lund taxonomy for urothelial carcinoma using the TCGA cohort. Sci Rep 2018;8(1):3737.

47. Seiler R, Ashab HAD, Erho N, et al. Impact of molecular subtypes in muscle-invasive bladder cancer on predicting response and survival after neoadjuvant chemotherapy. Eur Urol 2017;72(4):544–54.

48. Warrick JI, Sjödahl G, Kaag M, et al. Intratumoral heterogeneity of bladder cancer by molecular subtypes and histologic variants. Eur Urol 2019;75(1):18–22.

49. Hovelson DH, Udager AM, McDaniel AS, et al. Targeted DNA and RNA sequencing of paired urothelial and squamous bladder cancers reveals discordant genomic and transcriptomic events and unique therapeutic implications. Eur Urol 2018;74(6):741–53.

50. Sjodahl G, Eriksson P, Lövgren K, et al. Discordant molecular subtype classification in the basal-squamous subtype of bladder tumors and matched lymph-node metastases. Mod Pathol 2018;31(12):1869–81.

51. Sjodahl G, Eriksson P, Patschan O, et al. Molecular changes during progression from nonmuscle invasive to advanced urothelial carcinoma. Int J Cancer 2020;146(9):2636–47.

52. Lee SH, Hu W, Matulay JT, et al. Tumor evolution and drug response in patient-derived organoid models of bladder cancer. Cell 2018;173(2):515–28.e17.

53. Amin MB. Histological variants of urothelial carcinoma: diagnostic, therapeutic and prognostic implications. Mod Pathol 2009;22(Suppl 2):S96–118.

54. Cancer Genome Atlas Research N. Comprehensive molecular characterization of urothelial bladder carcinoma. Nature 2014;507(7492):315–22.

55. Wasco MJ, Daignault S, Zhang Y, et al. Urothelial carcinoma with divergent histologic differentiation (mixed histologic features) predicts the presence of locally advanced bladder cancer when detected at transurethral resection. Urology 2007;70(1):69–74.

56. Linder BJ, Boorjian SA, Cheville JC, et al. The impact of histological reclassification during pathology re-review–evidence of a Will Rogers effect in bladder cancer? J Urol 2013;190(5):1692–6.

57. Shah RB, Montgomery JS, Montie JE, et al. Variant (divergent) histologic differentiation in urothelial carcinoma is under-recognized in community practice: impact of mandatory central pathology review at a large referral hospital. Urol Oncol 2013;31(8):1650–5.

58. Maurer A, Ortiz-Bruechle N, Guricova K, et al. Comparative genomic profiling of glandular bladder tumours. Virchows Arch 2020;477(3):445–54.

59. Al-Ahmadie HA, Iyer G, Lee BH, et al. Frequent somatic CDH1 loss-of-function mutations in plasmacytoid variant bladder cancer. Nat Genet 2016;48(4):356–8.

60. Keck B, Stoehr R, Wach S, et al. The plasmacytoid carcinoma of the bladder–rare variant of aggressive urothelial carcinoma. Int J Cancer 2011;129(2):346–54.

61. Nigwekar P, Tamboli P, Amin MB, et al. Plasmacytoid urothelial carcinoma: detailed analysis of morphology with clinicopathologic correlation in 17 cases. Am J Surg Pathol 2009;33(3):417–24.

62. Dayyani F, Czerniak BA, Sircar K, et al. Plasmacytoid urothelial carcinoma, a chemosensitive cancer with poor prognosis, and peritoneal carcinomatosis. J Urol 2013;189(5):1656–61.

63. Kaimakliotis HZ, Monn MF, Cheng L, et al. Plasma-cytoid bladder cancer: variant histology with aggressive behavior and a new mode of invasion along fascial planes. Urology 2014;83(5):1112–6.

64. Palsgrove DN, Taheri D, Springer SU, et al. Targeted sequencing of plasmacytoid urothelial carcinoma reveals frequent TERT promoter mutations. Hum Pathol 2019;85:1–9.

65. Penson A, Camacho N, Zheng Y, et al. Development of Genome-Derived Tumor Type Prediction to Inform Clinical Cancer Care. JAMA Oncol 2021;6(1):84–91.

66. Schneider SA, Sukov WR, Frank I, et al. Outcome of patients with micropapillary urothelial carcinoma following radical cystectomy: ERBB2 (HER2) amplification identifies patients with poor outcome. Mod Pathol 2014;27(5):758–64.

67. Tschui J, Vassella E, Bandi N, et al. Morphological and molecular characteristics of HER2 amplified urothelial bladder cancer. Virchows Arch 2015;466(6):703–10.

68. Ching CB, Amin MB, Tubbs RR, et al. HER2 gene amplification occurs frequently in the micropapillary variant of urothelial carcinoma: analysis by dual-color in situ hybridization. Mod Pathol 2011;24(8):1111–9.

69. Isharwal S, Huang H, Nanjangud G, et al. Intratumoral heterogeneity of ERBB2 amplification and HER2 expression in micropapillary urothelial carcinoma. Hum Pathol 2018;77:63–9.

70. Fleischmann A, Rotzer D, Seiler R, et al. Her2 amplification is significantly more frequent in lymph node metastases from urothelial bladder cancer than in the primary tumours. Eur Urol 2011;60(2):350–7.

71. Ross JS, Wang K, Gay LM, et al. A high frequency of activating extracellular domain ERBB2 (HER2) mutation in micropapillary urothelial carcinoma. Clin Cancer Res 2014;20(1):68–75.

72. Guo CC, Dadhania V, Zhang L, et al. Gene expression profile of the clinically aggressive micropapillary variant of bladder cancer. Eur Urol 2016;70(4):611–20.

73. Shen P, Jing Y, Zhang R, et al. Comprehensive genomic profiling of neuroendocrine bladder cancer pinpoints molecular origin and potential therapeutics. Oncogene 2018;37(22):3039–44.

74. Yang G, Bondaruk J, Cogdell D, et al. Urothelial-to-neural plasticity drives progression to small cell bladder cancer. iScience 2020;23(6):101201.

75. Lopez-Beltran A, Pacelli A, Rothenberg HJ, et al. Carcinosarcoma and sarcomatoid carcinoma of the bladder: clinicopathological study of 41 cases. J Urol 1998;159(5):1497–503.

76. Sanfrancesco J, McKenney JK, Leivo MZ, et al. Sarcomatoid urothelial carcinoma of the bladder: analysis of 28 cases with emphasis on clinicopathologic features and markers of epithelial-to-mesenchymal transition. Arch Pathol Lab Med 2016;140(5):543–51.

77. Sung MT, Wang M, MacLennan GT, et al. Histogenesis of sarcomatoid urothelial carcinoma of the urinary bladder: evidence for a common clonal origin with divergent differentiation. J Pathol 2007; 211(4):420–30.

78. Guo CC, Majewski T, Zhang L, et al. Dysregulation of EMT drives the progression to clinically aggressive sarcomatoid bladder cancer. Cell Rep 2019;27(6): 1781–93.e4.

79. Genitsch V, Kollar A, Vandekerkhove G, et al. Morphologic and genomic characterization of urothelial to sarcomatoid transition in muscle-invasive bladder cancer. Urol Oncol 2019;37(11):826–36.

80. Lin O, Cardillo M, Dalbagni G, et al. Nested variant of urothelial carcinoma: a clinicopathologic and immunohistochemical study of 12 cases. Mod Pathol 2003;16(12):1289–98.

81. Wasco MJ, Daignault S, Bradley D, et al. Nested variant of urothelial carcinoma: a clinicopathologic and immunohistochemical study of 30 pure and mixed cases. Hum Pathol 2010;41(2):163–71.

82. Comperat E, McKenney JK, Hartmann A, et al. Large nested variant of urothelial carcinoma: a clinicopathological study of 36 cases. Histopathology 2017;71(5):703–10.

83. Cox R, Epstein JI. Large nested variant of urothelial carcinoma: 23 cases mimicking von Brunn nests and inverted growth pattern of noninvasive papillary urothelial carcinoma. Am J Surg Pathol 2011;35(9): 1337–42.

84. Dhall D, Al-Ahmadie H, Olgac S. Nested variant of urothelial carcinoma. Arch Pathol Lab Med 2007; 131(11):1725–7.

85. Volmar KE, Chan TY, De Marzo AM, et al. Florid von Brunn nests mimicking urothelial carcinoma: a morphologic and immunohistochemical comparison to the nested variant of urothelial carcinoma. Am J Surg Pathol 2003;27(9):1243–52.

86. Weyerer V, Weisser R, Moskalev EA, et al. Distinct genetic alterations and luminal molecular subtype in nested variant of urothelial carcinoma. Histopathology 2019;75(6):865–75.

87. Weyerer V, Eckstein M, Compérat E, et al. Pure Large Nested Variant of Urothelial Carcinoma (LNUC) is the prototype of an FGFR3 mutated aggressive urothelial carcinoma with luminal-papillary phenotype. Cancers (Basel) 2020;12(3):763.

88. Johnson SM, et al. Nested variant of urothelial carcinoma is a luminal bladder tumor with distinct coexpression of the basal marker cytokeratin 5/6. Am J Clin Pathol 2020;155(4):588–96.

89. Cerami E, Gao J, Dogrusoz U, et al. The cBio cancer genomics portal: an open platform for exploring multidimensional cancer genomics data. Cancer Discov 2012;2(5):401–4.

90. Gao J, Aksoy BA, Dogrusoz U, et al. Integrative analysis of complex cancer genomics and clinical profiles using the cBioPortal. Sci Signal 2013; 6(269):pl1.

Molecular Pathology of Ovarian Epithelial Neoplasms

Predictive, Prognostic, and Emerging Biomarkers

Zehra Ordulu, MD[a,b], Jaclyn Watkins, MD[b],
Lauren L. Ritterhouse, MD, PhD[b,*]

KEYWORDS

- Ovarian carcinoma • Epithelial • High-grade serous • Low-grade serous • Endometrioid
- Mucinous • BRCA • Homologous recombination • Molecular

Key points

- The mutational landscape of ovarian epithelial tumors may have morphologic correlates, as exemplified by BRCA1/2 associated HGSC with solid, endometrioid, and transitional morphology.

- The molecular profile of ovarian tumors may assist in their systematic classification by elucidating their pathogenesis. Carcinosarcomas were previously categorized as mixed epithelial–mesenchymal tumors; however, now they are considered as epithelial origin based on their mutational profile.

- The spectrum of mutations detected in ovarian tumors can provide insights into tumor evolution. While benign mucinous tumors start with a KRAS mutation or CDKN2A inactivation, mucinous carcinomas acquire additional copy number alterations and more likely to have TP53 mutations.

- The decisions for therapy might significantly be influenced by the molecular background of the tumors. Homologous recombination deficiency in high-grade serous carcinomas and their response to PARP inhibitors or platinum based therapy is the most advanced example, however, other pathways are also entering into clinical practice.

- The detection of homologous recombination deficiency status can be done via different methodologies, albeit the resistance mechanisms challenge the currently used technologies. Eventually a functionality based method might trump the etiology and/or mutation-status based technologies that are in routine practice today.

ABSTRACT

This review focuses on the diagnostic, prognostic, and predictive molecular biomarkers in ovarian epithelial neoplasms in the context of their morphologic classifications. Currently, most clinically actionable molecular findings are reported in high-grade serous carcinomas; however, the data on less common tumor types are rapidly accelerating. Overall, the advances in genomic knowledge over the last decade highlight the significance of integrating molecular findings with morphology in ovarian epithelial tumors for a wide-range of clinical applications, from assistance in diagnosis to predicting response to therapy.

OVERVIEW

Ovarian cancer is the eighth most common cancer diagnosis and cause of cancer-related death in

---

[a] Department of Pathology, Brigham and Women's Hospital, Harvard Medical School, Boston, MA, USA;
[b] Department of Pathology, Massachusetts General Hospital, Harvard Medical School, Boston, MA 02124, USA
* Corresponding author.
E-mail address: lritterhouse@mgh.harvard.edu

Surgical Pathology 14 (2021) 415–428
https://doi.org/10.1016/j.path.2021.05.006
1875-9181/21/© 2021 Elsevier Inc. All rights reserved.

women.[1] There is a gradual decreasing trend in its incidence with multiple contributory factors, including oral contraceptive use, increased parity, breastfeeding, and, more recently, risk-reducing surgery in women with germline BRCA1/2 mutations.[2,3] The expanding knowledge in molecular features of ovarian cancer has not only been useful for cancer prophylaxis in the setting of screening for hereditary syndromes, but has also shifted the paradigm of clinical decision-making from solely morphology-based diagnosis to the use of molecular signatures for prognostic and therapeutic implications. Even though the concept of splitting versus lumping[4,5] of ovarian epithelial tumors in the setting of their molecular pathogenesis has been controversial, emerging data continue to support the idea that the integration of molecular and morphologic findings remains essential for clinical management. Herein, predictive and prognostic molecular biomarkers in epithelial tumors of the ovary, as well as their syndromic associations, are reviewed in parallel to their most recent World Health Organization (WHO) classification.[6]

HISTOLOGIC SUBTYPES OF EPITHELIAL TUMORS

SEROUS TUMORS

High-Grade Serous Carcinoma

The most common histologic type of ovarian cancer is high-grade serous carcinoma (HGSC),[3] which is traditionally characterized by variably sized papillary architecture with slit-like spaces and high-grade nuclei. Although HGSC is commonly referred to as ovarian, it is now established that the vast majority arise from serous tubal intraepithelial carcinoma, which is commonly located at the fimbriated end of the fallopian tube.[7]

With large-scale genomic studies, the definition of HGSC has expanded to tumors with high-grade nuclei and TP53 mutations,[8,9] introducing a range of morphologies including those with solid, endometrioid, and transitional features (Fig. 1). In addition to TP53 mutations, HGSCs have extensive copy number alterations and aneuploidy, indicating genomic instability. Recurrent copy number alterations include amplifications of oncogenes such as CCNE1, MYC and MECOM, as well as the deletion of tumor suppressors such as PTEN, RB1, and NF1. Of note, recurrent mutations in NF1 (4%–6%), RB1 (2%–6%), and PTEN (<1%) are also observed and, when including larger deletions and structural alterations, their inactivation rates in HGSC become significantly frequent (NF1: 20%, RB1: 17%, PTEN: 7%).[8,10] Approximately 30% of HGSCs have BRCA1/2 alterations, including 20% with BRCA1/ 2 mutations (approximately 15% germline, 5% somatic) and 11% with BRCA1 epigenetic silencing via hypermethylation.[8] BRCA1/2 genes are members of the homologous recombination DNA repair (HRR) pathway, and altogether HRR pathway gene mutations are seen in approximately 50% of HGSC.[11] Other HRR pathway alterations involve Fanconi anemia genes (PALB2, FANCA, FANCI, FANCL, and FANCC), core RAD genes (RAD50, RAD51, RAD51B, RAD51C, and RAD54L), and DNA damage response genes (ATM, ATR, CHEK1, and CHEK2) (Table 1). Morphologically, it has been shown that the tumors with HRR pathway gene mutations are more likely to have solid, endometrioid, and transitional–like characteristics (see Fig. 1).[12,13] In addition, germline alterations in HRR pathway genes are responsible for predisposition to HGSC. Germline BRCA1/BRCA2 alterations account for the majority of inherited cases of HGSC (through hereditary breast and ovarian cancer syndrome), whereas germline mutations in other HRR genes, including BRIP1, ATM, RAD51C, and RAD51D,[14,15] are less common etiologies, cumulatively contributing to approximately 2% of HGSC.

Key points 1: HGSC genomic alterations

- Most common mutations and/or epigenetic alterations:

  ○ TP53 (>95%)

  ○ HRR pathway (50%: BRCA1/2 [30%], Fanconi anemia genes [5%], DNA damage response genes—ATM [2%] and ATR [2%], core RAD genes—hypermethylation of RAD51C [3%])

  ○ NF1 (mutation, 4%–6%; overall inactivation, 20%)

  ○ RB1 (mutation, 5%; overall inactivation, 17%), and

  ○ CDK12 (3%)

- Thirty percent of HGSC with BRCA1/2 alterations: 15% germline, 5% somatic, 11% epigenetic silencing via hypermethylation

- Most common structural alterations: Amplification of CCNE1 (20%), MYC, MECOM, and EMSY; deletion/breakage of PTEN, RB1, NF1, and RAD51B

- Germline predisposition mutations in HRR pathway (BRCA1/2 [15% of HGSC]), non-BRCA1/2 (2% of HGSC: BRIP1, ATM, RAD51C, and RAD51D)

The HRR pathway is responsible for repairing DNA damage caused by double-strand breaks (DSBs)

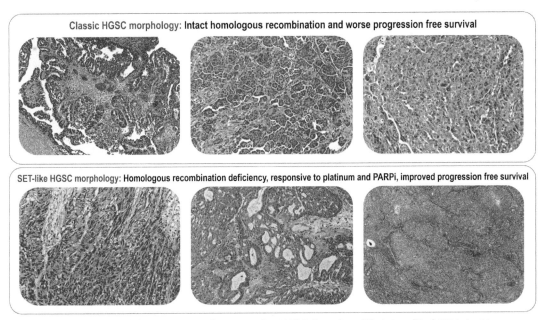

Fig. 1. Clinicopathological characteristics of extrauterine HGSCs based on HR status. (*Top*) HR-intact tumors usually have classic morphology (papillary [*left*] and micropapillary [*middle*] architecture, and slit-like spaces [*right*]). (*Bottom*) HRD tumors are more likely to have solid, endometrioid, and transitional (SET)–like morphology (solid [*left*], pseudoendometrioid [*middle*], and transitional pattern [*right*]).

Table 1
Comparison of genetic alterations, prognostic and predictive biomarkers in ovarian serous carcinomas

	HGSC	%	LGSC	%
Recurrently mutated genes	*TP53*	>95%	*KRAS*	25%
	HRR pathway	50%	*BRAF*	8%
	BRCA1/2	30%	*NRAS*	8%
	FANC genes	5%	*EIFAX*	15%
	ATM	2%	*USP9X*	11%
	ATR	2%		
	RAD51C met.	3%		
	NF1			
	Mutation	4%–6%		
	Overall inactivation	20%		
	RB1			
	Mutation	5%		
	Overall inactivation	17%		
Mutational signature	HRD	50%		
Copy number alterations	High-level genome wide changes		Low-level copy number changes	
Prognostic and predictive biomarkers	HRD: platinum and PARPi responsive HR-intact, *CCNE1* amplified: chemoresistant		Early stage: *BRAF>KRAS* Clinically aggressive: *KRAS>BRAF*	

Abbreviations: HGSC, high-grade serous carcinoma; HR, homologous recombination; HRD, homologous recombination deficiency; HGSC, high-grade serous carcinoma.

(**Fig. 2**). In response to damage resulting in DSBs, cells use HRR as the central pathway for DSB repair because it is a high-fidelity pathway in comparison with alternatives, such as Polθ/PARP1–mediated nonhomologous end joining.[16] Germline and somatic mutations or epigenetic modifications of HRR pathway genes may result in homologous recombination deficiency (HRD), leading to the use of more error-prone alternative repair pathways. In addition, there may be indirect mechanisms for HRD, such as *PTEN* deficiency, resulting in *RAD51* downregulation,[17] amplification of *EMSY* resulting in inactivation of BRCA2[18] or inactivating mutations of *CDK12* (3%),[8] leading to decreased expression of *BRCA1* and other HRR genes.[19] In HRD tumor cells, the error-prone alternative repair mechanisms creates genomic alterations that have been termed genomic scars. Owing to their defect in repairing DSBs, these tumors have been shown to have increased sensitivity to platinum-based chemotherapy and to poly (ADP-ribose) polymerase inhibitors (PARPi).[20–22] homologous recombination (HR)-intact tumors are more likely to be therapy-resistant and have a poor prognosis. In particular HGSC with *CCNE1* amplifications (20%) are reported to be mutually exclusive with *BRCA1/2* pathway disruption and are associated with a poor prognosis.[10]

The current National Comprehensive Cancer Network Guidelines for ovarian cancer (version 2.2020)[23] recommend that all patients with ovarian, fallopian tube, or primary peritoneal cancer undergo a genetic risk evaluation and germline and somatic testing, because germline and/or somatic *BRCA1/2* status informs maintenance therapy. Additionally, the National Comprehensive

Cancer Network guidelines recommend that, in the absence of *BRCA1/2* mutation, HRD status may provide information on the magnitude of benefit of PARPi. Several assays testing HRD status have entered clinical practice as predictive biomarkers[24] to optimize PARPi use given the sensitivity of HRD tumors to PARPi. Currently, most HRD assays are focusing on DNA-level changes and evaluate germline and/or somatic HRR pathway gene mutations,[25] and/or screen for genomic scars, which is evidence of genomic instability in HRD tumors (see **Fig. 2**). Genomic scars can be assessed through different scoring systems analyzing genomic loss of heterozygosity percentage, large-scale genomic transitions, telomeric allelic imbalance, or screening for HRD-related mutational signatures.[26–29]

HRD genomic scar metrics are limited in that they represent a permanent signature present within the tumor genome that may not be reflective of the current dynamic DNA repair status of the tumor. A common mechanism of acquired resistance to therapy in HRD tumors is the restoration of BRCA function by means of genetic reversion, in which secondary mutations within HRR genes restore the previously impaired protein function.[30,31] This acquired resistance mechanism is considered the most common for *BRCA1/2* mutated tumors.[32] In this setting, the initial *BRCA* mutation may imprint a genomic scar, but through genetic reversion the tumor becomes HR intact, resulting in decreased sensitivity to PARPi (**Fig. 3**). An emerging research field in this setting is establishing a functional assay analyzing HRD status at RNA and/or protein levels, which might

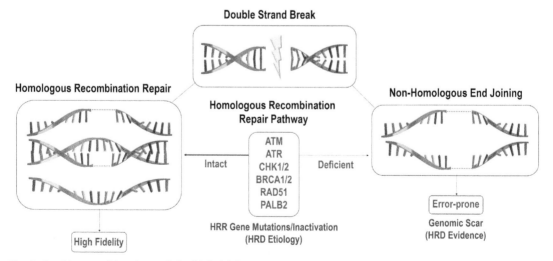

Fig. 2. Double strand break repair by high-fidelity HR repair or error-prone nonhomologous end joining. HRD status can be tested through analyzing different mechanisms, including the etiology of HRD status (mutations/inactivation in HRR pathway genes) or screening for prior HRD evidence (genomic scar).

Key points 2: HRD

- HRD etiology: Mutations/epigenetic alterations in HRR genes or indirect effect on HRR pathway (amplification of *EMSY*, inactivation of *PTEN* or *CDK12*)

- Clinical testing: Germline and somatic *BRCA1/2* testing for all ovarian, fallopian tube, and primary peritoneal cancer, which can inform maintenance therapy. In the absence of a *BRCA1/2* mutation, HRD status may provide information on the magnitude of benefit of PARPi therapy

  o HRD scores: Assess for genomic scars in DNA (genomic loss of heterozygosity, large-scale genomic transitions, telomeric allelic imbalance, screening for HRD-related mutational signature)

- Primary resistance to PARPi: HR intact, in particular *CCNE1* amplified

- The most common acquired resistance to PARPi in *BRCA1/2*–mutated tumors are reversion mutations

- Limitations in current HRD scores:

  o The genomic scar is not a functional assay and does not assess current status of HRR pathway

Key points 3: HGSC: other potential prognostic and predictive markers

- Transcriptional profile groups

  o Favorable: Immunoreactive and differentiated

  o Unfavorable: Mesenchymal and proliferative

- DNA methylation profile: Hypermethylation of *TAP1* promoter region in 6p21.3 (unfavorable)

- Programmed cell death ligand 1 expression (equivocal), presence of CD8+ tumor infiltrating lymphocytes (favorable); immunotherapy

- *HER2* amplification: 4%, no significant difference in survival; anti-HER2 therapy

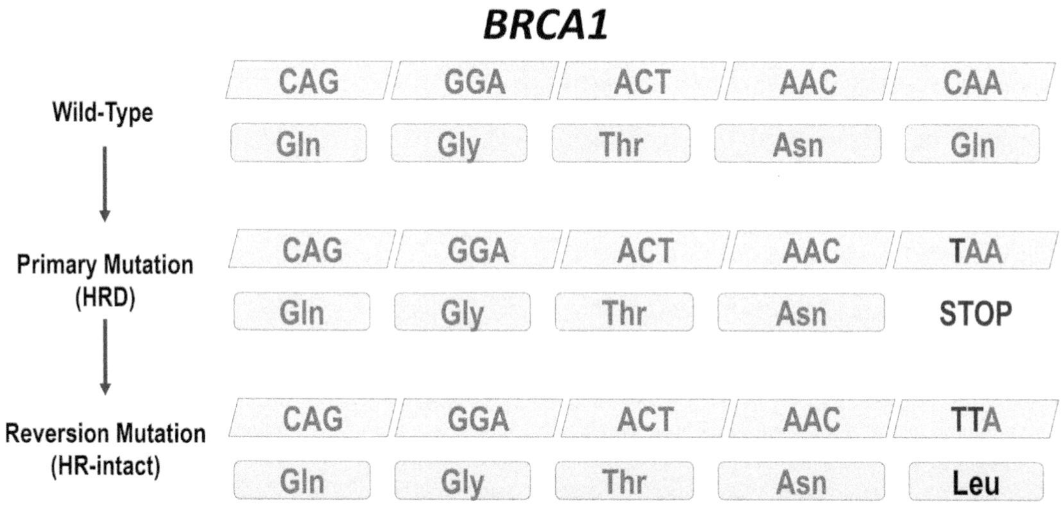

overcome the limitations of the current genomic HRD assays.

Subtyping of HGSCs based on their transcriptional profile (differentiated, immunoreactive, mesenchymal, and proliferative) is also proposed to be useful in the prediction of clinical behavior, with differentiated and immunoreactive groups being associated with favorable outcomes and mesenchymal and proliferative groups with a worse prognosis.[8,33,34] Other potential prognostic and predictive markers in HGSC include programmed cell death ligand 1 expression (equivocal), the presence of CD8+ tumor-infiltrating lymphocytes (favorable), *HER2* amplification (for anti-HER2 therapy) and DNA methylation profile (hypermethylation of *TAP1* promoter region in 6p21.3; unfavorable).[35–42]

Fig. 3. Schematic diagram of acquisition of reversion mutations in HRD tumors with primary mutation in HRR pathway, which would subsequently result in restoration of HR-intact status. In this example a primary mutation caused by a nonsense *BRCA1* mutation resulting in a premature stop codon, is reversed by a missense mutation in the same codon in a recurrence following platinum based chemotherapy.

Serous Tumors Other than High-Grade Serous Carcinoma

Low-grade serous carcinomas (LGSCs) have papillary architecture with low-grade nuclei and at least focally prominent nucleoli. Unlike HGSC, almost all LGSC arise from benign or borderline serous tumors (SBTs). Certain features of SBT have been associated with a more aggressive disease course, including presence of micropapillary architecture, microinvasion, and bilaterality.[43]

In contrast with HGSCs, LGSCs are genomically stable with fewer copy number alterations and low mutation rates. Copy number alterations are detected in up to 86.5% of LGSC, the most common being the loss of 1p36.33 (54.1%).[44] The mutations commonly involve MAPK pathway genes (KRAS [25%], BRAF [8%], and NRAS [8%]), as well as EIFAX (15%) and USP9X (11%), which are linked to the mechanistic target of rapamycin pathway.[45–47] (Table 1) It has been reported that clinically aggressive LGSCs tend to have KRAS rather than BRAF mutations, whereas tumors with BRAF mutations are associated with earlier stage disease.[48–50] Unlike HGSC, LGSC have an indolent clinical course and are usually resistant to chemotherapy.[51] Therefore, targeting the activating mutations detected in MAPK and mechanistic target of rapamycin pathways may be beneficial for patients with chemotherapy resistant advanced/recurrent disease.[52–54]

Mutations in KRAS and BRAF have been reported in approximately 85% of SBTs and their associated benign cystadenoma counterparts, indicating an early event in the development of LGSC.[55] Although BRAF mutations occur exclusively in SBTs with conventional morphology, a micropapillary morphology is more frequently seen in BRAF and KRAS wild-type tumors.[56] Progression of SBTs and/or LGSC into HGSC is rare, but has been reported.[57,58] Although virtually all HGSCs are considered TP53 mutated (>95%), recent studies analyzing TP53 wild-type HGSCs showed the presence of mixed low- to intermediate-grade morphology and KRAS, BRAF, or NRAS mutations, which may be further evidence for this transformation phenomenon.[59,60] In fact, one of these studies recommends further classification of TP53 wild-type HGSC into LGSC-like (40%) and usual HGSC-like (60%) categories.[60] In this study, LGSC-like tumors showed mixed low to intermediate grade morphology and/or KRAS, BRAF, or NRAS mutations (60%), whereas the usual HGSC-like tumors had grade 3 nuclei with morphology indistinguishable from TP53-mutated HGSC

and had evidence of TP53 dysfunction by immunohistochemistry (64%), showed MDM2 amplification (14%), RAD21 loss-off function fusion (14%), and ARID1B mutation (14%). Of note, both of these groups showed micropapillary morphology in a subset of cases (60% of LGSC-like and 25% of HGSC-like, 53% overall).

Key points 4: serous tumors other than HGSC: genomic alterations, prognostic and predictive biomarkers

- Benign serous tumors and SBT: KRAS or BRAF mutations (85%)
  - SBT with conventional morphology: BRAF > KRAS mutations
  - SBT with micropapillary morphology: KRAS and BRAF wild-type > BRAF/KRAS mutated
- LGSC: KRAS (25%), BRAF (8%), NRAS (8%), EIFAX (15%), and USP9X (11%) mutations
- Early stage LGSC: BRAF > KRAS mutations
- TP53 wild-type HGSC (<5%): approximately 50% have micropapillary features
  - LGSC-like (40%): Mixed low- to intermediate-grade morphology and/or KRAS, BRAF, or NRAS mutations (60%)
  - Usual HGSC-like (60%): Grade 3 nuclei with TP53 mutated HGSC-like morphology, TP53 dysfunction by immunohistochemistry (64%), MDM2 amplification (14%), RAD21 loss-of-function fusion (14%), ARID1B mutation (14%)
- Involvement of MAPK and mechanistic target of rapamycin pathways could qualify for targeted therapy

---

MUCINOUS TUMORS

The most recent WHO guidelines (2020) describe primary mucinous carcinomas of the ovary as tumors with gastrointestinal epithelium.[6,] The majority of these carcinomas arise from mucinous borderline tumors, with a smaller subset arising from mature cystic teratomas or Brenner tumors with gastrointestinal type cells.[6] It is suggested that the molecular evolution of mucinous ovarian tumors follows a tumor progression model,[61–64] such that benign tumors start with either a KRAS mutation or CDKN2A inactivation, whereas mucinous borderline tumors are more likely to have both with additional copy number changes. Finally, mucinous carcinomas acquire additional copy number alterations (in particular amplification of 9p13.3) and are more likely to have *TP53* mutations. Overall, the inactivation of *CDNK2A* (76%) and *KRAS* mutations (64%) are the most common alterations in mucinous adenocarcinomas and considered a major driver for their tumorigenesis, followed by *HER2* amplifications (20%). The latter are reported to be mutually exclusive with *KRAS* mutations, and occur almost always together with *TP53* mutations.[61,65] Other less frequent mutations in mucinous carcinomas include *RNF43*, *BRAF*, *PIK3CA*, and *ARID1A* (8%–12%) (**Table 2**). Mucinous carcinomas without *KRAS* or *HER2* alterations may represent tumors arising from less frequent precursors, such as mature cystic teratomas.[66] Among the molecular changes detected in mucinous carcinomas, an increased fraction of the genome altered by copy number changes is considered to be the key driver for worse prognosis owing to its association with increased tumor grade and progression.[61]

Key points 5: mucinous tumors: genomic alterations, prognostic, and predictive biomarkers

- Benign mucinous tumors: *KRAS* mutations or *CDKN2A* inactivation

- Mucinous borderline tumor: *KRAS* mutations and *CDKN2A* inactivation, as well as copy number alterations

- Mucinous adenocarcinomas

  ○ Most commonly altered genes: *KRAS* (64%) or *HER2* amplification (20%) (mutually exclusive), *CDKN2A* (76%), *TP53* (64%), increased copy number alterations in comparison with noncarcinoma counterparts (especially amplification of 9p13)

  ○ Less frequent mutations: *RNF43*, *BRAF*, *PIK3CA* and *ARID1A* (8%–12%)

- High copy number alteration burden is proposed to be a poor prognostic factor

- Involvement of MAPK pathway and *HER2* could qualify for targeted therapy

---

Table 2
Comparison of genetic alterations, prognostic and predictive biomarkers in nonserous ovarian carcinomas

	Mucinous	%	Endometrioid[a]	%	Clear Cell	%
Recurrently mutated genes	*KRAS*	64%	*CTNNB1*	30%–50%	*ARID1A*	50%–75%
	CDKN2A	76%	*PIK3CA*	15%–40%	*PIK3CA*	40%–50%
	TP53	64%	*ARID1A*	30%–35%	*KRAS*	15%
			PTEN	20%–30%	*PPP2R1A*	15%
			KRAS	10%–30%	*TERT*	15%
			TP53	10%–25%	*ARID1B*	10%
					TP53	5%–20%
					PTEN	1%–5%
Mutational signature			Ultra-mutated (*POLE*)	3%–10%	MMR deficiency	3%
			Hyper-mutated (MSI)	10%–20%		
			TP53-mutated	10%–25%		
			NSMP	60%–70%		
Copy number alterations	*HER2* amp.	20%			*HER2* amp.	15%
Prognostic and predictive biomarkers	High copy number alteration burden: Poor prognosis *HER2* and MAPK: Targeted therapy		*TP53*-mutated: complex genome and poor outcome *POLE mutated*: Ultra-mutated and favorable outcome *CTNNB1*-mutated: low genomic complexity and favorable outcome *Hyper-* or ultra-mutated: Immunotherapy WNT, MAPK and PI3K: Targeted therapy		MMR deficiency: Immunotherapy *HER2* and PI3K/AKT/ mechanistic target of rapamycin pathway: targeted therapy	

Abbreviations: amp, amplification; MMR: Mismatch repair; MSI, Microsatellite instability; NSMP, No specific molecular profile.
[a] Seromucinous carcinomas are now considered a part of endometrioid carcinoma spectrum and therefore are not categorized separately.

ENDOMETRIOID TUMORS

The majority of endometrioid carcinomas in the ovary arise from endometriosis, and less frequently from benign or borderline endometrioid tumors, mainly adenofibromas.[6] They show shared mutations (endometriosis, *PIK3CA*, *ARID1A*, and *KRAS*[67–69]; and borderline endometrioid tumors, *CTNNB1*[70]). Concurrent endometrial hyperplasia or carcinoma have been reported in up to 25% of cases, with a majority showing a clonal relationship between endometrial and ovarian endometrioid adenocarcinomas.[71,72] The term pseudometastasis has been proposed for this phenomenon, because synchronous organ-confined endometrial and ovarian carcinomas have favorable outcome.[73] Of note, in the current WHO classification, seromucinous carcinomas (may be referred to as mixed Müllerian carcinomas[74]), composed of serous and endocervical-type mucinous epithelium, are now considered a subtype of endometrioid adenocarcinomas owing to their morphologic and molecular overlap.[6,75] This terminology remains controversial and benign counterparts of seromucinous carcinomas have recently been described, which are commonly associated with endometriosis.[76,77] Borderline seromucinous tumors show *ARID1A* alterations[78] and *KRAS* mutations,[79] overlapping with endometrial and endometriosis-associated tumors, although *KRAS* alterations can be seen in mucinous borderline (intestinal epithelium) and serous tumors, as discussed elsewhere in this article.

Ovarian endometrioid adenocarcinomas are proposed to have 4 molecular subtypes akin to TCGA classification of their endometrial counterparts.[6,80–84] Hypermutated with microsatellite instability (10%–20%), ultramutated with *POLE* mutations (3%–10%), *TP53* mutated (10%–25%), and no specific molecular profile (60%–70%). Overall, the most common alterations seen in endometrial carcinomas are mutations in *CTNNB1* (30%–50%), *PIK3CA* (15%–40%), *ARID1A* (30%–35%), *PTEN* (20%–30%), *KRAS* (10%–30%), and *TP53* (10%–25%),[6,80–83] as well as mismatch repair deficiency (10%–20%) (see **Table 2**).[85,86] *TP53*-mutated cases have greater genomic complexity with frequent copy number alterations and poor prognosis, whereas *POLE*-mutated and mismatch repair (MMR)-abnormal tumors have excellent survival rates.[80] In addition, *CTNNB1*-mutated cases have low genomic complexity and a favorable outcome, unlike their endometrial counterparts, which confer a worse prognosis.[87–91] The high rates of genomic disruption of the WNT, MAPK, and PI3K pathways have the potential to inform therapeutic strategies, whereas hypermutated and ultramutated carcinomas with microsatellite instability and/or an increased tumor mutational burden may be responsive to immune checkpoint inhibition. In addition, Lynch syndrome (hereditary nonpolyposis colorectal cancer) owing to germline alterations in MMR genes (MMR: *MLH1*, *PMS2*, *MSH2*, and *MSH6*) increases predisposition to endometriosis-related ovarian carcinomas, most commonly the endometrioid variant.[92,93]

Key points 6: endometrioid tumors: genomic alterations and prognostic and predictive biomarkers

- Endometriosis-associated tumors: *PIK3CA*, *ARID1A*, and *KRAS* mutations

- Borderline endometrioid tumors: *CTNNB1* (90%) mutations

- Endometrioid adenocarcinomas

  ○ Most commonly mutated genes: *CTNNB1* (30%–50%), *PIK3CA* (15%–40%), *ARID1A* (30%–35%), *PTEN* (20%–30%), *KRAS* (10%–30%), and *TP53* (10%–25%)

  ○ Molecular subgroups: Hypermutated with microsatellite instability (10%–20%), ultramutated with *POLE* mutations (3%–10%), *TP53* mutated (10%–25%), and no specific molecular profile (60%–70%)

- *TP53* mutated: Complex genome with copy number changes and poor outcome

- *CTNNB1* mutated: Low genomic complexity and favorable outcome

- Hypermutated or ultramutated: Excellent survival, predictive biomarkers for response to immune checkpoint inhibition

- Germline predisposition with MMR gene mutations (Lynch syndrome, hereditary nonpolyposis colorectal cancer syndrome)

- Seromucinous carcinomas are now considered a subtype of endometrioid adenocarcinomas owing to their molecular resemblance

---

CLEAR CELL TUMORS

Clear cell carcinomas are most commonly associated with endometriosis (in the form of endometriotic cyst), and less frequently with clear cell borderline tumors, both having mutations in *PIK3CA* and *ARID1A*.[69,94,95] The genomic landscape of clear cell carcinomas has significant overlap with endometrioid adenocarcinomas, although with different alteration frequencies. The most common mutations involve *ARID1A* (50%–75%), *PIK3CA* (40%–50%), *KRAS* (15%), *PPP2R1A* (15%), *TERT* (15%), *ARID1B* (10%), *TP53* (5%–20%), and *PTEN* (1%–5%).[96–99] In addition, *HER2* amplifications (15%)[100] and MMR deficiency (3%)[85,101,102] are also detected (see **Table 2**). One study using the PROMISE algorithm for endometrial carcinoma[103] showed 7% had abnormal TP53 expression (copy number-high group), 2% had abnormal MMR expression, and none had a pathogenic *POLE* mutation.[104] Those with abnormal TP53 expression were associated with adverse outcomes. Although less common than endometrioid adenocarcinomas, germline mutations in MMR genes may also predispose to ovarian clear cell adenocarcinomas.[92,93]

Key points 7: clear cell tumors genomic alterations, prognostic and predictive biomarkers

- Endometriosis and clear cell borderline tumors: *PIK3CA* and *ARID1A* mutations

- Clear cell carcinomas

  ○ *ARID1A* (50%–75%), *PIK3CA* (40%–50%), *KRAS* (15%), *PPP2R1A* (15%), *TERT* (15%), *ARID1B* (10%), *TP53* (5%–20%), and *PTEN* (1%–5%) mutations

  ○ *TP53* mutated: Adverse outcome

  ○ *HER2* amplifications (15%) and MMR deficiency (3%)

- Germline predisposition with MMR gene mutations (Lynch syndrome, hereditary nonpolyposis colorectal cancer syndrome)

BRENNER TUMORS

Brenner tumors show transitional epithelium and are frequently associated with mucinous neoplasms. Benign and borderline Brenner tumors (BBT) and the associated mucinous epithelium, show mutually exclusive *MYC* amplification and RAS mutations (*HRAS* and *KRAS*).[105] Progression of benign to BBT is associated with *CDKN2A* loss, and, to a lesser extent, *KRAS* and *PIK3CA* mutations.[106] Malignant Brenner tumors show *MDM2 and CCND1* amplification and do not harbor *TERT or TP53* mutations unlike urothelial transitional carcinomas indicating a different molecular pathogenesis despite their morphologic resemblance.[107,108]

MESONEPHRIC-LIKE CARCINOMAS

Mesonephric-like carcinomas are proposed to either arise from mesonephric remnants or Müllerian tumors with mesonephric differentiation. These tumors show recurrent alterations similar to those seen in mesonephric carcinomas of the cervix, including *KRAS* mutations and gains of 1q, chromosomes 10 and 12. However, they also exhibit *PIK3CA* mutations, which are not detected in mesonephric carcinomas but rather seen in Müllerian carcinomas.[109] In addition, when seen together with SBTs or LGSCs, both components show *NRAS* or *KRAS* mutations.[110–112] Therefore, overall, a Müllerian origin with mesonephric differentiation is favored for mesonephric-like carcinomas of the ovary.

UNDIFFERENTIATED AND DEDIFFERENTIATED CARCINOMAS AND CARCINOSARCOMAS

Dedifferentiated carcinoma is composed of undifferentiated and differentiated carcinoma components, and has been shown to be associated with inactivation of chromatin remodeling genes and MMR deficiency.[6,113] Even though carcinosarcomas have a biphasic morphology, they are considered of epithelial origin[6] owing to the concordant mutations in carcinomatous and sarcomatous components, most frequently *TP53* in ovarian carcionosarcomas.[114,115]

Key points 8: Brenner tumors, mesonephric-like, undifferentiated and dedifferentiated carcinomas, carcinosarcomas genomic alterations

- Brenner tumors

  ○ Benign and BBT: RAS (*HRAS* or *KRAS*) mutations and *MYC* amplification (mutually exclusive)

  ○ Progression from benign to BBT: CDKN2A loss > *KRAS* and *PIK3A* mutations

  ○ Malignant Brenner tumor: *MDM2* and *CCND1* amplification (and no *TP53* or *TERT* mutations, unlike their morphologic mimic urothelial transitional carcinoma)

- Mesonephric-like carcinomas

  ○ Alterations seen in mesonephric carcinomas of the cervix: *KRAS* mutations and gains of 1q, chromosomes 10 and 12

  ○ Alterations seen in Müllerian carcinomas: *PIK3CA*, *NRAS*, and *KRAS* mutations

  ○ Overall, favored to be of Müllerian origin with mesonephric differentiation

- Undifferentiated and dedifferentiated carcinomas

- o Inactivation of chromatin remodeling genes (*ARID1A*/B and *SMARCA4*/A2/B2)
- o MMR deficiency
- Carcinosarcomas
- o Epithelial origin (high-grade carcinoma with sarcomatous differentiation), both components with *TP53* mutations

CLINICS CARE POINTS

- The genomic signature of ovarian epithelial tumors may be used as diagnostic, prognostic and predictive biomarker.
- TP53 mutations usually correlate with complex genomic signature and poor outcome.
- Homologous recombination deficiency status in high-grade serous ovarian carcinomas is associated with response to poly ADP-ribose polymerase (PARP) inhibition or platinum based therapy.
- In the setting of homologous recombination deficiency status, mechanisms of resistance, especially reversion mutations, should be taken into consideration.
- The mutational status of the tumors may make the patients eligible for targeted therapy (WNT, MAPK, PI3K, HER2 etc) particularly in advanced cases that do not respond to first line treatment.
- In particular settings such as ultra- or hypermutated status, patients may be eligible for immunotherapy.

DISCLOSURE

L.L. Ritterhouse has received honoraria/consulting fees from Abbvie, Personal Genome Diagnostics, Bristol Myers Squibb, Loxo Oncology, Amgen, and Merck.

REFERENCES

1. Bray F, Ferlay J, Soerjomataram I, et al. Global cancer statistics 2018: GLOBOCAN estimates of incidence and mortality worldwide for 36 cancers in 185 countries. CA Cancer J Clin 2018;68(6):394–424.
2. Petrucelli N, Daly MB, Feldman GL. Hereditary breast and ovarian cancer due to mutations in BRCA1 and BRCA2. Genet Med 2010;12(5):245–59.
3. Cabasag CJ, Arnold M, Butler J, et al. The influence of birth cohort and calendar period on global trends in ovarian cancer incidence. Int J Cancer 2020;146(3):749–58.
4. Hsu CY, Kurman RJ, Vang R, et al. Nuclear size distinguishes low- from high-grade ovarian serous carcinoma and predicts outcome. Hum Pathol 2005;36(10):1049–54.
5. Kurman RJ, Shih Ie M. The dualistic model of ovarian carcinogenesis: revisited, revised, and expanded. Am J Pathol 2016;186(4):733–47.
6. WHO Classification of Tumors Editorial Board. WHO classification of tumours: female genital tumours. vol. 4. 5th edition. Lyon (France): International Agency for Research on Cancer; 2020.
7. Kindelberger DW, Lee Y, Miron A, et al. Intraepithelial carcinoma of the fimbria and pelvic serous carcinoma: evidence for a causal relationship. Am J Surg Pathol 2007;31(2):161–9.
8. Cancer Genome Atlas Research Network. Integrated genomic analyses of ovarian carcinoma. Nature 2011;474(7353):609–15.
9. Shih Ie M, Kurman RJ. Ovarian tumorigenesis: a proposed model based on morphological and molecular genetic analysis. Am J Pathol 2004;164(5):1511–8.
10. Patch AM, Christie EL, Etemadmoghadam D, et al. Whole-genome characterization of chemoresistant ovarian cancer. Nature 2015;521(7553):489–94.
11. Pennington KP, Walsh T, Harrell MI, et al. Germline and somatic mutations in homologous recombination genes predict platinum response and survival in ovarian, fallopian tube, and peritoneal carcinomas. Clin Cancer Res 2014;20(3):764–75.
12. Soslow RA, Han G, Park KJ, et al. Morphologic patterns associated with BRCA1 and BRCA2 genotype in ovarian carcinoma. Mod Pathol 2012;25(4):625–36.
13. Ritterhouse LL, Nowak JA, Strickland KC, et al. Morphologic correlates of molecular alterations in extrauterine Mullerian carcinomas. Mod Pathol 2016;29(8):893–903.
14. Suszynska M, Ratajska M, Kozlowski P. BRIP1, RAD51C, and RAD51D mutations are associated with high susceptibility to ovarian cancer: mutation prevalence and precise risk estimates based on a pooled analysis of ~30,000 cases. J Ovarian Res 2020;13(1):50.
15. Minion LE, Dolinsky JS, Chase DM, et al. Hereditary predisposition to ovarian cancer, looking beyond BRCA1/BRCA2. Gynecol Oncol 2015;137(1):86–92.
16. Ceccaldi R, Liu JC, Amunugama R, et al. Homologous-recombination-deficient tumours are dependent on Poltheta-mediated repair. Nature 2015;518(7538):258–62.

17. Mendes-Pereira AM, Martin SA, Brough R, et al. Synthetic lethal targeting of PTEN mutant cells with PARP inhibitors. EMBO Mol Med 2009;1(6–7): 315–22.

18. Hollis RL, Churchman M, Michie CO, et al. High EMSY expression defines a BRCA-like subgroup of high-grade serous ovarian carcinoma with prolonged survival and hypersensitivity to platinum. Cancer 2019;125(16):2772–81.

19. Bajrami I, Frankum JR, Konde A, et al. Genome-wide profiling of genetic synthetic lethality identifies CDK12 as a novel determinant of PARP1/2 inhibitor sensitivity. Cancer Res 2014;74(1):287–97.

20. Kondrashova O, Topp M, Nesic K, et al. Methylation of all BRCA1 copies predicts response to the PARP inhibitor rucaparib in ovarian carcinoma. Nat Commun 2018;9(1):3970.

21. Tan DS, Rothermundt C, Thomas K, et al. "BRCA-ness" syndrome in ovarian cancer: a case-control study describing the clinical features and outcome of patients with epithelial ovarian cancer associated with BRCA1 and BRCA2 mutations. J Clin Oncol 2008;26(34):5530–6.

22. Yang D, Khan S, Sun Y, et al. Association of BRCA1 and BRCA2 mutations with survival, chemotherapy sensitivity, and gene mutator phenotype in patients with ovarian cancer. JAMA 2011;306(14):1557–65.

23. National Comprehensive Cancer Network. Ovarian Cancer (Version 2.2020). Available at: https://www.nccn.org/professionals/physician_gls/pdf/ovarian.pdf. Accessed January 13, 2021.

24. Miller RE, Leary A, Scott CL, et al. ESMO recommendations on predictive biomarker testing for homologous recombination deficiency and PARP inhibitor benefit in ovarian cancer. Ann Oncol 2020;31(12):1606–22.

25. Wagle N, Berger MF, Davis MJ, et al. High-throughput detection of actionable genomic alterations in clinical tumor samples by targeted, massively parallel sequencing. Cancer Discov 2012;2(1):82–93.

26. Swisher EM, Lin KK, Oza AM, et al. Rucaparib in relapsed, platinum-sensitive high-grade ovarian carcinoma (ARIEL2 Part 1): an international, multicentre, open-label, phase 2 trial. Lancet Oncol 2017;18(1):75–87.

27. Davies H, Glodzik D, Morganella S, et al. HRDetect is a predictor of BRCA1 and BRCA2 deficiency based on mutational signatures. Nat Med 2017; 23(4):517–25.

28. Mirza MR, Monk BJ, Herrstedt J, et al. Niraparib maintenance therapy in platinum-sensitive, recurrent ovarian cancer. N Engl J Med 2016;375(22): 2154–64.

29. Popova T, Manie E, Rieunier G, et al. Ploidy and large-scale genomic instability consistently identify basal-like breast carcinomas with BRCA1/2 inactivation. Cancer Res 2012;72(21):5454–62.

30. Lord CJ, Ashworth A. Mechanisms of resistance to therapies targeting BRCA-mutant cancers. Nat Med 2013;19(11):1381–8.

31. Norquist B, Wurz KA, Pennil CC, et al. Secondary somatic mutations restoring BRCA1/2 predict chemotherapy resistance in hereditary ovarian carcinomas. J Clin Oncol 2011;29(22):3008–15.

32. Konstantinopoulos PA, Ceccaldi R, Shapiro GI, et al. Homologous recombination deficiency: exploiting the fundamental vulnerability of ovarian cancer. Cancer Discov 2015;5(11):1137–54.

33. Konecny GE, Wang C, Hamidi H, et al. Prognostic and therapeutic relevance of molecular subtypes in high-grade serous ovarian cancer. J Natl Cancer Inst 2014;106(10):dju249.

34. Verhaak RG, Tamayo P, Yang JY, et al. Prognostically relevant gene signatures of high-grade serous ovarian carcinoma. J Clin Invest 2013;123(1): 517–25.

35. Strickland KC, Howitt BE, Shukla SA, et al. Association and prognostic significance of BRCA1/2-mutation status with neoantigen load, number of tumor-infiltrating lymphocytes and expression of PD-1/PD-L1 in high grade serous ovarian cancer. Oncotarget 2016;7(12):13587–98.

36. Bodelon C, Killian JK, Sampson JN, et al. Molecular classification of epithelial ovarian cancer based on methylation profiling: evidence for survival heterogeneity. Clin Cancer Res 2019; 25(19):5937–46.

37. Schmoeckel E, Hofmann S, Fromberger D, et al. Comprehensive analysis of PD-L1 expression, HER2 amplification, ALK/EML4 fusion, and mismatch repair deficiency as putative predictive and prognostic factors in ovarian carcinoma. Virchows Arch 2019;474(5):599–608.

38. Darb-Esfahani S, Kunze CA, Kulbe H, et al. Prognostic impact of programmed cell death-1 (PD-1) and PD-ligand 1 (PD-L1) expression in cancer cells and tumor-infiltrating lymphocytes in ovarian high grade serous carcinoma. Oncotarget 2016;7(2): 1486–99.

39. Pfisterer J, Du Bois A, Bentz EK, et al. Prognostic value of human epidermal growth factor receptor 2 (Her-2)/neu in patients with advanced ovarian cancer treated with platinum/paclitaxel as first-line chemotherapy: a retrospective evaluation of the AGO-OVAR 3 Trial by the AGO OVAR Germany. Int J Gynecol Cancer 2009;19(1):109–15.

40. Wang C, Cicek MS, Charbonneau B, et al. Tumor hypomethylation at 6p21.3 associates with longer time to recurrence of high-grade serous epithelial ovarian cancer. Cancer Res 2014;74(11): 3084–91.

41. Li J, Wang J, Chen R, et al. The prognostic value of tumor-infiltrating T lymphocytes in ovarian cancer. Oncotarget 2017;8(9):15621–31.

42. Wang L. Prognostic effect of programmed death-ligand 1 (PD-L1) in ovarian cancer: a systematic review, meta-analysis and bioinformatics study. J Ovarian Res 2019;12(1):37.

43. Longacre TA, McKenney JK, Tazelaar HD, et al. Ovarian serous tumors of low malignant potential (borderline tumors): outcome-based study of 276 patients with long-term (> or =5-year) follow-up. Am J Surg Pathol 2005;29(6):707–23.

44. Van Nieuwenhuysen E, Busschaert P, Laenen A, et al. Loss of 1p36.33 frequent in low-grade serous ovarian cancer. Neoplasia 2019;21(6):582–90.

45. Jones S, Wang TL, Kurman RJ, et al. Low-grade serous carcinomas of the ovary contain very few point mutations. J Pathol 2012;226(3):413–20.

46. Hunter SM, Anglesio MS, Ryland GL, et al. Molecular profiling of low grade serous ovarian tumours identifies novel candidate driver genes. Oncotarget 2015;6(35):37663–77.

47. Romero I, Leskela S, Mies BP, et al. Morphological and molecular heterogeneity of epithelial ovarian cancer: therapeutic implications. EJC Suppl 2020; 15:1–15.

48. Wong KK, Tsang YT, Deavers MT, et al. BRAF mutation is rare in advanced-stage low-grade ovarian serous carcinomas. Am J Pathol 2010;177(4):1611–7.

49. Tsang YT, Deavers MT, Sun CC, et al. KRAS (but not BRAF) mutations in ovarian serous borderline tumour are associated with recurrent low-grade serous carcinoma. J Pathol 2013;231(4):449–56.

50. Grisham RN, Iyer G, Garg K, et al. BRAF mutation is associated with early stage disease and improved outcome in patients with low-grade serous ovarian cancer. Cancer 2013;119(3):548–54.

51. Kaldawy A, Segev Y, Lavie O, et al. Low-grade serous ovarian cancer: a review. Gynecol Oncol 2016;143(2):433–8.

52. Farley J, Brady WE, Vathipadiekal V, et al. Selumetinib in women with recurrent low-grade serous carcinoma of the ovary or peritoneum: an open-label, single-arm, phase 2 study. Lancet Oncol 2013; 14(2):134–40.

53. Combe P, Chauvenet L, Lefrere-Belda MA, et al. Sustained response to vemurafenib in a low grade serous ovarian cancer with a BRAF V600E mutation. Invest New Drugs 2015;33(6):1267–70.

54. Stover EH, Feltmate C, Berkowitz RS, et al. Targeted next-generation sequencing reveals clinically actionable BRAF and ESR1 mutations in low-grade serous ovarian carcinoma. JCO Precis Oncol 2018;2018.

55. Ho CL, Kurman RJ, Dehari R, et al. Mutations of BRAF and KRAS precede the development of ovarian serous borderline tumors. Cancer Res 2004;64(19):6915–8.

56. Chui MH, Xing D, Zeppernick F, et al. Clinicopathologic and molecular features of paired cases of metachronous ovarian serous borderline tumor and subsequent serous carcinoma. Am J Surg Pathol 2019;43(11):1462–72.

57. Garg K, Park KJ, Soslow RA. Low-grade serous neoplasms of the ovary with transformation to high-grade carcinomas: a report of 3 cases. Int J Gynecol Pathol 2012;31(5):423–8.

58. Quddus MR, Rashid LB, Hansen K, et al. High-grade serous carcinoma arising in a low-grade serous carcinoma and micropapillary serous borderline tumour of the ovary in a 23-year-old woman. Histopathology 2009;54(6):771–3.

59. Zarei S, Wang Y, Jenkins SM, et al. Clinicopathologic, immunohistochemical, and molecular characteristics of ovarian serous carcinoma with mixed morphologic features of high-grade and low-grade serous carcinoma. Am J Surg Pathol 2020;44(3):316–28.

60. Chui MH, Momeni Boroujeni A, Mandelker D, et al. Characterization of TP53-wildtype tubo-ovarian high-grade serous carcinomas: rare exceptions to the binary classification of ovarian serous carcinoma. Mod Pathol 2020;34(2):490–501.

61. Cheasley D, Wakefield MJ, Ryland GL, et al. The molecular origin and taxonomy of mucinous ovarian carcinoma. Nat Commun 2019;10(1):3935.

62. Hunter SM, Gorringe KL, Christie M, et al. Pre-invasive ovarian mucinous tumors are characterized by CDKN2A and RAS pathway aberrations. Clin Cancer Res 2012;18(19):5267–77.

63. Mackenzie R, Kommoss S, Winterhoff BJ, et al. Targeted deep sequencing of mucinous ovarian tumors reveals multiple overlapping RAS-pathway activating mutations in borderline and cancerous neoplasms. BMC Cancer 2015;15:415.

64. Cuatrecasas M, Villanueva A, Matias-Guiu X, et al. K-ras mutations in mucinous ovarian tumors: a clinicopathologic and molecular study of 95 cases. Cancer 1997;79(8):1581–6.

65. Anglesio MS, Kommoss S, Tolcher MC, et al. Molecular characterization of mucinous ovarian tumours supports a stratified treatment approach with HER2 targeting in 19% of carcinomas. J Pathol 2013;229(1):111–20.

66. Bouri S, Simon P, D'Haene N, et al. P53 and PIK3CA Mutations in KRAS/HER2 negative ovarian intestinal-type mucinous carcinoma associated with mature teratoma. Case Rep Obstet Gynecol 2020;2020:8863610.

67. Noe M, Ayhan A, Wang TL, et al. Independent development of endometrial epithelium and stroma within the same endometriosis. J Pathol 2018;245(3):265–9.

68. Wiegand KC, Shah SP, Al-Agha OM, et al. ARID1A mutations in endometriosis-associated ovarian carcinomas. N Engl J Med 2010;363(16):1532–43.

69. Bulun SE, Wan Y, Matei D. Epithelial mutations in endometriosis: link to ovarian cancer. Endocrinology 2019;160(3):626–38.

70. Oliva E, Sarrio D, Brachtel EF, et al. High frequency of beta-catenin mutations in borderline endometrioid tumours of the ovary. J Pathol 2006;208(5): 708–13.

71. Anglesio MS, Wang YK, Maassen M, et al. Synchronous endometrial and ovarian carcinomas: evidence of clonality. J Natl Cancer Inst 2016;108(6):djv428.

72. Schultheis AM, Ng CK, De Filippo MR, et al. Massively parallel sequencing-based clonality analysis of synchronous endometrioid endometrial and ovarian carcinomas. J Natl Cancer Inst 2016; 108(6):djv427.

73. Gilks CB, Kommoss F. Synchronous tumours of the female reproductive tract. Pathology 2018;50(2): 214–21.

74. Kurman RJ, Shih Ie M. Seromucinous tumors of the ovary. what's in a name? Int J Gynecol Pathol 2016; 35(1):78–81.

75. Rambau PF, McIntyre JB, Taylor J, et al. Morphologic reproducibility, genotyping, and immunohistochemical profiling do not support a category of seromucinous carcinoma of the ovary. Am J Surg Pathol 2017;41(5):685–95.

76. Watkins JC, Young RH. Mullerian mucinous cystadenomas of the ovary: a report of 25 cases of an unheralded benign ovarian neoplasm often associated with endometriosis and a brief consideration of neoplasms arising from the latter. Int J Gynecol Pathol 2021.

77. Ben-Mussa A, McCluggage WG. Ovarian seromucinous cystadenomas and adenofibromas: first report of a case series. Histopathology 2021; 78(3):445–52.

78. Wu CH, Mao TL, Vang R, et al. Endocervical-type mucinous borderline tumors are related to endometrioid tumors based on mutation and loss of expression of ARID1A. Int J Gynecol Pathol 2012;31(4): 297–303.

79. Kim KR, Choi J, Hwang JE, et al. Endocervical-like (Mullerian) mucinous borderline tumours of the ovary are frequently associated with the KRAS mutation. Histopathology 2010;57(4):587–96.

80. Parra-Herran C, Lerner-Ellis J, Xu B, et al. Molecular-based classification algorithm for endometrial carcinoma categorizes ovarian endometrioid carcinoma into prognostically significant groups. Mod Pathol 2017;30(12):1748–59.

81. Cybulska P, Paula ADC, Tseng J, et al. Molecular profiling and molecular classification of endometrioid ovarian carcinomas. Gynecol Oncol 2019; 154(3):516–23.

82. McConechy MK, Ding J, Senz J, et al. Ovarian and endometrial endometrioid carcinomas have distinct CTNNB1 and PTEN mutation profiles. Mod Pathol 2014;27(1):128–34.

83. Hollis RL, Thomson JP, Stanley B, et al. Molecular stratification of endometrioid ovarian carcinoma predicts clinical outcome. Nat Commun 2020; 11(1):4995.

84. Leskela S, Romero I, Rosa-Rosa JM, et al. Molecular heterogeneity of endometrioid ovarian carcinoma: an analysis of 166 cases using the endometrial cancer subrogate molecular classification. Am J Surg Pathol 2020;44(7):982–90.

85. Leskela S, Romero I, Cristobal E, et al. Mismatch repair deficiency in ovarian carcinoma: frequency, causes, and consequences. Am J Surg Pathol 2020;44(5):649–56.

86. Bennett JA, Pesci A, Morales-Oyarvide V, et al. Incidence of mismatch repair protein deficiency and associated clinicopathologic features in a cohort of 104 ovarian endometrioid carcinomas. Am J Surg Pathol 2019;43(2):235–43.

87. Gamallo C, Palacios J, Moreno G, et al. beta-catenin expression pattern in stage I and II ovarian carcinomas: relationship with beta-catenin gene mutations, clinicopathological features, and clinical outcome. Am J Pathol 1999;155(2):527–36.

88. Wang L, Rambau PF, Kelemen LE, et al. Nuclear beta-catenin and CDX2 expression in ovarian endometrioid carcinoma identify patients with favourable outcome. Histopathology 2019;74(3):452–62.

89. Nagy B, Toth L, Molnar P, et al. Nuclear beta-catenin positivity as a predictive marker of long-term survival in advanced epithelial ovarian cancer. Pathol Res Pract 2017;213(8):915–21.

90. Zyla RE, Olkhov-Mitsel E, Amemiya Y, et al. CTNNB1 mutations and aberrant beta-catenin expression in ovarian endometrioid carcinoma: correlation with patient outcome. Am J Surg Pathol 2021;45(1):68–76.

91. Rosen DG, Zhang Z, Chang B, et al. Low membranous expression of beta-catenin and high mitotic count predict poor prognosis in endometrioid carcinoma of the ovary. Mod Pathol 2010;23(1): 113–22.

92. Malander S, Rambech E, Kristoffersson U, et al. The contribution of the hereditary nonpolyposis colorectal cancer syndrome to the development of ovarian cancer. Gynecol Oncol 2006;101(2): 238–43.

93. Chui MH, Ryan P, Radigan J, et al. The histomorphology of Lynch syndrome-associated ovarian carcinomas: toward a subtype-specific screening strategy. Am J Surg Pathol 2014; 38(9):1173–81.

94. Yamamoto S, Tsuda H, Takano M, et al. PIK3CA mutations and loss of ARID1A protein expression are early events in the development of cystic ovarian clear cell adenocarcinoma. Virchows Arch 2012;460(1):77–87.

95. Yamamoto S, Tsuda H, Takano M, et al. Loss of ARID1A protein expression occurs as an early event in ovarian clear-cell carcinoma development

and frequently coexists with PIK3CA mutations. Mod Pathol 2012;25(4):615–24.

96. Friedlander ML, Russell K, Millis S, et al. Molecular profiling of clear cell ovarian cancers: identifying potential treatment targets for clinical trials. Int J Gynecol Cancer 2016;26(4):648–54.

97. Murakami R, Matsumura N, Brown JB, et al. Exome sequencing landscape analysis in ovarian clear cell carcinoma shed light on key chromosomal regions and mutation gene networks. Am J Pathol 2017;187(10):2246–58.

98. Shibuya Y, Tokunaga H, Saito S, et al. Identification of somatic genetic alterations in ovarian clear cell carcinoma with next generation sequencing. Genes Chromosomes Cancer 2018;57(2):51–60.

99. Wu RC, Ayhan A, Maeda D, et al. Frequent somatic mutations of the telomerase reverse transcriptase promoter in ovarian clear cell carcinoma but not in other major types of gynaecological malignancy. J Pathol 2014;232(4):473–81.

100. Tan DS, Iravani M, McCluggage WG, et al. Genomic analysis reveals the molecular heterogeneity of ovarian clear cell carcinomas. Clin Cancer Res 2011;17(6):1521–34.

101. Rambau PF, Duggan MA, Ghatage P, et al. Significant frequency of MSH2/MSH6 abnormality in ovarian endometrioid carcinoma supports histotype-specific Lynch syndrome screening in ovarian carcinomas. Histopathology 2016;69(2):288–97.

102. Bennett JA, Morales-Oyarvide V, Campbell S, et al. Mismatch repair protein expression in clear cell carcinoma of the ovary: incidence and morphologic associations in 109 cases. Am J Surg Pathol 2016;40(5):656–63.

103. Talhouk A, McConechy MK, Leung S, et al. Confirmation of ProMisE: a simple, genomics-based clinical classifier for endometrial cancer. Cancer 2017; 123(5):802–13.

104. Parra-Herran C, Bassiouny D, Lerner-Ellis J, et al. p53, mismatch repair protein, and POLE abnormalities in ovarian clear cell carcinoma: an outcome-based clinicopathologic analysis. Am J Surg Pathol 2019;43(12):1591–9.

105. Tafe LJ, Muller KE, Ananda G, et al. Molecular genetic analysis of ovarian Brenner tumors and associated mucinous epithelial neoplasms: high variant concordance and identification of mutually exclusive RAS driver mutations and MYC amplification. Am J Pathol 2016;186(3):671–7.

106. Kuhn E, Ayhan A, Shih Ie M, et al. The pathogenesis of atypical proliferative Brenner tumor: an immunohistochemical and molecular genetic analysis. Mod Pathol 2014;27(2):231–7.

107. Cuatrecasas M, Catasus L, Palacios J, et al. Transitional cell tumors of the ovary: a comparative clinicopathologic, immunohistochemical, and molecular genetic analysis of Brenner tumors and transitional cell carcinomas. Am J Surg Pathol 2009;33(4): 556–67.

108. Khani F, Diolombi ML, Khattar P, et al. Benign and malignant Brenner tumors show an absence of TERT promoter mutations that are commonly present in urothelial carcinoma. Am J Surg Pathol 2016;40(9):1291–5.

109. Mirkovic J, McFarland M, Garcia E, et al. Targeted genomic profiling reveals recurrent KRAS mutations in mesonephric-like adenocarcinomas of the female genital tract. Am J Surg Pathol 2018;42(2): 227–33.

110. McCluggage WG, Vosmikova H, Laco J. Ovarian combined low-grade serous and mesonephric-like adenocarcinoma: further evidence for a Mullerian origin of mesonephric-like adenocarcinoma. Int J Gynecol Pathol 2020;39(1):84–92.

111. Chapel DB, Joseph NM, Krausz T, et al. An ovarian adenocarcinoma with combined low-grade serous and mesonephric morphologies suggests a Mullerian origin for some mesonephric carcinomas. Int J Gynecol Pathol 2018;37(5): 448–59.

112. Dundr P, Gregova M, Nemejcova K, et al. Ovarian mesonephric-like adenocarcinoma arising in serous borderline tumor: a case report with complex morphological and molecular analysis. Diagn Pathol 2020;15(1):91.

113. Coatham M, Li X, Karnezis AN, et al. Concurrent ARID1A and ARID1B inactivation in endometrial and ovarian dedifferentiated carcinomas. Mod Pathol 2016;29(12):1586–93.

114. Jin Z, Ogata S, Tamura G, et al. Carcinosarcomas (malignant Mullerian mixed tumors) of the uterus and ovary: a genetic study with special reference to histogenesis. Int J Gynecol Pathol 2003;22(4): 368–73.

115. Brunetti M, Agostini A, Staurseth J, et al. Molecular characterization of carcinosarcomas arising in the uterus and ovaries. Oncotarget 2019;10(38): 3614–24.

Molecular Approach to Colorectal Carcinoma
Current Evidence and Clinical Application

Cameron Beech, MD[a], Jaclyn F. Hechtman, MD[b],*

KEYWORDS

- Colorectal carcinoma • Microsatellite instability • Lynch syndrome • Immunotherapy
- Epidermal growth factor receptor

Key points

- Colorectal carcinoma tumorigenesis is predicated on a predictable stepwise accumulation of mutations.
- Microsatellite instability remains an important molecular signature for colorectal carcinoma with implications for therapy and genetic testing.
- Extended RAS testing is crucial for stratifying patients for anti-epidermal growth factor receptor therapy.

Colorectal carcinoma is one of the most common cancer types in men and women, responsible for both the third highest incidence of new cancer cases and the third highest cause of cancer deaths. In the last several decades, the molecular mechanisms surrounding colorectal carcinoma's tumorigenesis have become clearer through research, providing new avenues for diagnostic testing and novel approaches to therapeutics. Laboratories are tasked with providing the most current information to help guide clinical decisions. In this review, we summarize the current knowledge surrounding colorectal carcinoma tumorigenesis and highlight clinically relevant molecular testing.

OVERVIEW

One of the central mechanisms surrounding colorectal carcinoma (CRC) tumorigenesis is the adenoma to carcinoma sequence.[1–5] This concept describes a stepwise accumulation of genetic changes from adenoma formation progressing toward invasive carcinoma.[3] Previously, CRC was grouped into microsatellite unstable or chromosomal instability pathways. The chromosomal instability pathway represents 85% of colorectal cancers, with chromosomal alterations including frequent gains of chromosome 8q, 13, and 20q and losses of chromosomes 8p, 17p, and 18q.[6] This pathway is also characterized by frequent genetic alterations in *TP53*, *KRAS*, and *APC*.[4] Recently, a group of experts put forth 4 consensus molecular subtypes (CMS) as another way to classify CRC (**Table 1**). These consist of microsatellite instability immune subtype with hypermutation, microsatellite instability, and strong immune activation (CMS1, 14%); canonical subtype with marked WNT and MYC signaling activation (CMS2, 37%); metabolic subtype with evident metabolic dysregulation (CMS3, 13%); and

---

[a] Department of Pathology, Yale New Haven Hospital, New Haven, CT, USA; [b] Molecular and GI Pathologist, NeoGenomics Laboratories, Fort Myers, FL, USA
* Corresponding author.
E-mail address: Jaclyn.hechtman@neogenomics.com

Surgical Pathology 14 (2021) 429–441
https://doi.org/10.1016/j.path.2021.05.007
1875-9181/21/© 2021 Elsevier Inc. All rights reserved.

Table 1
Proposed colorectal CMS

Subtype Numbers	CMS1	CMS2	CMS3	CMS4
Subtype name	MSI immune	Canonical	Metabolic	Mesenchymal
Prevalence	14%	37%	13%	23%
Molecular features	MSI-H, CIMP-H	Increased copy number alterations	Mixed MSI-H and MSS, CIMP-L	Increased copy number alterations
Mutations	BRAF p. V600 E		KRAS	
	Immune activation and infiltration	Wnt pathway and MYC activation	Metabolic deregulation	Tumor growth factor-beta activation, angiogenesis, stromal infiltration
Prognosis	Worse survival after progression/relapse			Worse progression-free and overall survival

Abbreviations: CIMP, CpG island methylator phenotype; MSI, microsatellite instability; MSS, microsatellite stable.

mesenchymal subtype with prominent transforming growth factor-β activation, stromal invasion and angiogenesis (CMS4, 23%).[7]

MISMATCH REPAIR DEFICIENCY AND MICROSATELLITE INSTABILITY

Approximately 15% of CRCs are mismatch repair deficient/microsatellite instability-high (MSI-H). These tumors are characterized by small insertions and deletions, particularly within repetitive DNA sequences known as microsatellites. The mismatch repair pathway is composed of a complex of proteins whose role is to maintain genomic integrity by editing newly synthesized DNA strands for errors during DNA replication. Four proteins are responsible for the majority of mismatch repair deficiency: MSH2, MSH6, PMS2, and MLH1. These proteins form heterodimers, with pairing of MSH2 with MSH6 and PMS2 with MLH1. Loss of expression of either MSH2 or MLH1 leads to instability and degradation of their respective partners (MSH6 or PMS2). However, loss of expression of MSH6 and PMS2 does not lead to loss of the heterodimer partners (**Table 2**). Mismatch repair deficiency can arise

Table 2
Mismatch repair IHC patterns and their interpretation

MLH1	PMS2	MSH2	MSH6	Interpretation
Loss	Loss	Retention	Retention	MLH1 promoter hypermethylation (usually sporadic) or germline mutation
Retention	Loss	Retention	Retention	PMS2 germline mutation
Retention	Retention	Loss	Loss	EPCAM or MSH2 germline mutation, rarely double somatic inactivation of MSH2
Retention	Retention	Retention	Loss	Not meaningful after neoadjuvant therapy (test pretreatment sample), MSH6 germline mutation, rarely double somatic inactivation of MSH6
Loss	Loss	Loss	Loss	Constitutional mismatch repair deficiency

from either germline mutations (Lynch syndrome) or sporadic inactivation of these proteins via somatic mutations or epigenetic alterations (*MLH1* promoter hypermethylation).

SPORADIC MISMATCH REPAIR DEFICIENCY

Sporadic mismatch repair deficiency occurs in approximately 12% of CRC, usually owing to *MLH1* promoter hypermethylation and subsequent loss of expression of MLH1 and its partner, PMS2.[8] *BRAF* V600 E mutations are enriched in tumors with *MLH1* promoter hypermethylation and have been shown to induce *MLH1* promoter hypermethylation via the upregulation of transcriptional regulator MAFG.[9] In contrast, somatic inactivation of MSH2 and MSH6 occurs in approximately 5% and less than 1% of sporadic CRC, respectively.[10]

LYNCH SYNDROME

Germline mutations within mismatch repair genes lead to Lynch syndrome, which is responsible for approximately 2% to 3% of CRC.[11] Germline mutation in *MSH2* and *MLH1* make up the majority of patients with Lynch syndrome, responsible for 70% of identified mutations.[12,13] In addition, germline deletions within the *EPCAM* gene, which is located 5′ to *MSH2*, can lead to hypermethylation and loss of MSH2 expression.[14,15]

The Lynch syndrome manifests when one of the mismatch repair protein alleles is inactivated by a germline mutation, followed by a somatic mutation, leading to an inactivation of the wild-type allele, known as the Knudson 2-hit hypothesis. Some patients have germline inactivation of both mismatch repair protein alleles, known as constitutional mismatch repair deficiency, and typically present with CRC at a much earlier age (mean age of onset 16 years).[16] The Lynch syndrome is associated with an increased risk for colorectal, gastric, hepatobiliary, renal, ovarian, and endometrial cancer.[17,18]

The Amsterdam criteria were developed as a screen for Lynch syndrome; however, they lacked sufficient sensitivity.[19] The Bethesda guidelines followed, which used histologic and clinical data.[20] A variety of histologic appearances have been described for CRC arising in the setting of mismatch repair deficiency, including various patterns of lymphocytic infiltrate (Crohn's disease-like, peritumoral, and intratumor lymphocytic infiltrate pattern), as well as a medullary growth pattern, and mucinous differentiation.[21,22] Ultimately, the Bethesda guidelines lacked the appropriate performance in identifying patients with the

Lynch syndrome. In 2009, the Evaluation of Genomic Applications in Practice and Prevention working group, a working group for the Centers for Disease Control and Prevention, recommended offering genetic testing for the Lynch syndrome for all patients with newly diagnosed CRC, a strategy that has been endorsed by the National Comprehensive Cancer Network.[23,24]

MISMATCH REPAIR AND MICROSATELLITE INSTABILITY TESTING

Testing for mismatch repair deficiency can be accomplished with immunohistochemistry (IHC) by assessing for complete loss of nuclear expression of at least 1 mismatch repair protein. Alternatively, testing for MSI can be performed by comparing nucleotide repeat lengths between tumor and normal tissue using polymerase chain reaction with a panel of 5 mononucleotide microsatellite loci (revised Bethesda guidelines)[20] or next-generation sequencing (NGS) (**Fig. 1**).

Comparing these tests, IHC has the advantages of being inexpensive, fast, working well in low tumor purity cases unlike polymerase chain reaction, and identifying the gene with loss of function. However, retained mismatch repair expression occurs within approximately 6% of MSI-H cancers, usually owing to missense mutations leading to altered protein function but retained antigenicity.[20,25,26] Additionally, clinically insignificant loss of MSH6 expression after neoadjuvant therapy in MSS cancers can occur.[27]

Several methods for assessment of MSI by NGS data are currently used by various laboratories. These methods require adequate tumor purity like polymerase chain reaction. One method, MSIsensor, was originally developed comparing matched tumor and normal samples using whole exome sequencing data, but has been applied to targeted cancer panels.[28,29] MSIsensor assesses mono- to penta-nucleotide microsatellite repeats and compares the distribution of repeat lengths across multiple loci between tumor and normal samples. A χ^2 test is used for each locus to identify loci that differ significantly in length to generate an MSIsensor score.[29] Another method, mSINGs, assesses microsatellites with mononucleotide repeats and compares their length with a population of normal controls, using a z-score to identify tumors with microsatellite length distributions different from the mean.[30] A third method, MANTIS, assesses mono- to penta-nucleotide microsatellite repeats in matched tumor and normal samples. Unlike other methods, MANTIS compares the normal tumor sample pair as an

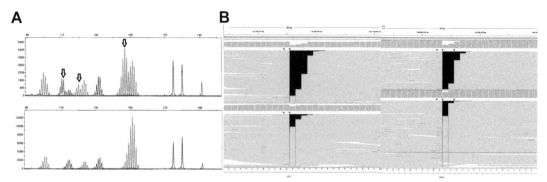

Fig. 1. (A) Polymerase chain reaction–based analysis reveals the distribution of microsatellite lengths at multiple microsatellite loci, comparing normal tissue (*bottom*) to tumor tissue (*top*). Differences in microsatellite lengths, highlighted by *arrows*, between tumor and normal tissue confirms microsatellite instability. (B) Integrated genomics viewer (IGV) of NGS data in a mononucleotide of a microsatellite stable tumor. *Top* is the tumor and the bottom is the corresponding normal. (C) IGV of NGS data of a microsatellite unstable tumor. *Top* is the tumor, with larger deletions in the mononucleotide tracts, and the bottom is the corresponding normal. Insertions and deletions are highlighted in black.

aggregate of loci instead of individual loci differences, which generates a general baseline in the normal for correction of sequencing errors. These methods perform similarly in identifying MSI; however, MANTIS has the highest overall sensitivity (MANTIS 97.18%, MSISensor 96.48%, mSINGS 76.06%) and specificity (MANTIS 99.68%, MSI-Sensor 98.73%, mSINGS 99.68%).[31] The advantage of these methods is they can be integrated into existing NGS pipelines for routine clinical testing.

PROGNOSTIC FEATURES OF MICROSATELLITE INSTABILITY-HIGH CANCER

MSI-H CRCs have an improved prognosis in comparison with MSS tumors, particularly in the stage II setting.[32–34] However, a number of studies have shown discordant results with regard to its role as a predictive biomarker for overall survival in stage III and stage IV CRC.[35–39]

THERAPEUTIC IMPLICATIONS OF MICROSATELLITE INSTABILITY-HIGH TUMORS

MICROSATELLITE INSTABILITY-HIGH AND 5-FLUOROURACIL

Fluorouracil–based chemotherapy is a well-accepted adjuvant therapy for patients with stage III disease, as well as for some patients with stage II disease with high-risk features. Several studies have shown that patients with MSI-H CRCs do not benefit from 5-fluorouracil–based adjuvant therapy in stage II and III CRC.[39–41]

MICROSATELLITE INSTABILITY AND IMMUNOTHERAPY

It has been shown that MSI-H status correlates with the presence of increased tumor-infiltrating lymphocytes.[42] Favorable survival outcomes and a lower risk of metastasis have been previous illustrated among MSI-high tumors, which have increased tumor-infiltrating lymphocytes, suggesting that MSI-H may be closely associated with a robust immune response.[43] Two inhibitors of programmed cell death-1 protein—pembrolizumab and nivolumab—have demonstrated improved survival benefits in patients with mismatch repair deficient/MSI-high metastatic and/or recurrent CRC, leading to their subsequent approval by the US Food and Drug Administration (FDA) for this patient cohort.[44,45] Most recently, the combination of ipilimumab, a monoclonal antibody against cytotoxic T-lymphocyte–associated protein 4, with nivolumab has been approved by the FDA for mismatch repair deficient/MSI-high CRC in patients previously treated with chemotherapy.[46]

TUMOR MUTATION BURDEN AND IMMUNOTHERAPY

Similar to MSI being used to help guide therapeutic decision-making, tumor mutation burden (TMB) has arisen as a biomarker for response to immunotherapy. TMB is the rate of somatic mutations within a particular cancer, commonly reported as the number of mutations per megabase. Tumors with a high mutational load are thought to have a greater immunogenicity. With the presence of a greater number of mutations, tumors may generate novel antigens known as neoantigens, whose presence leads to an adaptive immune response against the tumor.

Although TMB was initially estimated using whole-exome sequencing as the gold standard, targeted NGS panels have shown to yielded similar results.[47–49] One of the key determinants of accuracy of NGS for measuring TMB is the extent of genomic coverage, with up to 1 megabase or more than 300 genes suggested at a minimum for a comparable performance with whole exome sequencing.[50] Recently, in a landmark trial across multiple tumor types (KEYNOTE 158), programmed cell death-1 protein blockade by pembrolizumab led to the FDA approval of pembrolizumab for tumors with TMB-high status (>10 mutations/Mb), regardless of tumor type, for patients with metastatic or unresectable disease or in patients whose tumor has progressed after prior treatment.[51] Some studies have shown that approximately 8% of CRC are TMB-high. A large proportion of TMB-high CRC, roughly 65%, arise in the setting of MSI-H status. Practically all MSI-H CRC are TMB-high. POLE/D1 alterations are identified in 1% or less of MSI-H/TMB-high tumors; however, POLE alterations do seem to be enriched in MSS/TMB-high CRC. Interestingly, 3% of MSS tumors are TMB-H, suggesting that testing for TMB may help to identify patients for treatment with immunotherapy who may otherwise not be eligible.[52]

NEUROTROPHIC TYROSINE RECEPTOR KINASE

Neurotrophic tyrosine receptor kinase (NTRK) are a family of receptor tyrosine kinases consisting of TrkA (NTRK1), TrkB (NTRK2), and TrkC (NTRK3).[53] Under normal physiologic conditions, Trk proteins play a role with normal neural development and cell survival. Oncogenic fusions involving the C terminal kinase domain with an N-terminal fusion partner causes constitutive activation of the TRK pathway and drives tumorigenesis.[53–55] Although NTRK fusions are closely associated with a select group of tumors, including infantile fibrosarcoma, mesoblastic nephroma, and secretory carcinoma of breast and salivary glands, NTRK fusions occur in approximately 0.4% of CRC.[56–60]

Recently, it has been found that kinase fusions, including NTRK1-3, are enriched in MSI-H CRC, specifically in cases with MLH1 promoter hypermethylation and mismatch repair deficiency (Fig. 2).[61–63] Of 22 NTRK fusions identified in these recent studies in CRC, 20 were MSI-H and all tested positive for MLH1 deficiency and promoter hypermethylation. None of these patients had KRAS, NRAS, or BRAF mutations, or the Lynch syndrome.

Various approaches exist to identify NTRK fusion positive tumors, via assessment of DNA by targeted cancer panels by NGS and RNA fusion panels. Pan-cancer studies assessing immunohistochemical staining with pan-Trk IHC support their use to screen for tumor with NTRK fusion, offering considerable sensitivity (87.9%) and specificity (100% in CRC).[64] The sensitivity is lower for NTRK3 fusions at approximately 80%, often with focal or faint staining, whereas NTRK1 and NTRK2 fusions are readily detected by pan-Trk IHC with diffuse staining (Fig. 3). DNA-based NGS detects NTRK1 and NTRK2 fusions when kinase domain exons and introns are targeted with sufficient probe coverage. Fusions involving NTRK3 remain challenging to identify with DNA-based NGS approaches owing to the size of the introns of NTRK3, such that to provide sufficient coverage of these introns, a proposed assay would suffer in total depth of coverage owing to excessive sequencing.[65] The solution is RNA-based NGS, because RNA NGS assays work well to detect NTRK fusions given decent quality RNA.

EPIDERMAL GROWTH FACTOR RECEPTOR AND DOWNSTREAM SIGNALING PATHWAYS

The epidermal growth factor receptor (EGFR) pathway, including downstream Ras/Raf/MEK, are key drivers of CRC. EGFR is a receptor tyrosine kinase that, when bound to a ligand, leads to receptor dimerization and autophosphorylation of the cytoplasmic kinase domain, and subsequent activation of downstream signal transduction pathways (Fig. 4). Inhibitors of EGFR, including panitumumab and cetuximab, are approved for use in the setting of RAS wild-type metastatic CRC.

EPIDERMAL GROWTH FACTOR RECEPTOR AND THE RAS/RAF/MEK/ERK PATHWAY

The RAS family are GTP binding proteins that act downstream of EGFR receptor activation and function to propagate downstream signaling to influence cell survival. Although RAS genes share 82% to 90% of their genomic sequence, they differ in their frequency of pathogenic variants across different tumor types, with KRAS and NRAS occurring in approximately 44.7% and 7.5% of CRC, respectively.[66–69] Most RAS mutations occur in a few specific codons across the RAS

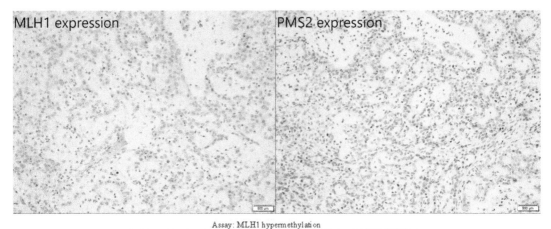

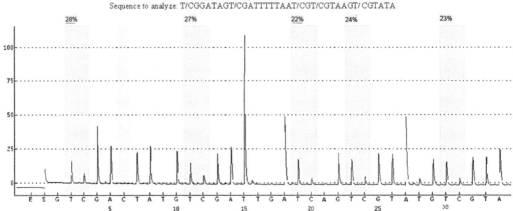

Fig. 2. (*A*) Photomicrograph of a CRC with loss of both MLH1 and PMS2 nuclear expression. (*B*) Analysis of MLH1 promoter methylation via pyrosequencing of the same patient's CRC. The *x*-axis represents the nucleotide order at the CpG site. The *y*-axis is the percentage of methylation represented by the ratio between signal intensities of C and T at each C in the CpG site, which is determined by the relative luminescence emitted following nucleotide base incorporation into the sequence. Shown is methylation within the MHL1 promoter region. (Adapted from https://oncologypro.esmo.org/oncology-in-practice/anti-cancer-agents-and-biological-therapy/targeting-ntrk-gene-fusions/case-studies/case-3; with permission.)

isoforms: codons 12 and 13 (exon 2), codons 59 and 61 (exon 3), and codons 117, and 146 (exon 4).[66]

Activating mutations within the RAS family lead to downstream signaling pathway activation. Multiple studies have shown that *KRAS/NRAS* activating mutations predict resistance to anti-EGFR therapy in metastatic CRC.[70–72] In 2017, the American Society for Clinical Pathology, College of American Pathologists, Association for Molecular Pathology, and the American Society of Clinical Oncology gave recommendations for biomarker testing for CRC and included extended RAS mutational assessment for patients with CRC before starting anti-EGFR therapy.[73] Extended RAS mutational analysis should include *KRAS* and *NRAS* codons 12 and 13 of exon 2, 59 and 61 of exon 3, and 117 and 146 of exon 4. Among CRC,

KRAS G12C alterations make up approximately 3% of tumors.[74–76] Recently, the early phase I/II KRYSTAL-1 (NCT03785249) trial examining the response of KRAS G12C inhibitor, MRTX849, across multiple solid tumors has shown promise and may offer additional therapeutic options for patients.[77]

BRAF is a serine/threonine protein kinase that functions downstream of RAS signaling. Activating mutations within *BRAF* occur in approximately 8% of metastatic CRC and 14% of stage II and stage III CRC. Prior studies assessing for the presence of *BRAF* V600 mutations in patients with CRC has shown inferior overall survival and progression free survival compared with BRAF wild type, especially in the setting of metastatic disease.[78–80] Studies have shown that patients with CRC with *BRAF* V600 mutations have a decreased response

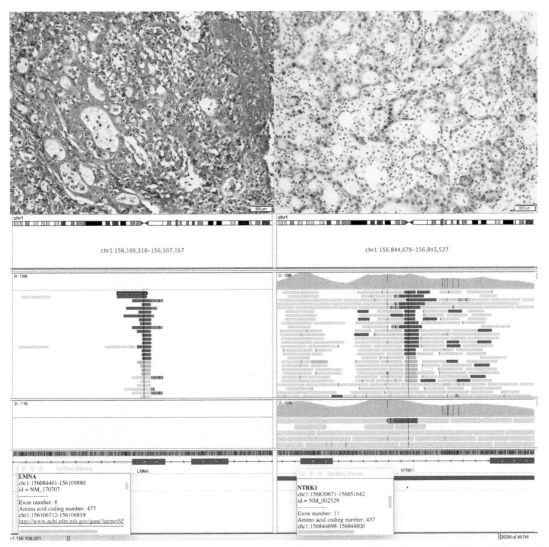

Fig. 3. Hematoxylin and eosin (*top left*) and Pan-TRK IHC (*top right*) and identification of the LMNA-NTRK1 fusion via MSK-IMPACT, a DNA-based NGS. The integrated genomics viewer (IGV) shows a structural variant involving LMNA exon 8 and NTRK1 exon 11 in the bottom. Antibody for IHC: clone EPR17341 available from Abcam, Cambridge, Massachusetts (www.abcam.com). (From https://oncologypro.esmo.org/oncology-in-practice/anti-cancer-agents-and-biological-therapy/targeting-ntrk-gene-fusions/case-studies/case-3; with permission.)

to EGFR inhibitors cetuximab and panitumumab, including decreased progression-free survival and overall survival.[78–82] However, many of these studies included nonrandomized cohorts, and follow-up metanalyses across multiple randomized studies have shown there to be insufficient evidence to suggest *BRAF* V600 mutant CRC responds differently to EGFR inhibitors than *BRAF* wild-type CRC.[83,84] Therefore, it is currently recommended to use *BRAF* V600 mutation testing for prognostic stratification for CRC but not as a predictive biomarker for response to EGFR inhibition.[73]

BRAF inhibitor therapy, which has been shown to have favorable response rates in other tumor types with V600E mutations, has not been shown to be effective in treating V600E mutant CRC when used as a monotherapy.[85–89] This difference may be partially explained by a compensatory activation of EGFR signaling, which has been described in *BRAF* V600E mutated CRC treated with BRAF inhibitors.[90] Several clinical trials have suggested that the combination of EGFR and BRAF inhibitor therapy can lead to an antitumoral response.[91–93] Mitogen-activated protein kinase kinases (MEK), which acts downstream of BRAF

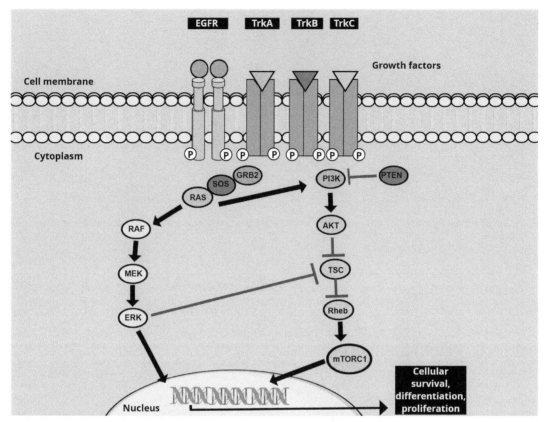

Fig. 4. The EGFR and NTRK signaling pathway. Signaling occurs when growth factors bind to the extracellular portion of the EGFR or Trk proteins. Two main downstream pathways can be activated, including the Ras/Raf/MEK/ERK and the PI3K/AKT/mTOR pathways, leading to increased cell survival, differentiation, and proliferation. Monoclonal antibodies directed against the extracellular domain can inhibit growth factor binding and downstream signaling.

to phosphorylate mitogen-activated protein kinase, has been suggested to be a suitable target for BRAF V600E mutated CRC. Several preclinical and clinical trials have supported the combined use of BRAF and MEK inhibitors over combined BRAF inhibitor and anti-EGFR therapy.[89,94,95] However, other studies using encorafenib, a BRAF inhibitor with a prolong pharmacodynamic activity, have shown that its combination with anti-EGFR therapy showed promising clinical activity.[96] The BEACON trial showed that a doublet regimen of encorafenib and cetuximab (anti-EGFR monoclonal antibody) and triplet regimen of encorafenib, binimetinib (MEK inhibitor), and cetuximab both led to a longer overall survival in comparison with standard therapy in patients with V600E mutated CRC that had progressed on other therapies.[97] Recently, the FDA approved the combination of encorafenib/cetuximab for *BRAF* V600E mutated previously treated metastatic CRC. Therefore, *BRAF* V600 testing helps to identify which patients may be eligible for combined BRAF inhibitor and anti-EGFR therapy.[98]

Circulating Tumor DNA in Colorectal Carcinoma

Monitoring circulating tumor DNA (ctDNA) is a potentially transformative assay for early diagnosis and monitoring of response to therapy.[99,100] The presence of ctDNA has been identified in approximately 50% of nonmetastatic and 90% of metastatic cancers across multiple tumor types.[101] Studies have shown that patients with CRC who have ctDNA after surgery have a greater risk for recurrence.[102,103] There are a number of trials ongoing to answer the question of what is the clinical usefulness of monitoring ctDNA in patients with CRC, including the II/III COBRA study, the CIRCULATE trial, and the DYNAMIC-II study, which are studying the role of ctDNA to predict recurrence. The II/III DYNAMIC-III study is being performed to understand the role of ctDNA to inform decisions about escalation or de-escalation of therapy.[104] At present, ctDNA remains an emerging biomarker whose usefulness as a noninvasive method to guide treatment decisions remains to be seen. Hopefully, future research will further characterize its role in monitoring disease in patients with CRC.

SUMMARY

The importance of molecular pathology to guide the management of patients with CRC is increasingly evident. Clinical laboratories are challenged with providing the most clinically actionable and up-to-date information to guide clinical care. In this era of molecular testing, tumor profiling by NGS has created new opportunities for a more personalized approach toward cancer care. Clearly molecular testing surrounding CRC tumorigenesis is becoming more complex, as well as more critical for daily patient care, thus a firm understanding of laboratory testing practices is a necessity for the practicing pathologist.

CLINICS CARE POINTS

- Microsatellite instability testing continues to have usefulness in the identification of patients with Lynch syndrome, as well as for predicting response to immunotherapy.

- TMB is an approved biomarker for immunotherapy eligibility.

- Extended RAS testing helps to determine which patients may respond to anti-EGFR therapy.

- *BRAF* testing determines which patients with CRC may respond to the combination of BRAF inhibition and anti-EGFR therapy, with or without MEK inhibition.

- Targetable kinase fusions are enriched in *MLH1* promoter methylated CRCs that are also negative for alternations in mitogen-activated protein kinase pathway and thus may represent a suitable therapy option in select patients.

- Future studies examining the role of ctDNA to predict tumor recurrence (COBRA study, CIRCULATE trial, and DYNAMIC-II study), as well as the KRYSTAL-1 trial examining response toward KRAS G12C inhibition, are pending and may offer additional diagnostic and therapeutic options for patients in the future.

DISCLOSURE

Cameron Beech has no disclosures. Jaclyn F. Hechtman reports research funding from Bayer, Lilly Oncology, Boehringer Ingelheim, and consulting fees from Axiom Healthcare Strategies and Bayer; honoraria from Bayer, Illumina, Cor2Ed, and WebMD.

REFERENCES

1. Siegel RL, Miller KD, Jemal A. Cancer statistics, 2020. CA Cancer J Clin 2020. https://doi.org/10.3322/caac.21590.

2. Fearon ER, Vogelstein B. A genetic model for colorectal tumorigenesis. Cell 1990. https://doi.org/10.1016/0092-8674(90)90186-I.

3. Vogelstein B, Fearon ER, Hamilton SR, et al. Genetic alterations during colorectal-tumor development. N Engl J Med 1988. https://doi.org/10.1056/NEJM198809013190901.

4. Network TCGA, Muzny DM, Bainbridge MN, et al. Comprehensive molecular characterization of human colon and rectal cancer. Nature 2012. https://doi.org/10.1038/nature11252.Comprehensive.

5. Fearon E. Molecular genetics of colorectal cancer annual review of pathology mechanisms of disease. Annu Rev 2011.

6. Habermann JK, Paulsen U, Roblick UJ, et al. Stage-specific alterations of the genome, transcriptome, and proteome during colorectal carcinogenesis. Genes Chromosom Cancer 2007. https://doi.org/10.1002/gcc.20382.

7. Guinney J, Dienstmann R, Wang X, et al. The consensus molecular subtypes of colorectal cancer. Nat Med 2015. https://doi.org/10.1038/nm.3967.

8. Aaltonen LA, Peltomäki P, Leach FS, et al. Clues to the pathogenesis of familial colorectal cancer. Science 1993. https://doi.org/10.1126/science.8484121.

9. Fang M, Ou J, Hutchinson L, et al. The BRAF oncoprotein functions through the transcriptional repressor MAFG to Mediate the CpG Island Methylator Phenotype. Mol Cell 2014. https://doi.org/10.1016/j.molcel.2014.08.010.

10. Cunningham JM, Kim CY, Christensen ER, et al. The frequency of hereditary defective mismatch repair in a prospective series of unselected colorectal carcinomas. Am J Hum Genet 2001. https://doi.org/10.1086/323658.

11. Hampel H, Frankel WL, Martin E, et al. Feasibility of screening for Lynch syndrome among patients with colorectal cancer. J Clin Oncol 2008. https://doi.org/10.1200/JCO.2008.17.5950.

12. Abdel-Rahman WM, Peltomäki P. Lynch syndrome and related familial colorectal cancers. Crit Rev Oncog 2008. https://doi.org/10.1615/CritRevOncog.v14.i1.10.

13. Vilar E, Gruber SB. Microsatellite instability in colorectal cancer: the stable evidence. Nat Rev Clin Oncol 2010. https://doi.org/10.1038/nrclinonc.2009.237.

14. Ligtenberg MJL, Kuiper RP, Chan TL, et al. Heritable somatic methylation and inactivation of MSH2 in families with Lynch syndrome due to deletion of the 3′ exons of TACSTD1. Nat Genet 2009. https://doi.org/10.1038/ng.283.

15. Kovacs ME, Papp J, Szentirmay Z, et al. Deletions removing the last exon of TACSTD1 constitute a distinct class of mutations predisposing to lynch syndrome. Hum Mutat 2009. https://doi.org/10.1002/humu.20942.

16. Wimmer K, Etzler J. Constitutional mismatch repair-deficiency syndrome: have we so far seen only the tip of an iceberg? Hum Genet 2008. https://doi.org/10.1007/s00439-008-0542-4.

17. Rustgi AK. The genetics of hereditary colon cancer. Genes Dev 2007. https://doi.org/10.1101/gad.1593107.

18. Lynch HT, De la Chapelle A. Hereditary colorectal cancer. N Engl J Med 2003. https://doi.org/10.1056/NEJMra012242.

19. Vasen HFA, Watson P, Mecklin JP, et al. New clinical criteria for hereditary nonpolyposis colorectal cancer (HNPCC, Lynch syndrome) proposed by the International Collaborative Group on HNPCC. Gastroenterology 1999. https://doi.org/10.1016/S0016-5085(99)70510-X.

20. Umar A, Boland CR, Terdiman JP, et al. Revised Bethesda Guidelines for hereditary nonpolyposis colorectal cancer (Lynch syndrome) and microsatellite instability. J Natl Cancer Inst 2004. https://doi.org/10.1093/jnci/djh034.

21. Messerini L, Mori S, Zampi G. Pathologic features of hereditary non-polyposis colorectal cancer. Tumori 1996. https://doi.org/10.1177/030089169608200204.

22. Jenkins MA, Hayashi S, O'Shea AM, et al. Pathology features in Bethesda guidelines predict colorectal cancer microsatellite instability: a population-based study. Gastroenterology 2007. https://doi.org/10.1053/j.gastro.2007.04.044.

23. Berg AO, Armstrong K, Botkin J, et al. Recommendations from the EGAPP Working Group: genetic testing strategies in newly diagnosed individuals with colorectal cancer aimed at reducing morbidity and mortality from Lynch syndrome in relatives. Genet Med 2009. https://doi.org/10.1097/GIM.0b013e31818fa2ff.

24. Gupta S, Provenzale D, Llor X, et al. NCCN Guidelines Insights: Genetic/Familial High-Risk Assessment: Colorectal, Version 2.2019. J Natl Compr Canc Netw 2019;17(9):1032–41.

25. Baudhuin LM, Burgart LJ, Leontovich O, et al. Use of microsatellite instability and immunohistochemistry testing for the identification of individuals at risk for Lynch syndrome. Fam Cancer 2005. https://doi.org/10.1007/s10689-004-1447-6.

26. Hechtman JF, Rana S, Middha S, et al. Retained mismatch repair protein expression occurs in approximately 6% of microsatellite instability-high cancers and is associated with missense mutations in mismatch repair genes. Mod Pathol 2020. https://doi.org/10.1038/s41379-019-0414-6.

27. Bao F, Panarelli NC, Rennert H, et al. Neoadjuvant therapy induces loss of MSH6 expression in colorectal carcinoma. Am J Surg Pathol 2010. https://doi.org/10.1097/PAS.0b013e3181f906cc.

28. Middha S, Zhang L, Nafa K, et al. Reliable pan-cancer microsatellite instability assessment by using targeted next-generation sequencing data. JCO Precis Oncol 2017. https://doi.org/10.1200/po.17.00084.

29. Niu B, Ye K, Zhang Q, et al. MSIsensor: microsatellite instability detection using paired tumor-normal sequence data. Bioinformatics 2014. https://doi.org/10.1093/bioinformatics/btt755.

30. Salipante SJ, Scroggins SM, Hampel HL, et al. Microsatellite instability detection by next generation sequencing. Clin Chem 2014. https://doi.org/10.1373/clinchem.2014.223677.

31. Kautto EA, Bonneville R, Miya J, et al. Performance evaluation for rapid detection of pan-cancer microsatellite instability with MANTIS. Oncotarget 2017. https://doi.org/10.18632/oncotarget.13918.

32. Sankila R, Aaltonen LA, Jarvinen HJ, et al. Better survival rates in patients with MLH1-associated hereditary colorectal cancer. Gastroenterology 1996. https://doi.org/10.1053/gast.1996.v110.pm8608876.

33. Thibodeau SN, Bren G, Schaid D. Microsatellite instability in cancer of the proximal colon. Science 1993. https://doi.org/10.1126/science.8484122.

34. Hveem TS, Merok MA, Pretorius ME, et al. Prognostic impact of genomic instability in colorectal cancer. Br J Cancer 2014. https://doi.org/10.1038/bjc.2014.133.

35. Guidoboni M, Gafà R, Viel A, et al. Microsatellite instability and high content of activated cytotoxic lymphocytes identify colon cancer patients with a favorable prognosis. Am J Pathol 2001. https://doi.org/10.1016/S0002-9440(10)61695-1.

36. Venderbosch S, Nagtegaal ID, Maughan TS, et al. Mismatch repair status and BRAF mutation status in metastatic colorectal cancer patients: a pooled analysis of the CAIRO, CAIRO2, COIN, and FOCUS studies. Clin Cancer Res 2014. https://doi.org/10.1158/1078-0432.CCR-14-0332.

37. Klingbiel D, Saridaki Z, Roth AD, et al. Prognosis of stage II and III colon cancer treated with adjuvant 5-fluorouracil or FOLFIRI in relation to microsatellite status: results of the PETACC-3 trial. Ann Oncol 2015. https://doi.org/10.1093/annonc/mdu499.

38. Wang B, Li F, Zhou X, et al. Is microsatellite instability-high really a favorable prognostic factor for advanced colorectal cancer? A meta-analysis. World J Surg Oncol 2019. https://doi.org/10.1186/s12957-019-1706-5.

39. Popat S, Hubner R, Houlston RS. Systematic review of microsatellite instability and colorectal cancer prognosis. J Clin Oncol 2005. https://doi.org/10.1200/JCO.2005.01.086.

40. Sargent DJ, Marsoni S, Monges G, et al. Defective mismatch repair as a predictive marker for lack of efficacy of fluorouracil-based adjuvant therapy in colon cancer. J Clin Oncol 2010. https://doi.org/10.1200/JCO.2009.27.1825.

41. Ribic CM, Sargent DJ, Moore MJ, et al. Tumor microsatellite-instability status as a predictor of benefit from fluorouracil-based adjuvant chemotherapy for colon cancer. N Engl J Med 2003. https://doi.org/10.1056/NEJMoa022289.

42. Smyrk TC, Watson P, Kaul K, et al. Tumor-infiltrating lymphocytes are a marker for microsatellite instability in colorectal carcinoma. Cancer 2001. https://doi.org/10.1002/1097-0142(20010615)91:12<2417.

43. Prall F, Dührkop T, Weirich V, et al. Prognostic role of CD8+ tumor-infiltrating lymphocytes in stage III colorectal cancer with and without microsatellite instability. Hum Pathol 2004. https://doi.org/10.1016/j.humpath.2004.01.022.

44. Overman MJ, McDermott R, Leach JL, et al. Nivolumab in patients with metastatic DNA mismatch repair-deficient or microsatellite instability-high colorectal cancer (CheckMate 142): an open-label, multicentre, phase 2 study. Lancet Oncol 2017. https://doi.org/10.1016/S1470-2045(17)30422-9.

45. Le DT, Uram JN, Wang H, et al. PD-1 blockade in tumors with mismatch-repair deficiency. N Engl J Med 2015. https://doi.org/10.1056/NEJMoa1500596.

46. Overman MJ, Lonardi S, Wong KYM, et al. Durable clinical benefit with nivolumab plus ipilimumab in DNA mismatch repair-deficient/microsatellite instability-high metastatic colorectal cancer. J Clin Oncol 2018. https://doi.org/10.1200/JCO.2017.76.9901.

47. Steuer CE, Ramalingam SS. Tumor mutation burden: leading immunotherapy to the era of precision medicine? J Clin Oncol 2018. https://doi.org/10.1200/JCO.2017.76.8770.

48. Vanderwalde A, Spetzler D, Xiao N, et al. Microsatellite instability status determined by next-generation sequencing and compared with PD-L1 and tumor mutational burden in 11,348 patients. Cancer Med 2018. https://doi.org/10.1002/cam4.1372.

49. Rizvi H, Sanchez-Vega F, La K, et al. Molecular determinants of response to anti-programmed cell death (PD)-1 and anti-programmed death-ligand 1 (PD-L1) blockade in patients with non-small-cell lung cancer profiled with targeted next-generation sequencing. J Clin Oncol 2018. https://doi.org/10.1200/JCO.2017.75.3384.

50. Chalmers ZR, Connelly CF, Fabrizio D, et al. Analysis of 100,000 human cancer genomes reveals the landscape of tumor mutational burden. Genome Med 2017. https://doi.org/10.1186/s13073-017-0424-2.

51. FDA. FDA approves pembrolizumab for adults and children with TMB-H solid tumors. Updated 6/17/2020. Available at: https://www.fda.gov/drugs/drug-approvals-and-databases/fda-approves-pembrolizumab-adults-and-children-tmb-h-solid-tumors. Accessed September 15, 2020.

52. Fabrizio DA, George TJ, Dunne RF, et al. Beyond microsatellite testing: assessment of tumor mutational burden identifies subsets of colorectal cancer who may respond to immune checkpoint inhibition. J Gastrointest Oncol 2018. https://doi.org/10.21037/jgo.2018.05.06.

53. Vaishnavi A, Le AT, Doebele RC. TRKing down an old oncogene in a new era of targeted therapy. Cancer Discov 2015. https://doi.org/10.1158/2159-8290.CD-14-0765.

54. Cocco E, Scaltriti M, Drilon A. NTRK fusion-positive cancers and TRK inhibitor therapy. Nat Rev Clin Oncol 2018. https://doi.org/10.1038/s41571-018-0113-0.

55. Kheder ES, Hong DS. Emerging targeted therapy for tumors with NTRK fusion proteins. Clin Cancer Res 2018. https://doi.org/10.1158/1078-0432.CCR-18-1156.

56. Martin-Zanca D, Hughes SH, Barbacid M. A human oncogene formed by the fusion of truncated tropomyosin and protein tyrosine kinase sequences. Nature 1986. https://doi.org/10.1038/319743a0.

57. Knezevich SR, McFadden DE, Tao W, et al. A novel ETV6-NTRK3 gene fusion in congenital fibrosarcoma. Nat Genet 1998. https://doi.org/10.1038/ng0298-184.

58. Tognon C, Knezevich SR, Huntsman D, et al. Expression of the ETV6-NTRK3 gene fusion as a primary event in human secretory breast carcinoma. Cancer Cell 2002. https://doi.org/10.1016/S1535-6108(02)00180-0.

59. Anderson J, Gibson S, Sebire NJ. Expression of ETV6-NTRK in classical, cellular and mixed subtypes of congenital mesoblastic nephroma. Histopathology 2006. https://doi.org/10.1111/j.1365-2559.2006.02400.x.

60. Skálová A, Vanecek T, Sima R, et al. Mammary analogue secretory carcinoma of salivary glands, containing the etv6-ntrk3 fusion gene: a hitherto undescribed salivary gland tumor entity. Am J Surg Pathol 2010. https://doi.org/10.1097/PAS.0b013e3181d9efcc.

61. Sato K, Kawazu M, Yamamoto Y, et al. Fusion kinases identified by genomic analyses of sporadic microsatellite instability–high colorectal cancers. Clin Cancer Res 2019. https://doi.org/10.1158/1078-0432.CCR-18-1574.

62. Chou A, Fraser T, Ahadi M, et al. NTRK gene rearrangements are highly enriched in MLH1/PMS2 deficient, BRAF wild-type colorectal carcinomas—a study of 4569 cases. Mod Pathol 2020. https://doi.org/10.1038/s41379-019-0417-3.

63. Cocco E, Benhamida J, Middha S, et al. Colorectal Carcinomas Containing Hypermethylated MLH1 Promoter and Wild-Type BRAF/KRAS Are Enriched for Targetable Kinase Fusions. Cancer Res 2019; 79(6):1047–53.

64. Solomon JP, Linkov I, Rosado A, et al. NTRK fusion detection across multiple assays and 33,997 cases: diagnostic implications and pitfalls. Mod Pathol 2020. https://doi.org/10.1038/s41379-019-0324-7.

65. Davies KD, Aisner DL. Wake up and smell the fusions: single-modality molecular testing misses drivers. Clin Cancer Res 2019. https://doi.org/10.1158/1078-0432.CCR-19-1361.

66. Prior IA, Lewis PD, Mattos C. A comprehensive survey of ras mutations in cancer. Cancer Res 2012. https://doi.org/10.1158/0008-5472.CAN-11-2612.

67. Papke B, Der CJ, Drugging RAS. Know the enemy. Science 2017. https://doi.org/10.1126/science.aam7622.

68. Jinesh GG, Sambandam V, Vijayaraghavan S, et al. Molecular genetics and cellular events of K-Ras-driven tumorigenesis. Oncogene 2018. https://doi.org/10.1038/onc.2017.377.

69. Cox AD, Fesik SW, Kimmelman AC, et al. Drugging the undruggable RAS: mission possible? Nat Rev Drug Discov 2014. https://doi.org/10.1038/nrd4389.

70. Sorich MJ, Wiese MD, Rowland A, et al. Extended RAS mutations and anti-EGFR monoclonal antibody survival benefit in metastatic colorectal cancer: a meta-analysis of randomized, controlled trials. Ann Oncol 2015. https://doi.org/10.1093/annonc/mdu378.

71. Douillard JY, Oliner KS, Siena S, et al. Panitumumab-FOLFOX4 treatment and RAS mutations in colorectal cancer. N Engl J Med 2013. https://doi.org/10.1056/NEJMoa1305275.

72. Van Cutsem E, Lenz HJ, Köhne CH, et al. Fluorouracil, leucovorin, and irinotecan plus cetuximab treatment and RAS mutations in colorectal cancer. J Clin Oncol 2015. https://doi.org/10.1200/JCO.2014.59.4812.

73. Sepulveda AR, Hamilton SR, Allegra CJ, et al. Molecular biomarkers for the evaluation of colorectal cancer: guideline from The American Society for Clinical Pathology, College of American Pathologists, Association for Molecular Pathology, and the American Society of Clinical Oncology. J Clin Oncol 2017. https://doi.org/10.1200/JCO.2016.71.9807.

74. Cerami E, Gao J, Dogrusoz U, et al. The cBio Cancer Genomics Portal: an open platform for exploring multidimensional cancer genomics data. Cancer Discov 2012. https://doi.org/10.1158/2159-8290.CD-12-0095.

75. Gao J, Aksoy BA, Dogrusoz U, et al. Integrative analysis of complex cancer genomics and clinical profiles using the cBioPortal. Sci Signal 2013. https://doi.org/10.1126/scisignal.2004088.

76. Araujo LH, Souza BM, Leite LR, et al. Molecular profile of KRAS G12C-mutant colorectal and non-small-cell lung cancer. BMC Cancer 2021. https://doi.org/10.1186/s12885-021-07884-8.

77. Mirati Therapeutics Inc. Phase 1/2 Study of MRTX849 in patients with cancer having a KRAS G12C mutation KRYSTAL-1. Available at: https://clinicaltrials.gov/ct2/show/NCT03785249. Accessed September 15, 2020.

78. Xu Q, Xu AT, Zhu MM, et al. Predictive and prognostic roles of BRAF mutation in patients with metastatic colorectal cancer treated with anti-epidermal growth factor receptor monoclonal antibodies: a meta-analysis. J Dig Dis 2013. https://doi.org/10.1111/1751-2980.12063.

79. Yuan ZX, Wang XY, Qin QY, et al. The prognostic role of BRAF mutation in metastatic colorectal cancer receiving anti-EGFR monoclonal antibodies: a meta-analysis. PLoS One 2013. https://doi.org/10.1371/journal.pone.0065995.

80. Yang ZY, Wu XY, Huang YF, et al. Promising biomarkers for predicting the outcomes of patients with KRAS wild-type metastatic colorectal cancer treated with anti-epidermal growth factor receptor monoclonal antibodies: a systematic review with meta-analysis. Int J Cancer 2013. https://doi.org/10.1002/ijc.28153.

81. Cui D, Cao D, Yang Y, et al. Effect of BRAF V600E mutation on tumor response of anti-EGFR monoclonal antibodies for first-line metastatic colorectal cancer treatment: a meta-analysis of randomized studies. Mol Biol Rep 2014. https://doi.org/10.1007/s11033-013-2974-8.

82. Mao C, Liao RY, Qiu LX, et al. BRAF V600E mutation and resistance to anti-EGFR monoclonal antibodies in patients with metastatic colorectal cancer: a meta-analysis. Mol Biol Rep 2011. https://doi.org/10.1007/s11033-010-0351-4.

83. Rowland A, Dias MM, Wiese MD, et al. Meta-analysis of BRAF mutation as a predictive biomarker of benefit from anti-EGFR monoclonal antibody therapy for RAS wild-type metastatic colorectal cancer. Br J Cancer 2015. https://doi.org/10.1038/bjc.2015.173.

84. Pietrantonio F, Petrelli F, Coinu A, et al. Predictive role of BRAF mutations in patients with advanced colorectal cancer receiving cetuximab and panitumumab: a meta-analysis. Eur J Cancer 2015.

85. Dummer R, Ascierto PA, Gogas HJ, et al. Encorafenib plus binimetinib versus vemurafenib or encorafenib in patients with BRAF-mutant melanoma (COLUMBUS): a multicentre, open-label, randomised phase 3 trial. Lancet Oncol 2018. https://doi.org/10.1016/S1470-2045(18)30142-6.

86. Kopetz S, Desai J, Chan E, et al. Phase II pilot study of vemurafenib in patients with metastatic BRAF-mutated colorectal cancer. J Clin Oncol 2015. https://doi.org/10.1200/JCO.2015.63.2497.

87. Khunger A, Khunger M, Velcheti V. Dabrafenib in combination with trametinib in the treatment of patients with BRAF V600-positive advanced or metastatic non-small cell lung cancer: clinical evidence and experience. Ther Adv Respir Dis 2018. https://doi.org/10.1177/1753466618767611.

88. Mao M, Tian F, Mariadason JM, et al. Resistance to BRAF inhibition in BRAF-mutant colon cancer can be overcome with PI3K inhibition or demethylating agents. Clin Cancer Res 2013. https://doi.org/10.1158/1078-0432.CCR-11-1446.

89. Corcoran RB, Atreya CE, Falchook GS, et al. Combined BRAF and MEK inhibition with dabrafenib and trametinib in BRAF V600-Mutant colorectal cancer. J Clin Oncol 2015. https://doi.org/10.1200/JCO.2015.63.2471.

90. Prahallad A, Sun C, Huang S, et al. Unresponsiveness of colon cancer to BRAF(V600E) inhibition through feedback activation of EGFR. Nature 2012. https://doi.org/10.1038/nature10868.

91. Corcoran RB, Ezzibdeh RM, Chhour P, et al. Combined BRAF, EGFR, and MEK inhibition in patients with BRAFV600E-mutant colorectal cancer. Cancer Discov 2018. https://doi.org/10.1016/j.biomaterials.2016.06.015.Tunable.

92. Hong DS, Morris VK, El Osta B, et al. Phase IB study of vemurafenib in combination with irinotecan and cetuximab in patients with metastatic colorectal cancer with BRAFV600E mutation. Cancer Discov 2016. https://doi.org/10.1158/2159-8290.CD-16-0050.

93. Yaeger R, Cercek A, O'Reilly EM, et al. Pilot trial of combined BRAF and EGFR inhibition in BRAF-mutant metastatic colorectal cancer patients. Clin Cancer Res 2015. https://doi.org/10.1158/1078-0432.CCR-14-2779.

94. Corcoran RB, Dias-Santagata D, Bergethon K, et al. BRAF gene amplification can promote acquired resistance to MEK inhibitors in cancer cells harboring the BRAF V600E mutation. Sci Signal 2010. https://doi.org/10.1126/scisignal.2001148.

95. Corcoran RB, Ebi H, Turke AB, et al. EGFR-mediated reactivation of MAPK signaling contributes to insensitivity of BRAF-mutant colorectal cancers to RAF inhibition with vemurafenib. Cancer Discov 2012. https://doi.org/10.1158/2159-8290.CD-11-0341.

96. Tabernero J, Geel RV, Guren TK, et al. Phase 2 results: Encorafenib (ENCO) and cetuximab (CETUX) with or without alpelisib (ALP) in patients with advanced BRAF- mutant colorectal cancer (BRAFm CRC). J Clin Oncol 2016. https://doi.org/10.1200/jco.2016.34.15_suppl.3544.

97. Kopetz S, Grothey A, Yaeger R, et al. Encorafenib, binimetinib, and cetuximab in BRAF V600E–mutated colorectal cancer. N Engl J Med 2019. https://doi.org/10.1056/NEJMoa1908075.

98. FDA. FDA approves encorafenib in combination with cetuximab for metastatic colorectal cancer with a BRAF V600E mutation. Available at: https://www.fda.gov/drugs/resources-information-approved-drugs/fda-approves-encorafenib-combination-cetuximab-metastatic-colorectal-cancer-braf--v600e-mutation. Accessed September 15, 2020.

99. Petit J, Carroll G, Gould T, et al. Cell-free DNA as a diagnostic blood-based biomarker for colorectal cancer: a systematic review. J Surg Res 2019. https://doi.org/10.1016/j.jss.2018.11.029.

100. Cree IA, Uttley L, Buckley Woods H, et al. The evidence base for circulating tumour DNA blood-based biomarkers for the early detection of cancer: a systematic mapping review. BMC Cancer 2017. https://doi.org/10.1186/s12885-017-3693-7.

101. Bettegowda C, Sausen M, Leary RJ, et al. Detection of circulating tumor DNA in early- and late-stage human malignancies. Sci Transl Med 2014. https://doi.org/10.1126/scitranslmed.3007094.

102. Diehl F, Schmidt K, Choti MA, et al. Circulating mutant DNA to assess tumor dynamics. Nat Med 2008. https://doi.org/10.1038/nm.1789.

103. Tie J, Wang Y, Tomasetti C, et al. Circulating tumor DNA analysis detects minimal residual disease and predicts recurrence in patients with stage II colon cancer. Sci Transl Med 2016. https://doi.org/10.1126/scitranslmed.aaf6219.

104. Dasari A, Morris VK, Allegra CJ, et al. ctDNA applications and integration in colorectal cancer: an NCI Colon and Rectal–Anal Task Forces whitepaper. Nat Rev Clin Oncol 2020. https://doi.org/10.1038/s41571-020-0392-0.

Molecular Pathology of Gastroesophageal Cancer

Matthew D. Stachler, MD, PhD[a],*, Ramon U. Jin, MD, PhD[b]

KEYWORDS

- Esophageal squamous cell carcinoma • Esophageal adenocarcinoma • Gastric adenocarcinoma
- Molecular pathology

Key points

- Esophageal squamous cell carcinoma and esophageal adenocarcinoma are separate entities with differing molecular pathology.
- Gastric adenocarcinomas can be classified into 4 distinct molecular subtypes that may suggest treatments unique to the subtypes.
- Esophageal adenocarcinoma and chromosomal unstable–type gastric adenocarcinoma are very similar to each other and likely constitute a spectrum of the same disease.

ABSTRACT

Upper gastroesophageal carcinomas consist of cancers arising from the esophagus and stomach. Squamous cell carcinomas and adenocarcinomas are seen in the esophagus and despite arising from the same organ have different biology. Gastric adenocarcinomas are categorized into 4 molecular subtypes: high Epstein-Barr virus load, microsatellite unstable cancers, chromosomal unstable (CIN) cancers, and genomically stable cancers. Genomically stable gastric cancers correlate highly with histologically defined diffuse-type cancers. Esophageal carcinomas and CIN gastric cancers often are driven by high-level amplifications of oncogenes and contain a high degree of intratumoral heterogeneity. Targeted therapeutics is an active area of research for gastroesophageal cancers.

OVERVIEW

Upper gastrointestinal cancers comprise malignancies of the esophagus and stomach. Although most gastrointestinal cancers are adenocarcinomas, esophageal cancers come in both adenocarcinoma and squamous cell carcinoma. Despite being derived from the same organ, esophageal adenocarcinoma (EAC) and esophageal squamous cell carcinoma (ESCC) are quite different at both cellular and molecular levels and should be treated as separate entities.[1] Traditionally, adenocarcinomas of the esophagus and stomach were considered two separate types of cancer and treated as such. Recent evidence has suggested, however, that EAC is very similar to intestinal-type gastric adenocarcinomas of the proximal stomach.[1,2] Although they are discussed separately, they should be considered as a spectrum of the same disease.[3] In the United States, gastroesophageal cancers represent a significant source of cancer morbidity and mortality with more than 45,000 new cases resulting in more than 26,000 deaths estimated for 2021.[4] The lack of early endoscopic surveillance guidelines and the often subtle clinical symptoms have resulted in many patients presenting at time of diagnosis with advanced metastatic disease and 5-year survival rates under 20%.[5] As understanding of these

[a] Department of Pathology, University of California San Francisco, 513 Parnassus Avenue HSW450B, San Francisco, CA 94143, USA; [b] Section of Hematology/Oncology, Department of Medicine, Baylor College of Medicine, 7200 Cambridge Street, Suite 7B, MS: BCM904, Houston, TX 77030, USA
* Corresponding author.
E-mail address: Matthew.Stachler@UCSF.edu

Surgical Pathology 14 (2021) 443–453
https://doi.org/10.1016/j.path.2021.05.008
1875-9181/21/© 2021 Elsevier Inc. All rights reserved.

complex cancers continues to improve, new more efficacious and better tolerated targeted therapies are being developed.

ESOPHAGEAL SQUAMOUS CELL CARCINOMA

ESCC arises in the upper and middle esophagus and has a widely varying regional incidence, with highest rates in China, South Africa, and South America.[6] Risk factors also vary according to region, but common ones include tobacco, diet, and alcohol.[6] The molecular alterations present in ESCC have been well studied. As in other squamous cell carcinomas, ESCCs typically have a moderately high mutation burden and frequent copy number alterations. A recent The Cancer Genome Atlas (TCGA) article,[1] as well as others,[7,8] describe frequent activation of the RAS and PI(3)K pathways, loss of cell-cycle regulation, chromatin remodeling dysregulation, and alterations in transcription factors/cell differentiation pathways. RAS and PI(3)K pathway alterations include frequent amplifications of EGFR and FGFR1 with ERBB2, KRAS, and MET less commonly amplified and common activating mutations in PIK2CA. PTEN, a negative regulator of PIK3CA, is inactivated through deletion or loss of function mutations in approximately 10% of cases. Commonly altered genes involved in cell-cycle regulation include very frequent deletions of CDKN2A (approximately 75% of ESCCs), deletions or mutations in RB1, and amplifications of CCND1 and/or CDK6. Genes involved in chromatin remodeling are altered in approximately a third of cases with mutations or deletions of SMARCA4, KDM6A, and KMT2D the most common. Transcription factors or other genes involved in cell differentiation also commonly are altered. Amplifications involving genomic regions that contain TP63/SOX2 are seen in approximately half of ESCCs with mutations in NOTCH1 and ZNF750 also somewhat common. Finally, a few other genes also commonly are altered. These include TP53 mutations in more than 80% of cases, MYC amplifications, and less commonly SMAD4 mutations or deletions.

ESCC arises from dysplastic (premalignant) lesions similar to other squamous cancers. Studies comparing ESCC and dysplasia adjacent to ESCC found remarkably similar aggregate mutational and copy number profiles, with areas of dysplasia having a similar frequency of events in genes commonly altered in ESCC.[9,10] Despite a similar frequency of alterations, when paired ESCC and dysplasia samples from the same patient were compared with each other, there still was a high degree of genomic heterogeneity as well as private, nonshared events. This suggests that fields of dysplasia may consist of an oligoclonal population, where 1 of these clones eventually develops an invasive phenotype to become ESCC. When dysplasia adjacent to ESCC was compared with dysplasia from patients without ESCC, 2 important differences were identified.[10] First, although TP53 mutations still were identified in patients with only dysplastic tissue, a second event affecting the alternative allele was very rare. This is in contrast to ESCC and dysplasia adjacent to ESCC, where finding 2 alterations of TP53 was extremely common. Second, the number of mutations and CNVs in patients with only dysplastic tissue was lower than both low-grade dysplasia and high-grade dysplasia taken adjacent to ESCC. These results raise the possibility of using molecular alterations to better stratify patients with esophageal squamous dysplasia into high and low risk.

ESOPHAGEAL ADENOCARCINOMA

EAC arises in the lower esophagus out of a field of columnar metaplasia that develops a varying degree of intestinal differentiation (called Barrett's esophagus [BE]). Although traditionally EAC was rare, with ESCC the predominate cancer type of the esophagus, there has been a dramatic rise in incidence of EAC within European and North American countries.[11–14] Combined with the low 5-year survival rate, this increase in incidence has driven an increased interest in understanding the molecular alterations that are present in this cancer. Several large studies have characterized the landscape of alterations present, including both by the TCGA[1] and the International Cancer Gene Consortium.[15] Like ESCC and many other cancers, pathways that commonly are altered in EAC include receptor tyrosine kinases (RTK) and their downstream signaling partners (Ras signaling), cell-cycle control, transcription factors/cell differentiation, chromatin remodeling, and transforming growth factor (TGF)-β signaling. Oncogenic activation through the RTK pathway typically occurs through amplification of ERBB2, EGFR, or KRAS which are present in approximately 25%, 15%, and 10% to 15% of cancers, respectively. Less commonly, amplifications can be seen in IGFR1, FGFR1, FGFR2, and MET. Additionally, amplifications in VEGFA are seen in 10% to 20% of EACs. Loss of cell-cycle regulation occurs through inactivation of CDKN2A in 75% of cases and amplifications of CCNE1, CCND1, and CDK6, all of which occur in 10% to 30% of EACs, with CCND1 reported to be the most commonly amplified.[16] The majority of CDKN2A inactivation in EAC occurs through promotor methylation and less commonly through deletions or mutations. The transcription factors GATA4 and GATA6, which both have a role in cellular differentiation and development, are amplified in approximately 20% of EACs each and usually (but not always) are mutually exclusive. Although not as common as in ESCC, loss of function alterations in genes involved in chromatin remodeling can be seen in EAC. The most commonly altered genes include SMARCA4 and ARID1A, both of which are altered in approximately 10% of cases. Deletions and loss of function mutations in SMAD4 and SMAD2, which are mediators of TGF-β signaling, are seen in approximately 25% of EACs. MYC amplifications can be seen in 20% to 30% of these cancers. Loss of normal TP53 function has been proposed to play a vital role in EAC progression and can be seen in approximately 75% of EACs with MDM2 amplifications seen in some of the TP53 wild-type cancers.[17]

EACs typically emerge from premalignant lesions within the lower esophagus, termed BE. BE, which is the replacement of the normally squamous lined esophagus with columnar epithelial cells that develop intestinal differentiation, is thought to form in response to injury induced by chronic bile and acid reflux and the resultant inflammation. The prevalence of BE is thought to be much higher than EAC and has been estimated to exist in 1% to 10% of adults in the United States.[18] The vast majority of those with BE never progresses to cancer, complicating the understanding of BE progression to EAC. In order to understand this process, several groups have either studied paired genomic profiles of EAC and adjacent BE or BE samples with known long-term follow-up to characterize the evolution of cancer from precursor lesions. These studies have identified that TP53 inactivation is a common early event that can occur in nondysplastic BE. This is followed by the development of aneuploidy, often including development of genome doubling.[17,19–25] Transformation of dysplastic lesions to EAC is thought to occur via acquisition of high-level focal amplifications of oncogenes (as described previously), often in the context of complex genomic disruptions.[17,26,27]

GASTRIC ADENOCARCINOMA

Gastric cancer is one of the world's leading causes of cancer mortality, with an estimated 783,000 deaths in 2018.[28,29] Similar to esophageal cancer, the incidence is highly variable according to geographic region. Most cases of gastric cancer are associated with Helicobacter pylori or Epstein-Barr virus (EBV) infection and a small subset are associated with germline mutations in CDH1 (E-cadherin) or mismatch repair genes (Lynch syndrome).[30,31] Gastric adenocarcinomas traditionally are classified by histology. The Lauren classification divides gastric cancer into diffuse and intestinal types whereas the World Health Organization uses papillary, tubular, mucinous, and poorly cohesive.[32,33] Recent comprehensive molecular characterization has suggested, however, a classification system based on genomic and methylation differences. TCGA Research Network gastric cancer study, suggests gastric cancers should be categorized in 4 molecular subtypes (Table 1).[2] Although more work needs to be done to better correlate the molecular findings with clinical parameters, these molecular subtypes provide more insight into the biology of the tumor and give some suggestions for targeted therapies. The first molecular subtype includes gastric cancers that are EBV positive. These tumors tend to have extensive DNA methylation of gene promotors and low overall mutation and copy number alteration rates and often are found in the gastric body or fundus. EBV-positive gastric adenocarcinomas almost always have CDKN2A promotor methylation and have high rates of PIK3CA and ARID1A mutations and low rates of TP53 mutations. Amplifications involving CD274 (programmed death ligand [PD-L] 1 protein), JAK2, and ERBB2 can be seen in approximately 15%, 12%, and 12% of EBV-positive gastric cancers, respectively. The second molecular subtype of gastric cancers are the microsatellite instability (MSI) gastric cancers. These cancers are characterized by hypermethylation with methylation of (and thus inactivation of) the MLH1 gene promotor. This leads to defective mismatch repair and highly elevated mutation rates. Prominent alterations in MSI gastric cancers include mutations in PIK3CA, ERBB3, KRAS, NRAS, PTEN, and RASA1. High-level amplifications are rare in MSI gastric cancers but occasionally are found involving PIK3CA. The third molecular subtype of gastric cancer is the genomically stable subgroup. These gastric cancers are EBV-negative and microsatellite stable with a low level of copy number alterations. This subgroup is enriched for the diffuse-type gastric cancers in the Lauren classification. As such, frequent alterations in CDH1 can be found. Other commonly altered genes include ARID1A and RHOA. Although copy number alterations are rare, activating amplifications or mutations in FGFR2, ERBB2, KRAS, NRAS, and PIK3CA can be seen in 5% to 10% of cancers for each gene. The fourth molecular subtype is the chromosomal instability (CIN) subtype that is characterized by a

Table 1
Molecular classification of gastric adenocarcinomas

Subgroup	Defining Characteristic	Methylation Status	Mutation Rates	Copy Number Variant Rates	Associations
EBV positive	High EBV burden	Extensive DNA promotor methylation (CIMP)	Low to moderate	Low to moderate	Enriched in gastric fundus and body
MSI	Microsatellite unstable	Hypermethylation with methylation of *MLH1* promotor	High	Low to moderate	Loss of mismatch repair through mutation (Lynch syndrome) or MLH1 promotor methylation
Genomically stable	Low degree of genomic complexity	Variable (moderate)	Low	Low	Enriched for diffuse-type cancers
CIN	High degree of genomic complexity	Variable (moderate)	Moderate	High	Enriched in proximal stomach

Abbreviations: CIMP, CpG island methylator phenotype.

high degree of copy number changes. This subtype is found more commonly in the proximal stomach and is very similar to EACs. Like EAC, the CIN gastric cancers have frequent *TP53* mutations, amplifications in the RTK/RAS pathway (*ERBB2*, *EGFR*, *FGFR2*, *ERBB3*, *MET*, *KRAS*, and *NRAS*) and in cell-cycle mediators (*CCNE1*, *CCND1*, and *CDK6*). Loss-of-function mutations in the β-catenin pathway (*APC* and *CTNNB1*) also can be seen.

Two different forms of metaplasia have been described in the stomach. The first, gastric intestinal metaplasia, is histologically similar to BE. In one study, genomic and methylation–based profiling of gastric intestinal metaplasia showed that it harbored several recurrent genomic alterations and methylation patterns different than normal gastric epithelium.[34] This study, which looked at a mix of metaplasia from patients with regressive/stable disease and a lower number of patients in which the metaplasia progressed to high-grade dysplasia or cancer, found an overall lower mutational and copy number burden compared with gastric adenocarcinomas. Despite this, recurrent hot spot mutations in *FBXW7* and rarer mutations in *TP53* and *ARID1A* still were identified. In addition, copy number gains of 8q involving the oncogene *MYC* were seen. When metaplasia from patients who progressed were compared with those who did not progress, a trend for increased numbers of mutations, copy number alterations, and shorter telomeres was seen in the intestinal metaplasia from progressors.

The second type of metaplasia is termed, spasmolytic polypeptide–expressing metaplasia (SPEM) or pseudopyloric metaplasia. The exact relationship of gastric intestinal metaplasia and SPEM to each other and to gastric cancers is controversial and an area of ongoing research. Few studies have looked at the genomic landscape of SPEM; however, Srivastava and colleagues performed paired targeted sequencing on a small number of gastric cancer patients who had concurrent intestinal metaplasia and SPEM.[35] In this study, they found SPEM to have a much lower number of mutations compared with the paired intestinal-type gastric adenocarcinomas whereas the regions of intestinal metaplasia had similar numbers of mutations as the cancers. Further studies are needed to better delineate the genomic progression of gastric precancerous lesions to the different subtypes of gastric cancer.

INTRATUMORAL GENOMIC HETEROGENEITY IN ESOPHAGEAL AND GASTRIC ADENOCARCINOMA

As described previously, both esophageal and CIN-type gastric adenocarcinoma develop from preneoplastic lesions where early *TP53* mutations are common. This is followed by the development of aneuploidy and significant disruption of normal chromosomes. It is through this process that most of these cancers get their source of oncogenic signaling, namely development of high-level amplifications of oncogenes late in the progression process. This is in contrast to gastrointestinal adenocarcinomas of other sites where activating mutations in important oncogenes occur relatively early in the progression process. For example, *KRAS* mutations in colon or pancreatic adenocarcinoma. This highly unstable state seen in esophageal and CIN-type gastric adenocarcinoma can lead to significant heterogeneity within the late preneoplastic lesion and the invasive cancer. Several recent studies have looked at multiregion primary and metastatic tumor sequencing and found a high degree of heterogeneity.[24,36] This heterogeneity potentially includes targetable oncogenic drivers. Pectasides and colleagues[24] found that between paired primary and metastatic samples nearly half of patients had discrepant pathogenic alterations. When they looked at samples with activating alterations in RTKs, a major focus of targeted therapy, more than half of patients had discrepant results between samples depending on the cohort utilized. This heterogeneity in important driver genes may be a major source for failure of precision medicine/targeted therapy in these diseases and points toward the need of careful sample selection for clinical testing. There is some suggestion that sequencing of plasma circulating tumor DNA may be a better predictor of response to targeted therapy.[24,37]

PRECISION MEDICINE IN UPPER GASTROINTESTINAL CANCERS

As understanding of the molecular mechanisms underpinning upper gastrointestinal cancers has improved, new more efficacious and better tolerated targeted therapies, including immunotherapeutics have advanced the landscape of treatment beyond cytotoxic chemotherapy, summarized in **Table 2**. To date, however, many of these therapies have shown only modest success. Therefore, improved understanding of the genomic heterogeneity and other mechanisms of resistance will be vitally important to further improve treatment strategies. These novel treatments and how they are tailored based on patient histology, anatomic location, and pathologic biomarkers are discussed.

The emergence of genomics and its clinical accessibility has changed the way cancer treatment is approached. Molecular characteristics of the cancer now are just as important in clinical oncology decision making as cancer anatomic location and histology. Specifically, for gastroesophageal cancers, detailed sequencing studies have revealed shared subtypes with common molecular pathogenesis.[1,2] Growth factor signaling pathway activation is a shared trait for the most prevalent CIN subtype of gastroesophageal cancer. Thus, targeting these signaling cascades has translated well clinically. The human epidermal growth factor receptor 2 (HER2/*ERBB2*) is overexpressed or amplified in 10% to 30% of gastroesophageal cancers.[47] The landmark ToGA trial examined the efficacy of targeting this pathway using trastuzumab, a monoclonal antibody against HER2, for HER2-positive (ie, 3+ staining on immunohistochemistry [IHC] or [fluorescence in situ hybridization positive]) gastroesophageal junction and stomach adenocarcinomas.[38] Although no esophageal cancer patients were included in this study, these results are applied to advanced esophageal cancer patients due to molecular similarities between gastric adenocarcinoma and EAC, and similar rates of HER2 positivity.[48] Addition of trastuzumab to chemotherapy in the first-line treatment setting significantly improved survival metrics and has now become standard-of-care treatment of HER2-positive patients.

In the second-line treatment setting, targeting the vascular endothelial growth factor (VEGF) signaling pathway has proved clinically efficacious. In particular, ramucirumab, a monoclonal antibody blocking human VEGF receptor 2 (*VEGFR2*) has been shown superior to single-agent chemotherapy in two large phase III clinical trials.[40,41] The first trial, REGARD, showed that monotherapy with ramucirumab was superior to placebo in the second-line setting for gastric or gastroesophageal junction adenocarcinomas.[40] The RAINBOW trial also showed clinical improvements with the addition of ramucirumab to single-agent paclitaxel chemotherapy in the second-line setting for gastric or gastroesophageal junction adenocarcinomas.[41] Again, as discussed previously, these results have been extrapolated to EACs given their similarities to gastric and gastroesophageal junction adenocarcinomas. Unlike trastuzumab, ramucirumab is approved to be used in gastroesophageal adenocarcinoma patient without an *a priori* biomarker test.

Currently, these 2 agents are the only targeted agents approved for advanced gastroesophageal cancers. Multiple other pathways have been examined but have not proved clinically efficacious.[49] Much work remains to not only develop better pathway targeting agents but also elucidate new ways to predict and select patients that most likely would benefit from these treatments. One new agent that recently has gained Food and Drug Administration (FDA) breakthrough therapy

Table 2
Approved targeted therapies for gastroesophageal cancer

Targeted Agent	Mechanism of Action	Biomarker	Clinical Trial	Histology	Line of Therapy	Anatomic Location	Efficacy
Trastuzumab (Herceptin)	Monoclonal antibody against human epidermal growth factor receptor 2 (HER2/ERBB2)	HER2-positive tumors (3+ staining on IHC or FISH positive)	ToGA[38]	Adenocarcinoma	First	Gastroesophageal junction and stomach	Improved survival
Fam-trastuzumab Deruxtecan (Enhertu)	Antibody drug conjugate targeting human epidermal growth factor receptor 2 (HER2/ERBB2)	HER2-positive tumors (3+ staining on IHC or 2+ staining on IHC and FISH positive)	DESTINY-Gastric01[39]	Adenocarcinoma	Third	Gastroesophageal junction and stomach	Improved survival
Ramucirumab (Cyramza)	Monoclonal antibody against human VEGFR2	None	REGARD[40]	Adenocarcinoma	Second	Gastroesophageal junction and stomach	Improved survival
			RAINBOW[41]	Adenocarcinoma	Second	Gastroesophageal junction and stomach	Improved survival

Drug	Mechanism	Biomarker	Trial	Histology	Line	Location	Outcome
Pembrolizumab (Keytruda)	Monoclonal antibody against PD-1 receptor	PD-L1 positive tumors (CPS 1 or higher)	KEYNOTE-061[42]	Adenocarcinoma (79%), tubular adenocarcinoma (10%), signet ring cell carcinoma (4%)	Third	Gastroesophageal junction and stomach	Did not improve survival in the second-line setting but better adverse event profile compared with paclitaxel monotherapy
		PD-L1 positive tumors (CPS 10 or higher)	KEYNOTE-181[43]	Squamous cell carcinoma and adenocarcinoma	Second (FDA approved only for squamous cell carcinoma histology in the second-line setting)	Esophagus and Siewert type 1 gastroesophageal junction	Improved survival
		MSI-HIGH tumors	KEYNOTE-061[42]	Adenocarcinoma (79%), tubular adenocarcinoma (10%), signet ring cell carcinoma (4%)	Second	Gastroesophageal junction and stomach	Improved survival
			KEYNOTE-158[44]	Any solid tumor	Second	Any solid tumor	Improved survival
		Tumor mutational burden (at least 10 mutations per megabase)	KEYNOTE-158[45]	Any solid tumor	Second	Any solid tumor	Improved survival
Nivolumab (Optivo)	Monoclonal antibody against PD-1 receptor	None	ATTRACTION-3[46]	Squamous cell carcinoma	Second	Esophagus	Improved survival

designation is Fam-trastuzumab deruxtecan, a HER2 antibody-drug conjugate that was shown to have clinical activity in a cohort of heavily pre-treated HER2-positive gastric/gastroesophageal junction adenocarcinoma patients.[39] This promising new agent demonstrates the potential of targeted agents to not only improve survival but also incur fewer treatment related toxicities compared with cytotoxic chemotherapies.

Given the chronic injurious nature that spurs formation of gastroesophageal cancers[50,51] (ie, smoking for ESCCs, acid reflux for EACs, and *Helicobacter pylori* infection for gastric adenocarcinomas), it is not surprising that these entities have been found to accumulate somatic mutations.[52] These genomic changes likely result in neoantigens, which ultimately are targeted by the immune system through cancer immunosurveillence.[53] Thus, immunotherapy and specifically targeting programmed death-1 (PD-1) receptor to block immunosuppressing ligands (PD-L1 and PDL-2) have resulted in new approved therapies for gastroesophageal cancer patients. The first agent, pembrolizumab, is approved in the United States to be used in concert with a combined positive score (CPS)[54] designed to preferentially select patients with higher PD-L1 levels and a higher probability of response. Specifically, for gastroesophageal adenocarcinomas, pembrolizumab is approved to be used for CPS score of 1 or higher in the third-line treatment setting based on results from KEYNOTE-061 study[42] showing no significant clinical efficacy for these patients as second-line therapy. Pembrolizumab also is approved to be used after progression on one or more prior treatments (ie, second-line treatment) for ESCCs that expresses high PD-L1 levels (CPS ≥10) based on the KEYNOTE-181 study.[43] In addition, pembrolizumab is approved to be used for tumor histology agnostic treatment of any solid tumor with defective mismatch repair (MSI-high) or high tumor mutation burden (≥10 mut/Mb).[42,44,45] A second immunotherapy with a similar mechanism of action, nivolumab, is approved in the United States in the second line to treat ESCCs regardless of PD-L1 levels based on results of the ATTRACTION-3 trial.[46] These immunotherapy treatments have not only provided new safer avenues to treat gastroesophageal cancer patients but also have changed the basic approaches to cancer treatment. Multiple trials have recently completed or are ongoing to investigate the efficacy of these agents as part of combination systemic therapy. The promise of immunotherapy is evidenced by multiple recent FDA approvals. In the metastatic setting, immunotherapy is now approved for use in combination with frontline chemotherapy based on results of

the CheckMate 649 [PMID: 34102137], ATTRACTION-4 [PMID: 30566590], and KEYNOTE-590 [PMID: 30735435] trials. In fact, the use of immunotherapy is now also favored in HER-2 positive patients [PMID: 33167735]. Furthermore, in the adjuvant setting after curative intent tri-modality therapy, immunotherapy has been approved based on the CheckMate 577 data [PMID: 33789008].

This article details examples of how understanding the molecular pathology of gastroesophageal cancers can have a direct impact on patient care. The complexity and heterogeneity of all cancers, including gastroesophageal cancers, mandate personalization of oncologic treatment. One-size-fits-all chemotherapy no longer is the ideal treatment of many of these patients. Elucidating the underlying pathogenesis of these diseases has resulted in and will continue to lead to important advancements in cancer diagnosis, prognosis, and individualized treatments.

CLINICS CARE POINTS

- ESCC and EAC are separate entities with differing molecular pathology.

- Gastric adenocarcinomas can be classified into 4 distinct molecular subtypes that may suggest treatments unique to the subtypes.

- EAC and CIN-type gastric adenocarcinoma are driven by a high degree of CIN and high-level amplifications of oncogenes, which leads to significant intratumor heterogeneity. This heterogeneity can lead to the wrong treatment being assigned if not testing the lesion that is wanted to treat.

- Targeted therapy in upper gastroesophageal cancers is an active area of research and is evolving rapidly.

DISCLOSURE

Dr. Stachler: NIH National Institute of Diabetes and Digestive and Kidney Diseases (K08 K08DK109209) and Doris Duke Charitable Foundation. Dr. Jin: NIH National Heart, Lung, and Blood Institute (T32HL007088), and the Barrett's Esophagus Translational Research Network (NCI U54CA163060).

REFERENCES

1. Cancer Genome Atlas Research Network, Analysis Working Group, Asan University, BC Cancer Agency, et al. Integrated genomic characterization of oesophageal carcinoma. Nature 2017;541(7636):169–75.
2. Bass AJ, Thorsson V, Shmulevich I, et al. Comprehensive molecular characterization of gastric adenocarcinoma. Nature 2014;513(7517):202–9.
3. Hayakawa Y, Sethi N, Sepulveda AR, et al. Oesophageal adenocarcinoma and gastric cancer: should we mind the gap? Nat Publ Gr 2016;16. https://doi.org/10.1038/nrc.2016.24.
4. Siegel RL, Miller KD, Fuchs HE, et al. Cancer statistics, 2021. CA Cancer J Clin 2021;71:7–33.
5. Amin M. American Joint Committee on Cancer., American Cancer Society.: AJCC Cancer Staging Manual. 8th edition. Chicago, IL: Springer Healthcare; 2017, editor-in-chief, MB. Amin, MD, FCAP ; editors, SB. Edge, MD, FACS and 16 others ; Donna M. Gress, RHIT, CTR - Technical editor ; Laura R. Meyer C-M editor., ed.
6. Abnet CC, Arnold M, Wei W-Q. Epidemiology of Esophageal Squamous Cell Carcinoma. Gastroenterology 2018;154(2):360–73.
7. Gao Y-B, Chen Z-L, Li J-G, et al. Genetic landscape of esophageal squamous cell carcinoma. Nat Genet 2014;46(10):1097–102.
8. Lin D-C, Hao J-J, Nagata Y, et al. Genomic and molecular characterization of esophageal squamous cell carcinoma. Nat Genet 2014;46(5):467–73.
9. Liu X, Zhang M, Ying S, et al. Genetic Alterations in Esophageal Tissues From Squamous Dysplasia to Carcinoma. Gastroenterology 2017;153(1):166–77.
10. Chen XX, Zhong Q, Liu Y, et al. Genomic comparison of esophageal squamous cell carcinoma and its precursor lesions by multi-region whole-exome sequencing. Nat Commun 2017;8(1). https://doi.org/10.1038/s41467-017-00650-0.
11. Devesa SS, Blot WJ, Fraumeni JF. Changing patterns in the incidence of esophageal and gastric carcinoma in the United States. Cancer 1998; 83(10):2049–53. Available at: http://www.ncbi.nlm.nih.gov/pubmed/9827707.
12. Brown LM, Devesa SS, Chow W-H. Incidence of adenocarcinoma of the esophagus among white Americans by sex, stage, and age. J Natl Cancer Inst 2008;100(16):1184–7.
13. Pohl H, Welch HG. The role of overdiagnosis and reclassification in the marked increase of esophageal adenocarcinoma incidence. J Natl Cancer Inst 2005;97(2):142–6.
14. McColl KEL. What is causing the rising incidence of esophageal adenocarcinoma in the West and will it also happen in the East? J Gastroenterol 2019; 54(8):669–73.
15. Secrier M, Li X, de Silva N, et al. Mutational signatures in esophageal adenocarcinoma define etiologically distinct subgroups with therapeutic relevance. Nat Genet 2016. https://doi.org/10.1038/ng.3659.
16. Liu Y, Sethi NS, Hinoue T, et al. Comparative Molecular Analysis of Gastrointestinal Adenocarcinomas. Cancer Cell 2018;33(4):721–35.e8.
17. Stachler MD, Taylor-Weiner A, Peng S, et al. Paired exome analysis of Barrett's esophagus and adenocarcinoma. Nat Genet 2015;47(9). https://doi.org/10.1038/ng.3343.
18. Ormsby AH, Kilgore SP, Goldblum JR. The Location and Frequency of Intestinal Metaplasia at the Esophagogastric Junction in 223 Consecutive Autopsies : Implications for Patient Treatment and Preventive Strategies in Barrett ' s Esophagus. Mod Pathol 2000;6(13):614–20.
19. Gu J, Ajani J a, Hawk ET, et al. Genome-wide catalogue of chromosomal aberrations in barrett's esophagus and esophageal adenocarcinoma: a high-density single nucleotide polymorphism array analysis. Cancer Prev Res (Phila) 2010;3(9): 1176–86.
20. Li X, Galipeau PC, Paulson TG, et al. Temporal and Spatial Evolution of Somatic Chromosomal Alterations: A Case-Cohort Study of Barrett's Esophagus. Cancer Prev Res 2014;7(1):114–27.
21. Li X, Galipeau PC, Sanchez CA, et al. Single nucleotide polymorphism-based genome-wide chromosome copy change, loss of heterozygosity, and aneuploidy in Barrett's esophagus neoplastic progression. Cancer Prev Res 2008; 1(6):413–23.
22. Weaver JMJ, Ross-Innes CS, Shannon N, et al. Ordering of mutations in preinvasive disease stages of esophageal carcinogenesis. Nat Genet 2014; 46(8):837–43.
23. Contino G, Vaughan TL, Whiteman D, et al. The Evolving Genomic Landscape of Barrett's Esophagus and Esophageal Adenocarcinoma. Gastroenterology 2017;153(3):657–73.e1.
24. Pectasides E, Stachler MD, Derks S, et al. Genomic heterogeneity as a barrier to precision medicine in gastroesophageal adenocarcinoma. Cancer Discov 2018;8(1). https://doi.org/10.1158/2159-8290.CD-17-0395.
25. Stachler MD, Camarda ND, Deitrick C, et al. Detection of Mutations in Barrett's Esophagus Before Progression to High-Grade Dysplasia or Adenocarcinoma. Gastroenterology 2018;155(1): 156–67.
26. Dulak AM, Stojanov P, Peng S, et al. Exome and whole genome sequencing of esophageal adenocarcinoma identifies recurrent driver events and mutational complexity. Nat Genet 2013;45(5): 1–21.

27. Dulak AM, Schumacher SE, van Lieshout J, et al. Gastrointestinal adenocarcinomas of the esophagus, stomach, and colon exhibit distinct patterns of genome instability and oncogenesis. Cancer Res 2012;72(17):4383–93.

28. Rawla P, Barsouk A. Epidemiology of gastric cancer: global trends, risk factors and prevention. Prz Gastroenterol 2019;14(1):26–38.

29. Bray F, Ferlay J, Soerjomataram I, et al. Global cancer statistics 2018: GLOBOCAN estimates of incidence and mortality worldwide for 36 cancers in 185 countries. CA Cancer J Clin 2018;68(6): 394–424.

30. Richards FM, McKee SA, Rajpar MH, et al. Germline E-cadherin gene (CDH1) mutations predispose to familial gastric cancer and colorectal cancer. Hum Mol Genet 1999;8(4):607–10.

31. Keller G, Grimm V, Vogelsang H, et al. Analysis for microsatellite instability and mutations of the DNA mismatch repair gene hMLH1 in familial gastric cancer. Int J Cancer 1996;68(5):571–6.

32. Fléjou J-F. [WHO Classification of digestive tumors: the fourth edition]. Ann Pathol 2011;31(5 Suppl): S27–31.

33. Lauren p. The two histological main types of gastric carcinoma: diffuse and so-called intestinal-type carcinoma. An attempt at a histo-clinical classification. Acta Pathol Microbiol Scand 1965; 64:31–49.

34. Huang KK, Ramnarayanan K, Zhu F, et al. Genomic and Epigenomic Profiling of High-Risk Intestinal Metaplasia Reveals Molecular Determinants of Progression to Gastric Cancer. Cancer Cell 2018; 33(1):137–50.e5.

35. Srivastava S, Huang KK, Rebbani K, et al. An LCM-based genomic analysis of SPEM, Gastric Cancer and Pyloric Gland Adenoma in an Asian cohort. Mod Pathol 2020;33(10):2075–86.

36. Lee HH, Kim SY, Jung ES, et al. Mutation heterogeneity between primary gastric cancers and their matched lymph node metastases. Gastric Cancer 2019;22(2):323–34.

37. Maron SB, Chase LM, Lomnicki S, et al. Circulating Tumor DNA Sequencing Analysis of Gastroesophageal Adenocarcinoma. Clin Cancer Res 2019; 25(23):7098–112.

38. Bang YJ, Van Cutsem E, Feyereislova A, et al. Trastuzumab in combination with chemotherapy versus chemotherapy alone for treatment of HER2-positive advanced gastric or gastro-oesophageal junction cancer (ToGA): a phase 3, open-label, randomised controlled trial. Lancet 2010;376:687–97.

39. Shitara K, Bang YJ, Iwasa S, et al. Trastuzumab Deruxtecan in Previously Treated HER2-Positive Gastric Cancer. N Engl J Med 2020;382:2419–30.

40. Fuchs CS, Tomasek J, Yong CJ, et al. Ramucirumab monotherapy for previously treated advanced gastric or gastro-oesophageal junction adenocarcinoma (REGARD): an international, randomised, multicentre, placebo-controlled, phase 3 trial. Lancet 2014;383:31–9.

41. Wilke H, Muro K, Van Cutsem E, et al. Ramucirumab plus paclitaxel versus placebo plus paclitaxel in patients with previously treated advanced gastric or gastro-oesophageal junction adenocarcinoma (RAINBOW): a double-blind, randomised phase 3 trial. Lancet Oncol 2014;15:1224–35.

42. Shitara K, Ozguroglu M, Bang YJ, et al. Pembrolizumab versus paclitaxel for previously treated, advanced gastric or gastro-oesophageal junction cancer (KEYNOTE-061): a randomised, open-label, controlled, phase 3 trial. Lancet 2018;392: 123–33.

43. Kojima T, Shah MA, Muro K, et al. Randomized Phase III KEYNOTE-181 Study of Pembrolizumab Versus Chemotherapy in Advanced Esophageal Cancer. J Clin Oncol 2020;38(35):4138–48.

44. Marabelle A, Le DT, Ascierto PA, et al. Efficacy of pembrolizumab in patients with noncolorectal high microsatellite instability/mismatch repair-deficient cancer: results from the phase II KEYNOTE-158 Study. J Clin Oncol 2020;38:1–10.

45. Marabelle A, Fakih M, Lopez J, et al. Association of tumour mutational burden with outcomes in patients with advanced solid tumours treated with pembrolizumab: prospective biomarker analysis of the multicohort, open-label, phase 2 KEYNOTE-158 study. Lancet Oncol 2020;21:1353–65.

46. Kato K, Cho BC, Takahashi M, et al. Nivolumab versus chemotherapy in patients with advanced oesophageal squamous cell carcinoma refractory or intolerant to previous chemotherapy (ATTRACTION-3): a multicentre, randomised, open-label, phase 3 trial. Lancet Oncol 2019;20:1506–17.

47. Gravalos C, Jimeno A. HER2 in gastric cancer: a new prognostic factor and a novel therapeutic target. Ann Oncol 2008;19:1523–9.

48. Yoon HH, Shi Q, Sukov WR, et al. Association of HER2/ErbB2 expression and gene amplification with pathologic features and prognosis in esophageal adenocarcinomas. Clin Cancer Res 2012;18: 546–54.

49. Samson P, Lockhart AC. Biologic therapy in esophageal and gastric malignancies: current therapies and future directions. J Gastrointest Oncol 2017;8: 418–29.

50. in RU, Mills JC. Are gastric and esophageal metaplasia relatives? The case for barrett's stemming from SPEM. Dig Dis Sci 2018;63:2028–41.

51. Jin RU, Mills JC. The cyclical hit model: how paligenosis might establish the mutational landscape in Barrett's esophagus and esophageal adenocarcinoma. Curr Opin Gastroenterol 2019;35(4): 363–70.

52. Martincorena I, Campbell PJ. Somatic mutation in cancer and normal cells. Science 2015;349: 1483–9.

53. Waldman AD, Fritz JM, Lenardo MJ. A guide to cancer immunotherapy: from T cell basic science to clinical practice. Nat Rev Immunol 2020;20(11):651–68.

54. Kulangara K, Zhang N, Corigliano E, et al. Clinical utility of the combined positive score for programmed death ligand-1 expression and the approval of pembrolizumab for treatment of gastric cancer. Arch Pathol Lab Med 2019;143: 330–7.

Molecular Pathology of Breast Tumors
Diagnostic and Actionable Genetic Alterations

Dara S. Ross, MD*, Fresia Pareja, MD, PhD

KEYWORDS

- Breast cancer • Biomarkers • Estrogen receptor • HER2 • Mutation profiling • Resistance
- Mechanisms of resistance

Key points

- Pioneering gene expression studies and next-generation sequencing have revealed several intrinsic subtypes and various molecular profiles of invasive breast cancer, paving the way for personalized medical treatment.

- Few special histologic subtypes of breast tumors harbor pathognomonic or disease defining genetic alterations, many of which have the potential to be used diagnostically.

- The identification of genetic alterations and subsequent dysregulation of signaling pathways in breast cancer have led to the identification of actionable therapeutic targets, including *ERBB2* amplification, neurotrophic receptor tyrosine kinase (*NTRK*) fusions, and *PIK3CA* mutations.

- Somatic alterations identified in metastatic breast cancer associated with resistance to endocrine therapy include *ESR1* and *ERBB2* activating mutations, *NF1* loss-of-function genetic alterations, and alterations in other MAPK pathway genes and estrogen receptor transcriptional regulators.

- Exploration of new therapeutic options is ongoing.

Breast cancer is a heterogenous disease with various histologic subtypes, molecular profiles, behaviors, and response to therapy. After the histologic assessment and diagnosis of an invasive breast carcinoma, the use of biomarkers, multigene expression assays and mutation profiling may be used. With improved molecular assays, the identification of somatic genetic alterations in key oncogenes and tumor suppressor genes are playing an increasingly important role in many areas of breast cancer care. This review summarizes the most clinically significant somatic alterations in breast tumors and how this information is used to facilitate diagnosis, provide potential treatment options, and identify mechanisms of resistance.

OVERVIEW

Breast cancer is one of the leading causes of cancer-related death in women worldwide. In the United States alone 276,480 new cases of invasive breast cancer and 42,170 deaths are estimated in women for 2020.[1] Because invasive breast cancer is a biologically and clinically heterogeneous disease, the use of biomarker testing after histologic evaluation and diagnosis, including immunohistochemistry (IHC), fluorescence or bright field in situ hybridization, multigene expression assays, and mutation profiling, can help to further characterize tumors and identify targeted therapies. Biomarkers can be predictive (associated with whether a patient will respond to a given therapy), prognostic (associated with a patient's overall

Funding: F.P. is partially funded by a National Institutes of Health/National Cancer Institute K12 CA184746 grant and a National Institutes of Health/ National Cancer Institute P50 CA247749 01 grant.
Department of Pathology, Memorial Sloan Kettering Cancer Center, 1275 York Avenue, New York, NY 10065, USA
* Corresponding author.
E-mail address: rossd@mskcc.org

Surgical Pathology 14 (2021) 455–471
https://doi.org/10.1016/j.path.2021.05.009
1875-9181/21/© 2021 Elsevier Inc. All rights reserved.

clinical outcome) or both. Estrogen receptor (ER), progesterone receptor (PR), and human epidermal growth factor receptor 2 (HER2) are predictive biomarkers in breast cancer and the American Society of Clinical Oncology/College of American Pathologists guidelines recommend testing on every primary invasive breast cancer, recurrence, and metastasis to guide therapy.[2,3] Several companion diagnostic tests for the detection of HER2 amplification in particular are approved by the US Food and Drug Administration (FDA) for the safe and effective use of corresponding targeted therapies. Multigene expression assays provide prognostic and therapy-predictive information that complement breast cancer staging and the biomarker information described elsewhere in this article.

With the development of improved molecular profiling assays, the identification of "driver" and "actionable" somatic genetic alterations (ie, mutations, copy number alterations, insertions or deletions, and rearrangements) in key oncogenes and tumor suppressor genes now play an essential role in the diagnosis and treatment of many tumors, including breast cancer. Pioneering gene expression studies paved the way for personalized medical treatment with the identification of intrinsic molecular subtypes of breast cancer[4] and next-generation sequencing (NGS) has provided further categorization by demonstrating different molecular profiles for each group,[5] ultimately broadening our understanding of the disease and its heterogenous nature. Common approaches to NGS include whole-genome sequencing, whole-exome sequencing, targeted exome sequencing, and hotspot sequencing. In addition to NGS, alternate methods of detection for genomic alterations include single gene assays (SGA) such as Sanger sequencing, IHC, fluorescence in situ hybridization (FISH), and bright field in situ hybridization. This review provides a brief summary of the molecular classification of breast cancer and its application to clinical practice, in addition to an overview of the most clinically significant somatic genetic alterations in breast tumors at the present time, including how these alterations are detected and how this information can be used to facilitate histologic classification, provide targeted treatment options, and identify mechanisms of resistance.

MOLECULAR CLASSIFICATION OF BREAST CANCER

The heterogeneity of breast tumors was displayed classically with pioneering gene expression studies

that gave rise to the molecular classification of breast cancer into intrinsic subtypes, including luminal A and luminal B, which both predominantly express ER, basal like, which is mostly ER, PR, and HER2 negative, and HER2 enriched.[4,6] Notably, the molecular intrinsic subtypes showed concordance with classification based on the ER, PR, and HER2 IHC expression with the addition of Ki67 and basal cytokeratins.[7,8] Heterogeneity within each intrinsic subtype exists. For instance, even though most breast cancers classified as HER2 positive by IHC and/or FISH correspond with the HER2-enriched molecular subtype, a subset of them are classified into other intrinsic subtypes.[9] Upon subsequent examination, Lehmann and colleagues[10] put forward a triple-negative breast cancer (TNBC) molecular taxonomy that included 6 classes associated with enrichment in different gene networks, including (i) basal-like 1 (cell division and DNA damage response), (ii) basal-like 2 (growth factors), (iii) immunomodulatory (immune signaling), (iv) mesenchymal (epithelial to mesenchymal transition), (v) mesenchymal stem-like (mesenchymal stem cells), and (vi) luminal androgen receptor (AR) (luminal genes and AR). Importantly, the different TNBC molecular classes were found to differ at the genetic level[11] and possibly display different therapeutic vulnerabilities. For instance, luminal AR tumors display an enrichment in mutations typically identified in luminal tumors, including genes involved in the PI3K pathway,[11] indicating a potential benefit from pharmacologic inhibition reported by in vitro studies,[12] whereas the gene expression levels of PD-1 and PD-L1 were found to be increased in the immunomodulatory subtype compared with other TNBC, suggesting that these tumors might be sensitive to checkpoint inhibitors.[11] Further studies to refine the taxonomy of breast cancer and its incorporation in molecularly stratified clinical trials are ongoing.

KEY DIAGNOSTIC SOMATIC ALTERATIONS IN BREAST TUMORS

The heterogenous nature of breast cancer is quite evident histologically; although most breast cancers are classified as invasive ductal carcinoma of no special type or invasive lobular carcinoma (ILC), more than 20 other special histologic subtypes are recognized, which taken together make up to one-fifth of all breast tumors.[13] Recent studies on special histologic subtypes of breast cancer have revealed that a subset of them harbor pathognomonic or disease-defining genetic alterations, many of which

Table 1
Diagnostic somatic alterations in breast tumors

Gene	Alteration	Description	Detection Methods	Significance
CDH1	Truncating mutations, loss of heterozygosity, promoter hypermethylation	Located on 16q22, encodes E-cadherin, an intercellular adhesion protein	IHC, SGA, NGS	Diagnostic for lobular carcinoma
ETV6-NTRK3	Translocation	t(12;15) (p13;q25) leading to ETV6-NTRK3 gene fusion	FISH, NGS, pan-TRK IHC	Diagnostic for secretory carcinoma
MYB-NFIB MYBL1 MYB	Translocation Rearrangements Gene amplification	t(6;9) (q22–23;p23–24), leading to MYB-NF1B gene fusion. Gene fusions involving MYBL1 and MYB gene amplification	FISH, NGS, MYB IHC	Diagnostic for adenoid cystic carcinoma
IDH2	R172 hotspot mutations, co-occurring with mutations in genes of the PI3K-AKT pathway	Maps to 15q26.1 and encodes for a mitochondrial isocitrate dehydrogenase	IHC, SGA, NGS	Highly sensitive and specific for tall cell carcinomas with reversed polarity
HRAS	Q61 hotspot mutations, frequently coexisting with mutations in genes of the PI3K-AKT pathway	Located on 11p15.5, encodes for a GTPase	IHC, SGA, NGS	Moderately sensitive and highly specific for ER–negative adenomyoepitheliomas
HMGA2 or PLAG1	Rearrangements	Fusion genes involving HMGA2 (12q14.3; transcriptional regulator) or PLAG1 (8q12.1; transcription factor)	FISH, NGS	Diagnostic for pleomorphic adenomas of various anatomic locations, including breast
CRTC1-MAML2	Translocation	t(11;19) (q14–21; p12–13) resulting in the CRTC1-MAML2 gene fusion	FISH, NGS	Diagnostic of mucoepidermoid carcinomas in different anatomic locations, including breast

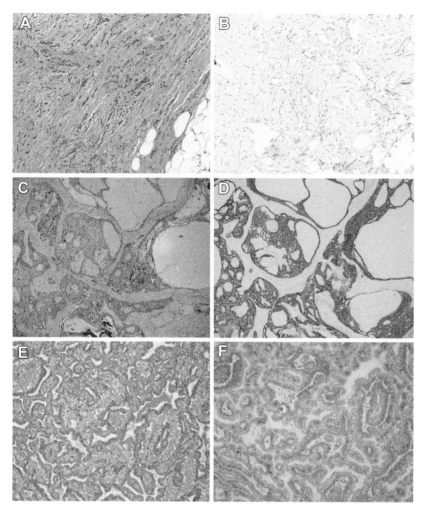

Fig. 1. Diagnostic alterations in breast tumors demonstrated by IHC. *A* and *B*, ILC. Hematoxylin and eosin (H&E) (*A*) and E-cadherin IHC stain (*B*) showing loss of membranous staining in the tumor. *C* and *D*, Adenomyoepithelioma. H&E (*C*) and IHC (*D*) showing positive staining for *RAS* Q61R mutation. *E* and *F*, tall cell carcinoma with reversed polarity. H&E (*E*) and IHC (*F*) showing positive staining for *IDH2* R172 mutation. E-cadherin IHC (clone 36, Ventana, Tucson, AZ), RAS Q61R IHC (clone SP174, Abcam, Cambridge, MA), IDH2 R172S IHC (clone 11C8B1, NewEast Biosciences, Malvern, PA).

have the potential to be used diagnostically[14] (**Table 1**).

CDH1 MUTATIONS IN INVASIVE LOBULAR CARCINOMA

ILC is the most frequent special histologic subtype of breast cancer, constituting approximately 15% of all cases.[13] The hallmark genetic alteration in ILC are mutations, and less frequently promoter hypermethylation, of *CDH1* which encodes E-cadherin, a cell–cell adhesion protein.[15,16] The cytoplasmic tail of E-cadherin is bound by different catenins and linked to the actin cytoskeleton.[17] Hence, *CDH1* functional inactivation, which is frequently associated with loss of heterozygosity of the wild-type allele,[15] results in the classic morphology of ILC characterized by a discohesive growth pattern.[13] Besides *CDH1* mutations, ILC shows an enrichment in mutations involving *TBX3, FOXA1, ERBB2, PIK3CA,* and *PTEN*.[15]

IHC assessment of E-cadherin is commonly used in the diagnostic workup of ILC and shows loss of membranous expression (**Figs. 1**A, B). Nonetheless, a subset of ILCs harboring *CDH1* inactivation might retain protein expression (ie, aberrant E-cadherin immunoreactivity),[18,19] indicating that, although E-cadherin IHC is diagnostic in most ILCs, it must be interpreted in conjunction with morphology. In addition, although not generally used for initial diagnostic purposes, *CDH1* alterations can also be assessed by SGA or NGS.

MYB GENETIC ALTERATIONS IN ADENOID CYSTIC CARCINOMAS

Breast adenoid cystic carcinomas (ACC) are rare tumors that are morphologically indistinguishable from those arising in the salivary glands and other anatomic locations.[13] These tumors are characterized by a tubular, cribriform, or trabecular architecture and composed of epithelial and myoepithelial cells.[13] Similar to ACC arising in other organs, most breast ACC harbor the *MYB–NFIB* gene fusion.[20,21] Less frequently, breast ACC harbor *MYB* gene amplification or gene fusions involving *MYBL1*,[22] supporting the notion that these tumors are underpinned by activation of the MYB signaling pathway. The identification of rearrangements involving *MYB* or *MYBL1* can be detected by FISH (**Fig. 2**A, B) or NGS, and *MYB* alterations can also be assessed by IHC, assisting in the diagnosis of this entity.

ETV6–NTRK3 GENE FUSION IN SECRETORY CARCINOMA

Secretory carcinomas are rare breast tumors associated with a favorable clinical outcome.[13] They display a distinctive histology characterized by microcystic, solid, and tubular growth patterns, cells with vacuolated cytoplasm, and intracellular and extracellular secretions.[13] Akin to the mammary analogue secretory carcinoma of the salivary gland, secretory carcinomas of the breast harbor the *ETV6–NTRK3* fusion,[23,24] which may be detected by FISH (see **Fig. 2**C, D), NGS, or IHC pan-TRK antibodies in a sensitive and specific manner.[25,26]

HRAS Q61 HOTSPOT MUTATIONS IN ADENOMYOEPITHELIOMAS

Breast adenomyoepitheliomas are biphasic epithelial and myoepithelial tumors that include a spectrum of lesions, ranging from benign to malignant with a propensity for recurrence or distant metastasis, and ER-positive and ER-negative cases.[13,27] The genetic makeup of adenomyoepitheliomas varies according to the ER status.[28] ER-positive adenomyoepitheliomas are characterized by recurrent mutations affecting *PIK3CA* or *AKT1*, whereas ER-negative tumors harbor recurrent *HRAS* Q61 hotspot mutations, frequently co-occurring with mutations in the PI3K–AKT pathway.[28] Given that *HRAS* Q61 hotspot mutations are otherwise extremely rare in breast tumors, their detection by NGS or SGA is a useful tool for the diagnosis of these tumors in the breast. *HRAS* Q61R mutations in particular may be also detected by IHC with moderate sensitivity and high specificity[29] (see **Fig. 1**C, D).

IDH2 R172 HOTSPOT MUTATIONS IN TALL CELL CARCINOMAS WITH REVERSED POLARITY

Tall cell carcinomas with reversed polarity are an exquisitely rare histologic subtype of breast cancer with a distinctive phenotype. These tumors display solid and papillary growth patterns with tall cells displaying reversed polarization. Tall cell carcinomas with reversed polarity are also called breast tumors resembling the tall cell variant of papillary thyroid carcinoma, given their nuclear grooves and clear nuclei.[30] Tall cell carcinomas with reversed polarity are characterized by *IDH2* mutations affecting the R172 hotspot, which were found to frequently coexist with mutations in PI3K–AKT pathway genes.[31–33] Although *IDH2* mutations have been reported in cancers arising in other organ systems, such as gliomas, sinonasal undifferentiated carcinomas, chondrosarcomas, and myeloproliferative neoplasms, they are specific to tall cell carcinomas with reversed polarity in the context of breast tumors.[31] Detection of the *IDH2* R172 hotspot mutation is possible not only by NGS or SGA, but also by IHC using mutation specific antibodies[34] (see **Fig. 1**E, F).

HMGA2 OR *PLAG1* REARRANGEMENTS IN PLEOMORPHIC ADENOMAS

Breast pleomorphic adenomas are morphologically indistinguishable from those arising in the salivary glands, featuring admixed epithelial and myoepithelial components intermixed with myxochondroid stroma.[35,36] Their diagnosis in the breast is challenging given their rare occurrence and overlapping morphologic features with metaplastic carcinoma.[35] The genetic underpinning of breast pleomorphic adenomas mirrors that of their salivary gland counterparts.[37] Indeed, *HMGA2–WIF1* and *CTNNB1–PLAG1* gene fusions have also been reported in breast pleomorphic adenomas.[37] Hence, the analysis of these rearrangements by FISH (see **Fig. 2**E, F) or NGS may be useful ancillary studies in the diagnostic workup of these rare breast tumors.

CRTC1–MAML2 GENE FUSION IN MUCOEPIDERMOID CARCINOMAS

Mucoepidermoid carcinomas are common salivary gland tumors that rarely arise in other anatomic sites, including the breast, but display characteristic histologic features regardless of their anatomic location.[35,38] Because breast mucoepidermoid carcinomas morphologically resemble their salivary gland counterparts, they are composed of a mixture of mucous-secreting cells, squamous cells, and intermediate cells.[39] Their diagnosis in the breast, however, poses significant challenges, because they display overlapping histologic features with other triple-negative entities, such as metaplastic squamous cell

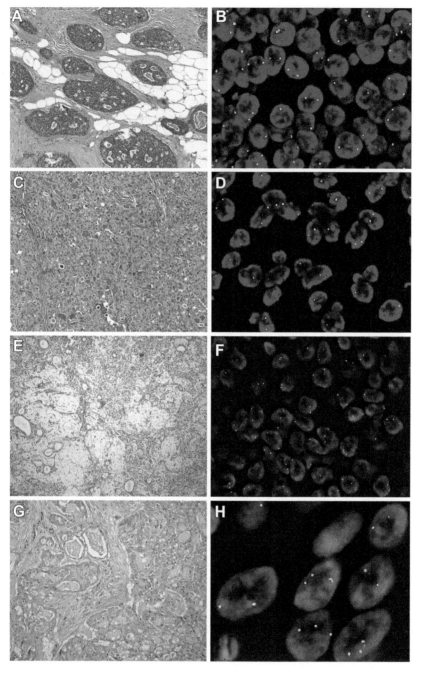

Fig. 2. Diagnostic alterations in breast tumors demonstrated by FISH. *A* and *B*, ACC. H&E [Original magnification x100] (*A*) and MYB dual color break apart FISH probe [Original magnification x1000] (*B*), with translocation affecting the 6q23.3 locus harboring the *MYB* gene, as indicated by one orange/green fusion (non-rearranged) signal, one orange signal, and one separate green signal. *C* and *D*, Secretory carcinoma. H&E [Original magnification x100] (*C*) and *NTRK3* break apart FISH probe [Original magnification x1000] (*D*) with translocation affecting the 15q25.3-q26.1 locus as indicated by one orange/green fusion (non-rearranged) signal, one orange signal, and one separate green signal. *E* and *F*, Pleomorphic adenoma. H&E [Original magnification x100] (*E*) and *PLAG1* dual color break apart FISH probe [Original magnification x1000] (*F*) with translocation affecting the 8q12.1 locus harboring the *PLAG1* gene, as indicated by one orange/green fusion (non-rearranged) signal, one orange signal, and one separate green signal. *G* and *H*, Mucoepidermoid carcinoma. H&E [Original magnification x200] (*G*) and CRTC1-MAML2 FISH fusion probe [Original magnification x1000] (*H*). H&E, hematoxylin and eosin. MYB breakapart probe, Zytovision nuc ish(MYBx2) (5′MYB sep 3′MYBx1). NTRK3 breakapart probe, Empire Genomics nuc ish(NTRK3x2) (3′NTRK3 sep 5′NTRK3x1). PLAG1 dual-color break-apart probes (red, 5′ PLAG1; green, 3′ PLAG1). CRTC1-MAML2 FISH fusion probe (red, 3′MAML2; orange 5′MAML2; green CRTC1).

carcinoma and secretory carcinoma.[13,40] Recently, the presence of the *CRTC1–MAML2* gene fusion,[41,42] the characteristic genetic alteration of mucodepidermoid carcinomas, has been reported in the breast.[37,40] Hence, the detection of the *CRTC1–MAML2* fusion by FISH (see **Fig. 2**G, H) or NGS might aid in distinguishing these exceedingly rare breast tumors.

KEY ACTIONABLE SOMATIC ALTERATIONS IN BREAST CANCER

Genetic alterations and subsequent dysregulation of signaling pathways involving hormones (ie, ER, PR, and AR), growth factors (ie, HER2 and FGFR1), cell cycle regulation (ie, cyclin D1, CDK4, CDK6, RB1, and TP53), PI3K/AKT/MTOR and RAS/RAF/MAPK underlie the pathogenesis of breast cancer. Various levels of evidence scales have emerged using information from the FDA, the National Comprehensive Cancer Network guidelines, clinical trials, and the literature to classify the genomic alterations in these signaling pathways according to their likelihood of being actionable therapeutic targets.[43–48] OncoKB in particular is a precision oncology knowledge base containing treatment information that is classified using the levels of evidence system that assigns clinical actionability to individual mutations. Potentially actionable alterations in a specific cancer type are assigned to 1 of 4 levels based on evidence that the mutation is a predictive biomarker to FDA-approved or investigational agents. Standard therapeutic implications include FDA-recognized biomarkers and standard care biomarkers that are predictive of response to an FDA-approved drug in a specific indication (levels 1 and 2A, respectively). Investigational therapeutic implications include FDA-approved biomarkers predictive of response to an FDA-approved drug detected in an off-label indication (level 2B), FDA- or non–FDA-recognized biomarkers that are predictive of response to novel targeted agents that have shown promising results in clinical trials (level 3A), and non–FDA-recognized biomarkers that are predictive of response to novel targeted agents on the basis of compelling biologic data (level 4).[48] For the purpose of this review, the most clinically relevant alterations in breast cancer at the present time are described and categorized according to the OncoKB designated levels of evidence for actionability (**Table 2**). In addition, the most significant clinical trial identifiers from ClinicalTrials.gov are referenced for each alteration.

US FOOD AND DRUG ADMINISTRATION–APPROVED AND NATIONAL COMPREHENSIVE CANCER NETWORK–RECOMMENDED BIOMARKERS

ERBB2 Amplification

HER2 is a transmembrane tyrosine kinase receptor encoded by the *ERBB2* gene. Approximately 20% to 30%[49,50] of all breast cancers are classified as HER2 positive as a result of *ERBB2* gene amplification and the subsequent overexpression of the HER2 protein on the tumor cell surface. Detection methods include IHC, which detects the expression of the HER2 protein, and FISH and bright field ISH, which both detect amplification of the *ERBB2* gene, and many assays are FDA-approved companion diagnostic tests.[51] The American Society of Clinical Oncology/College of American Pathologists have issued guidelines for the testing, interpretation, and reporting of HER2 IHC and HER2 ISH in breast cancer.[3] Given the advances in molecular diagnostics, NGS assays can also be used to provide data on HER2 copy number alterations.[52]

HER2 amplification in breast cancer serves as an independent prognostic factor associated with a shorter disease-free survival, but it is also predictive of response to HER2-directed therapy in the neoadjuvant, adjuvant, or metastatic settings.[3] Five drugs are FDA approved for the treatment of HER2-positive breast cancer, including the monoclonal antibodies trastuzumab and pertuzumab, the antibody–drug conjugate trastuzumab emtansine (T-DM1), and the tyrosine kinase inhibitors lapatinib and neratinib.[53] The joint analysis of overall survival from NSABP B-31 and NCCTG N9831 showed the addition of trastuzumab to chemotherapy (paclitaxel after doxorubicin and cyclophosphamide) in early stage HER2-positive breast cancer results in a substantial and durable improvement in survival owing to a sustained and marked decrease in cancer recurrence (NCT00045032, NCT00004067, NCT00 005970, NCT00021255).[54–57] Additional anti-HER2 agents have shown significant disease-free survival gains compared with 1 year of trastuzumab alone. The APHINITY study showed that the addition of pertuzumab to adjuvant trastuzumab and chemotherapy significantly improved the rates of invasive disease-free survival among patients with HER2-positive, operable breast cancer (NCT01358877).[58] For patients with residual HER2-positive disease after neoadjuvant therapy, the risk of recurrence of invasive breast cancer or death was 50% lower with the use of T-DM1 than with trastuzumab alone (NCT01772472).[59] Data from the phase III ExteNET study (NCT00878709) showed that extended adjuvant treatment with neratinib in early-stage, HER2-positive breast cancer after postoperative trastuzumab led to improved disease-free survival.[60]

NTRK Gene Fusions

The NTRK gene family is composed of 3 proto-oncogenes *NTRK1*, *NTRK2*, and *NTRK3*, which encode 3 membrane-bound kinase receptors,

Table 2
Actionable somatic genetic alterations in invasive breast cancer

Gene (Chromosome)	Protein Function	Type	Alteration		Detection Methods	OncoKB Level of Evidence	Targeted Therapy	Clinical Trials Identifier
			Most common	Frequency				
FDA-approved and/or NCCN recommended biomarker								
ERBB2/HER2 (17q12)	Transmembrane tyrosine kinase receptor	Amplification	N/A	20%–30%	IHC, FISH, bright-field ISH, NGS	1	Monoclonal antibodies: trastuzumab, pertuzumab Monoclonal antibody–drug conjugate: ado-trastuzumab emtansine Tyrosine kinase inhibitors: lapatinib, neratinib	NCT00045032 NCT00004067 NCT00005970 NCT00021255 NCT01358877 NCT01772472 NCT00878709 NCT02400476 NCT01808573
NTRK1 (1q23), *NTRK2* (9q21), *NTRK3* (15q25)	Membrane-bound tyrosine kinase receptors	Fusion	ETV6-NTRK3, LMNA-NTRK1	<1%	FISH, IHC NGS	1	Selective TRK inhibitors: larotrectinib entrectinib	NCT02122913 NCT02637687 NCT02576431
PIK3CA (3q26)	Catalytic subunit of PI3-kinase (p110α)	Activating mutation[a]	Exon 9, helical domain: E542K, E545K/A/Q, Exon 20, kinase domain: H1047R/L/Y	30%–40%	SGA, NGS	1	PI3-kinase targeted inhibitors: alpelisib (in combination with ER-antagonist fulvestrant)	NCT02437318 NCT01870505
Investigational biomarkers with compelling clinical evidence								
ERBB2/HER2 (17q12)	Transmembrane tyrosine kinase receptor	Activating mutation[b] In-frame insertion	S310F/Y, L755S, D769H/Y, V777L Y772_A775dup G778_P780dup	1.6%–4.0%	SGA, NGS	3A	Irreversible pan-HER tyrosine kinase inhibitor: neratinib	NCT01953926

AKT1 (14q32)	Intracellular serine/threonine kinase	Activating mutation	E17K	5%	SGA, NGS	3A	Pan-AKT kinase inhibitor: AZD5363 ATP-competitive selective inhibitor: ipatasertib	NCT01226316 NCT03337724 NCT01895946
PTEN (10q23)	Tumor suppressor, lipid and protein phosphatase	Loss of function, truncated and inactivating mutations, homozygous deletions[c]	T319*, R130*/G/P/Q	5%–6%	SGA, NGS	4	GSK2636771 and AZD8186	NCT01458067, NCT03218826, NCT01884285
Resistance alterations[abc]								
ESR1 (6q25)	ER transcription and ERα expression	Activating mutation	E380Q, L536H/P/R, Y537S/C/D/N, D538 G	30%–40%	SGA, NGS	3A	Alternate to estrogen deprivation therapies, including AZD9496 and fulvestrant	NCT03079011

Abbreviations: bright-field ISH, bright field in situ hybridization; NCCN, National Comprehensive Cancer Network; PARP, poly(ADP-ribose) polymerase; TRK, tropomyosin receptor kinase.

[a] Patients with *PIK3CA*-mutated hormone-receptor positive/HER2 negative metastatic breast cancer may display resistance to chemotherapy.

[b] *ERBB2* activating mutations can also serve as a resistance alteration to antiestrogen therapy.

[c] Loss-of-function genetic alterations in *PTEN* have been identified as a mechanism of resistance to the PI3-kinase inhibitor alpelisib.

TrkA, TrkB, and TrkC, respectively. Upon neuro-trophin binding, the kinase receptors phosphory-late themselves and members of the MAPK, PI3K and phospholipase C-γ pathways. *NTRK* gene fusions can lead to constitutively activated chimeric TRK fusion proteins, which result in cell proliferation and tumor growth.[61] Assays designed to detect *NTRK* gene fusions include FISH, IHC (pan-TRK IHC), and NGS (DNA and RNA based). FISH had classically been the standard assay for fusion detection; however, it does not establish whether rearrangement results in an oncogenic fusion or the fusion gene partner. Pan-TRK IHC has been demonstrated as a sensitive and specific assay to identify and/or confirm the presence of *NTRK1-3* fusions and specific staining patterns by IHC have been described for some of the most common NTRK fusion partners (*LMNA1*, *TPM3/4*, and *ETV6*).[26] Because IHC can detect wild-type NTRK proteins in addition to fusion proteins in some tissues (namely, smooth muscles, testes, and neural components), confirmation of a positive result with molecular testing (ie, NGS) may be indicated.[26] DNA-based NGS can characterize some fusions precisely, depending on the gene panel; however, RNA-based NGS is favored because it can determine if the fusion is in-frame and the fusion partner.

Kinase fusions in general are extremely rare in breast tumors, occurring in approximately 0.6% of patients and seem to be enriched in postprogression specimens after endocrine therapy.[62] Of the kinase fusions, NTRK gene fusions are of particular interest in breast owing to their FDA-approved targeted therapy; larotrectinib and entrectinib are selective TRK inhibitors FDA approved for pediatric and adult TRK-fusion–positive solid tumors, regardless of tumor origin, in patients without a known acquired resistance mutation (NCT02122913, NCT02637687, and NCT02576431).[63,64] Although the ETV6–NTRK3 fusion is used for diagnosis in secretory carcinoma of the breast as described elsewhere in this article, this fusion can also be targetable, as was successfully described in a case report of a 14-year-old girl with refractory secretory breast carcinoma.[65]

PIK3CA Mutations

Phosphatidylinositol-3-kinase (PI3K) is composed of a regulatory subunit (p85α) and a catalytic subunit (p110α) and it is the catalytic subunit that is encoded by the *PIK3CA* gene. PI3K is recruited to the plasma membrane by intracellular signals from multiple receptor tyrosine kinases, including EGFR, HER2, RET, MET, and VEGFR, among others. Upon stimulation, PI3K-p110α converts its lipid substrate PIP2 (phosphatidylinositol-4,5-bisphosphate) to PIP3 (phosphatidylinositol-3,4,5-bisphosphate), which activates several signaling cascades, including the AKT/mTOR pathway. Activating mutations in *PIK3CA* induce hyperactivation of p110α, impacting the downstream signaling of the AKT/mTOR pathway and promoting cell survival and proliferation.[66]

The Cancer Genome Atlas Network has shown that somatic *PIK3CA* mutations are more commonly seen the luminal intrinsic subtypes (45% of luminal A, 29% of luminal B) and in 39% of HER2-enriched tumors.[5] In the setting of early breast cancer, *PIK3CA* mutations have been reported in 32% of patients and show significant associations with ER positivity, increasing age, lower tumor grade, and smaller tumor size.[67] Genomic sequencing in hormone receptor–positive metastatic breast tumors in particular have identified recurrent, oncogenic alterations of *PIK3CA* in more than 36% of cases.[68] The most common mutations affecting *PIK3CA* cluster around 2 domains: exon 9, affecting amino acids 542 to 546 of the helical domain, and exon 20, affecting amino acid 1047 of the kinase domain.

The FDA approved the PI3K inhibitor alpelisib based on the phase III randomized trial SOLAR-1 (NCT02437318). Alpelisib is approved for use in combination with fulvestrant (a selective ER degrader) to treat postmenopausal women as well as men with *PIK3CA*-mutated, hormone receptor–positive, and HER2-negative advanced or metastatic breast cancer that have progressed during or after treatment with hormonal therapy.[69] The FDA has also approved the companion diagnostic test therascreen PIK3CA RGQ PCR Kit, to detect *PIK3CA* mutations in tissue and/or a liquid biopsies.[51]

INVESTIGATIONAL BIOMARKERS

ERBB2 Mutations

ERBB2 activating mutations have been identified in approximately 1.6% to 4.0% of invasive breast carcinomas. The frequency of *ERBB2* mutations vary according to the histologic subtype of breast cancer assessed, being reportedly higher in ILC.[70,71] These mutations seem to be independently associated with *HER2* amplification status, occurring in both HER2-positive and HER2-negative breast tumors.[70,72–74] Bose and colleagues[70] showed that *HER2* somatic mutations identified in breast cancer clustered around exon 8, affecting amino acids 309 to 310 of the extracellular domain, and exons 19 to 20, affecting amino acids 755 to 781 of the tyrosine kinase domain. Functional studies by Bose and colleagues of 13

HER2 mutations revealed that 7 of these mutations were activating, including G309A, D769H/Y, V777L, P780-Y781insGSP, V842I, and R896C. In addition, in vitro models used to test the impact of these mutations on the response to HER2-targeted agents, including trastuzumab, lapatinib, and neratinib, confirmed that the *HER2* L755S mutation is likely to result in resistance to the reversible tyrosine kinase inhibitor lapatinib, but cells harboring this mutation remain sensitive to the irreversible inhibitor neratinib.[70]

In the multihistology, phase II basket trial SUMMIT, the activity of neratinib was tested in patients affected by solid tumors with somatic *ERBB2/3* mutations. Breast cancer was the second most common tumor type and neratinib exhibited the greatest degree of activity in these patients (n = 25 total, objective response rate at week 8 of 32%; 95% confidence interval, 15%–54%) with responses observed in patients with missense mutations involving the extracellular and kinase domains, as well as insertions in the kinase domain (NCT01953926).[75]

BRCA1/2 Mutations

BRCA1 (breast cancer susceptibility gene 1) and *BRCA2* (breast cancer susceptibility gene 2) are both tumor suppressor genes involved in cell growth, cell division, and repair of damaged DNA repair during homologous recombination. Few breast cancers (approximately 3%) are attributable to germline mutations in *BRCA1/2*[13]; however, with NGS becoming more common, the identification of somatic *BRCA1/2* mutations are increasing. Poly (ADP-ribose) polymerase (PARP) is a critical enzyme involved in the repair of DNA single-strand breaks via the base excision pathway. PARP inhibitors such as olaparib or talazoparib lead to an accumulation of double-strand DNA breaks, resulting in activation of homologous recombination repair, which can compensate for the lack of activity of the base excision pathway and repair DNA damage.[76] However, patients with mutations in *BRCA1/2* and subsequent defects in the homologous recombination DNA repair pathway cannot repair these double-strand DNA damages caused by PARP inhibitors, and the tumor cell eventually dies.

PARP inhibitor therapy has applications beyond *BRCA1/2* germline-mutated tumors. There is evidence for the use of PARP inhibitors in patients with metastatic ovarian cancer and somatic *BRCA1/2* mutations; however, data and recommendations for this targeted therapy in metastatic breast cancer are still needed. In December 2016, the FDA approved the PARP inhibitor rucaparib as monotherapy for patients with advanced ovarian cancer who had been treated with 2 or more chemotherapies and a deleterious germline and/or somatic *BRCA* mutation based on ARIEL2 (NCT01891344) and Study 10 (NCT01482715).[77,78] Olaparib Expanded is a phase II study of olaparib monotherapy in patients with metastatic breast cancer with germline or somatic mutations in DNA repair genes, or somatic mutations in *BRCA1* or *BRCA2* (NCT03344965), but treatment in this setting is still undergoing investigation.

AKT1 and PTEN Alterations

Genetic alterations in breast cancer involving both *AKT* and *PTEN* lead to the dysregulation of the PI3K/AKT/MTOR pathway. The AKT kinase family includes 3 structurally related intracellular serine–threonine kinases—AKT1, AKT2, and AKT3—that serve as critical downstream effectors in the PI3K pathway. PTEN, in contrast, serves as a tumor suppressor, dephosphorylating PIP3, and preventing activation of AKT; loss of PTEN function leads to activation of AKT/MTOR signaling. Large-scale genomic profiling of human cancers identified activating mutations in *AKT1* in approximately 5% of breast cancers, with AKT1 E17K being the most frequent hotspot.[79–81] Somatic *PTEN* mutations occur in approximately 5% to 6% of breast cancers.[82]

AZD5363 is a potent, selective inhibitor of AKT1, AKT2, and AKT3. In a recent basket trial, AZD5363 was assessed in patients with advanced/metastatic breast, gynecologic or other solid cancers bearing either a *AKT1/PIK3CA* or *PTEN* mutation; 20 patients with breast cancer were enrolled with a hot spot *AKT1* E17K mutant tumor and the median progression-free survival was 5.5 months (95% confidence interval, 2.9–6.9 months) (NCT01226316).[83]

RESISTANCE ALTERATIONS IN BREAST CANCER

Resistance to targeted therapy is a major clinical challenge in the treatment of breast cancer. Various resistance mechanisms for all tumor types exist, including primary (intrinsic) resistance and secondary (acquired) resistance after treatment. Tissue biopsy upon progression of disease and analysis of circulating tumor DNA in plasma is becoming more common to explore the mechanisms of resistance. Somatic alterations in metastatic breast tumors associated with resistance to endocrine therapy, in particular, have been identified (see **Table 2**) and the exploration of new therapeutic options in this setting is ongoing.

ESR1 encodes ER-α, which functions as a ligand-activated transcription factor that is expressed in approximately 75% of invasive breast cancers. ER is a weak prognostic but a strong predictive biomarker, and antiestrogen therapy is an effective treatment for women with ER-positive breast cancer,[84,85] including estrogen deprivation therapy (aromatase inhibitors, gonadotropin-releasing hormone agonists) and direct inhibitors of ER (selective ER modulators and selective ER degraders). Despite the benefits of these drugs, *ESR1* mutations involving the ligand-binding domain can develop, resulting in a constitutively active receptor and acquired resistance to estrogen deprivation therapies.[86] The exact prevalence rate of *ESR1* mutations varies in the literature, depending on the cohort assessed. In studies assessing tissue samples and circulating tumor DNA, activating *ESR1* mutations have been reported in up to 30% to 40% of patients with hormone-resistant, ER-positive metastatic breast cancer previously treated with aromatase inhibitors.[87–89]The most common *ESR1* mutations are D538G and Y537S, which are reported as being associated with a worse overall prognosis.[89]

Because only a fraction of patients with breast cancer with endocrine-resistant tumors have *ESR1* mutations, Razavi and colleagues[68] explored additional mechanisms of resistance to hormonal therapy. In this large study with sequencing data from breast tumors previously exposed to hormonal therapy, there was an enrichment in *ERBB2* activating mutations, *NF1* loss-of-function mutations, and alterations in other MAPK pathway genes (*EGFR* and *KRAS*) and ER transcriptional regulators (*MYC*, *CTCF*, *FOXA1*, and *TBX3*).[68] Of note, mutations in *ESR1*, *ERRB2*, and *NF1* were mostly mutually exclusive. The incorporation of these findings into clinical practice is ongoing.

Additional mutations associated with resistance to endocrine therapy have been identified by sequencing of metastatic lesions. Loss-of-function *PTEN* mutations have been identified as a mechanism of resistance to the PI3K inhibitor alpelisib.[90] The amplification and overexpression of the growth factor *FGFR1* may contribute to poor prognosis in luminal A and B breast cancers and lead to subsequent endocrine therapy resistance.[91] In terms of cell cycle regulation, the cyclin D1-CDK4/6-Rb pathway has been implicated in resistance to endocrine therapy as well. Targeted CDK4/6 inhibitors (palbociclib, ribociclib, and abemaciclib) that act upstream of Rb are now routinely used in clinical practice for ER-positive breast cancer however inactivating mutations of *RB1* (<5%), which is wild type in the majority of ER-positive breast cancers,[5] will result in resistance to this targeted therapy. The AR pathway has also emerged as a potential therapeutic target in breast cancer, TNBC in particular (NCT02605486, NCT03090165, NCT02457910, NCT02750358). In prostate cancer, resistance to androgen deprivation therapy is frequently associated with the emergence of androgen-independent splice variants of AR and women with breast cancer may be prone to a similar mechanism of resistance.[92]

EMERGING MOLECULAR MARKERS AND FUTURE TRENDS

Novel methodologies, such as the assessment of mutational signatures, analysis of circulating tumor DNA in plasma and artificial intelligence are providing a greater understanding of the biology of breast cancer. Among the mutational signatures documented in breast cancer[93] are those related to aging (signatures 1 and 5), the activity of APOBEC cytidine deaminases (signatures 2 and 13), homologous recombination deficiency (signatures 3 and 8), or mismatch repair deficiency (signatures 6, 20, and 26), as well as signatures of cryptic origin (signatures 17, 18, and 30).[93] The assessment of mutational signatures has potential clinical implications. For instance, HRDetect is a mutational signature-based predictor of BRCA1 and BRCA2 deficiency that could aid in the identification of tumors that are selectively sensitive to PARP inhibitors, as briefly mentioned elsewhere in this article.[94] Efforts are also focusing on the detection of immune processes through the assessment of signatures that could facilitate triaging of patients that could benefit from immunotherapy,[95] which is another evolving treatment in breast cancer. Predictive biomarkers for immune checkpoint inhibitors in breast cancer currently include PD-L1 expression by IHC. The phase III IMpassion130 study led to the FDA approval of atezolizumab, a monoclonal antibody against PD-L1, in combination with the chemotherapy drug nab-paclitaxel for patients with metastatic TNBC whose tumors are infiltrated with immune cells that express PD-L1 detected by IHC using the Ventana SP142 assay.[96] In addition, although the incidence of microsatellite instability in breast cancer is rare (approximately 1%),[97] because mismatch repair-deficient tumors are more responsive to PD-1 blockade with pembrolizumab[98] the identification of microsatellite instability status can be determined by IHC, polymerase chain reaction, or some NGS panels. Liquid biopsies are quickly becoming a strategy to overcome the difficulties of sampling metastatic lesions and have the potential to identify genetic alterations in minimal residual disease,[99] drivers of resistance,[100] and genetic predictors of response to targeted therapies.[101]

Overall, the molecular classification of breast cancer and how this is incorporated into clinical practice is still evolving. Molecular profiling with new assays and larger gene panels on a wider spectrum of samples (primary/metastatic, tissue/plasma) continues to broaden our understanding of this heterogenous disease and to identify novel targetable biomarkers. Clinical trials in combination with genomics, transcriptomics and artificial intelligence in addition to traditional histologic examination will unlock the many facets of precision medicine in breast cancer.

CLINICS CARE POINTS

- *ERBB2* amplification in breast cancer serves as a strong prognostic and predictive biomarker, with several FDA-approved companion diagnostic tests for detection and subsequent treatment of HER2-positive disease.

- Tumors driven by *NTRK* gene fusions show durable responses to treatment with TRK inhibitors. Assays designed to detect *NTRK* fusions include FISH, pan-TRK IHC, and NGS. RNA-based NGS in particular can determine if the *NTRK* fusion is oncogenic and the fusion gene partner.

- PIK3CA mutations are more commonly seen in the luminal intrinsic subtypes of breast cancer. The FDA-approved PI3K inhibitor (alpelisib) is indicated for use in combination with fulvestrant in postmenopausal women, and men, with PIK3CA-mutated, hormone receptor positive, and HER2-negative advanced/metastatic breast cancer progressing during/after treatment with antiestrogen therapy.

- ESR1 activating mutations involving the ligand-binding domain should be tested for in patients with ER-positive breast cancer progressing on antiestrogen treatment as detection warrants selection of alternate therapies.

DISCLOSURE

The authors have nothing to disclose.

REFERENCES

1. Siegel RL, Miller KD, Jemal A. Cancer statistics, 2020. CA Cancer J Clin 2020;70(1):7–30.
2. Allison KH, Hammond MEH, Dowsett M, et al. Estrogen and progesterone receptor testing in breast cancer: ASCO/CAP guideline update. J Clin Oncol 2020;38(12):1346–66.
3. Wolff AC, Hammond MEH, Allison KH, et al. Human epidermal growth factor receptor 2 testing in breast cancer: American Society of Clinical Oncology/College of American Pathologists Clinical Practice Guideline Focused Update. J Clin Oncol 2018; 36(20):2105–22.
4. Sorlie T, Perou CM, Tibshirani R, et al. Gene expression patterns of breast carcinomas distinguish tumor subclasses with clinical implications. Proc Natl Acad Sci U S A 2001;98(19):10869–74.
5. Cancer Genome Atlas N. Comprehensive molecular portraits of human breast tumours. Nature 2012;490(7418):61–70.
6. Perou CM, Sorlie T, Eisen MB, et al. Molecular portraits of human breast tumours. Nature 2000; 406(6797):747–52.
7. Senkus E, Kyriakides S, Ohno S, et al. Primary breast cancer: ESMO Clinical Practice Guidelines for diagnosis, treatment and follow-up. Ann Oncol 2015;26(Suppl 5):v8–30.
8. Aleskandarany MA, Green AR, Benhasouna AA, et al. Prognostic value of proliferation assay in the luminal, HER2-positive, and triple-negative biologic classes of breast cancer. Breast Cancer Res 2012;14(1):R3.
9. Cheang MC, Martin M, Nielsen TO, et al. Defining breast cancer intrinsic subtypes by quantitative receptor expression. Oncologist 2015;20(5):474–82.
10. Lehmann BD, Bauer JA, Chen X, et al. Identification of human triple-negative breast cancer subtypes and preclinical models for selection of targeted therapies. J Clin Invest 2011;121(7):2750–67.
11. Bareche Y, Venet D, Ignatiadis M, et al. Unravelling triple-negative breast cancer molecular heterogeneity using an integrative multiomic analysis. Ann Oncol 2018;29(4):895–902.
12. Asghar US, Barr AR, Cutts R, et al. Single-cell dynamics determines response to CDK4/6 inhibition in triple-negative breast cancer. Clin Cancer Res 2017;23(18):5561–72.
13. WHO Classification of Tumors Editorial Board. Breast tumours. WHO classification of tumors. 5th Ed. Lyon: IARC; 2019.
14. Pareja F, Weigelt B, Reis-Filho JS. Problematic breast tumors reassessed in light of novel molecular data. Mod Pathol 2021;34(Suppl 1):38–47.

15. Ciriello G, Gatza ML, Beck AH, et al. Comprehensive molecular portraits of invasive lobular breast cancer. Cell 2015;163(2):506–19.

16. Caldeira JR, Prando EC, Quevedo FC, et al. CDH1 promoter hypermethylation and E-cadherin protein expression in infiltrating breast cancer. BMC Cancer 2006;6:48.

17. Aberle H, Schwartz H, Kemler R. Cadherin-catenin complex: protein interactions and their implications for cadherin function. J Cell Biochem 1996;61(4):514–23.

18. Da Silva L, Parry S, Reid L, et al. Aberrant expression of E-cadherin in lobular carcinomas of the breast. Am J Surg Pathol 2008;32(5):773–83.

19. Grabenstetter A, Mohanty AS, Rana S, et al. E-cadherin immunohistochemical expression in invasive lobular carcinoma of the breast: correlation with morphology and CDH1 somatic alterations. Hum Pathol 2020;102:44–53.

20. D'Alfonso TM, Mosquera JM, MacDonald TY, et al. MYB-NFIB gene fusion in adenoid cystic carcinoma of the breast with special focus paid to the solid variant with basaloid features. Hum Pathol 2014;45(11):2270–80.

21. Persson M, Andren Y, Mark J, et al. Recurrent fusion of MYB and NFIB transcription factor genes in carcinomas of the breast and head and neck. Proc Natl Acad Sci U S A 2009;106(44):18740–4.

22. Kim J, Geyer FC, Martelotto LG, et al. MYBL1 rearrangements and MYB amplification in breast adenoid cystic carcinomas lacking the MYB-NFIB fusion gene. J Pathol 2018;244(2):143–50.

23. Tognon C, Knezevich SR, Huntsman D, et al. Expression of the ETV6-NTRK3 gene fusion as a primary event in human secretory breast carcinoma. Cancer Cell 2002;2(5):367–76.

24. Skalova A, Vanecek T, Sima R, et al. Mammary analogue secretory carcinoma of salivary glands, containing the ETV6-NTRK3 fusion gene: a hitherto undescribed salivary gland tumor entity. Am J Surg Pathol 2010;34(5):599–608.

25. Harrison BT, Fowler E, Krings G, et al. Pan-TRK immunohistochemistry: a useful diagnostic adjunct for secretory carcinoma of the breast. Am J Surg Pathol 2019;43(12):1693–700.

26. Hechtman JF, Benayed R, Hyman DM, et al. Pan-Trk immunohistochemistry is an efficient and reliable screen for the detection of NTRK fusions. Am J Surg Pathol 2017;41(11):1547–51.

27. Nadelman CM, Leslie KO, Fishbein MC. "Benign," metastasizing adenomyoepithelioma of the breast: a report of 2 cases. Arch Pathol Lab Med 2006;130(9):1349–53.

28. Geyer FC, Li A, Papanastasiou AD, et al. Recurrent hotspot mutations in HRAS Q61 and PI3K-AKT pathway genes as drivers of breast adenomyoepitheliomas. Nat Commun 2018;9(1):1816.

29. Pareja F, Toss MS, Geyer FC, et al. Immunohistochemical assessment of HRAS Q61R mutations in breast adenomyoepitheliomas. Histopathology 2020;76(6):865–74.

30. Masood S, Davis C, Kubik MJ. Changing the term "breast tumor resembling the tall cell variant of papillary thyroid carcinoma" to "tall cell variant of papillary breast carcinoma". Adv Anat Pathol 2012;19(2):108–10.

31. Chiang S, Weigelt B, Wen HC, et al. IDH2 mutations define a unique subtype of breast cancer with altered nuclear polarity. Cancer Res 2016;76(24):7118–29.

32. Zhong E, Scognamiglio T, D'Alfonso T, et al. Breast tumor resembling the tall cell variant of papillary thyroid carcinoma: molecular characterization by next-generation sequencing and histopathological comparison with tall cell papillary carcinoma of thyroid. Int J Surg Pathol 2019;27(2):134–41.

33. Bhargava R, Florea AV, Pelmus M, et al. Breast tumor resembling tall cell variant of papillary thyroid carcinoma: a solid papillary neoplasm with characteristic immunohistochemical profile and few recurrent mutations. Am J Clin Pathol 2017;147(4):399–410.

34. Pareja F, da Silva EM, Frosina D, et al. Immunohistochemical analysis of IDH2 R172 hotspot mutations in breast papillary neoplasms: applications in the diagnosis of tall cell carcinoma with reverse polarity. Mod Pathol 2020;33(6):1056–64.

35. Foschini MP, Morandi L, Asioli S, et al. The morphological spectrum of salivary gland type tumours of the breast. Pathology 2017;49(2):215–27.

36. Pia-Foschini M, Reis-Filho JS, Eusebi V, et al. Salivary gland-like tumours of the breast: surgical and molecular pathology. J Clin Pathol 2003;56(7):497–506.

37. Pareja F, Da Cruz Paula A, Gularte-Merida R, et al. Pleomorphic adenomas and mucoepidermoid carcinomas of the breast are underpinned by fusion genes. NPJ Breast Cancer 2020;6:20.

38. Basbug M, Akbulut S, Arikanoglu Z, et al. Mucoepidermoid carcinoma in a breast affected by burn scars: comprehensive literature review and case report. Breast Care (Basel) 2011;6(4):293–7.

39. Di Tommaso L, Foschini MP, Ragazzini T, et al. Mucoepidermoid carcinoma of the breast. Virchows Arch 2004;444(1):13–9.

40. Bean GR, Krings G, Otis CN, et al. CRTC1-MAML2 fusion in mucoepidermoid carcinoma of the breast. Histopathology 2019;74(3):463–73.

41. Tonon G, Modi S, Wu L, et al. t(11;19)(q21;p13) translocation in mucoepidermoid carcinoma creates a novel fusion product that disrupts a Notch signaling pathway. Nat Genet 2003;33(2):208–13.

42. Behboudi A, Enlund F, Winnes M, et al. Molecular classification of mucoepidermoid carcinomas-

prognostic significance of the MECT1-MAML2 fusion oncogene. Genes Chromosomes Cancer 2006;45(5):470–81.

43. Andre F, Mardis E, Salm M, et al. Prioritizing targets for precision cancer medicine. Ann Oncol 2014; 25(12):2295–303.

44. Van Allen EM, Wagle N, Stojanov P, et al. Whole-exome sequencing and clinical interpretation of formalin-fixed, paraffin-embedded tumor samples to guide precision cancer medicine. Nat Med 2014;20(6):682–8.

45. Dienstmann R, Jang IS, Bot B, et al. Database of genomic biomarkers for cancer drugs and clinical targetability in solid tumors. Cancer Discov 2015; 5(2):118–23.

46. Sukhai MA, Craddock KJ, Thomas M, et al. A classification system for clinical relevance of somatic variants identified in molecular profiling of cancer. Genet Med 2016;18(2):128–36.

47. Condorelli R, Mosele F, Verret B, et al. Genomic alterations in breast cancer: level of evidence for actionability according to ESMO Scale for Clinical Actionability of molecular Targets (ESCAT). Ann Oncol 2019;30(3):365–73.

48. Chakravarty D, Gao J, Phillips SM, et al. OncoKB: a precision oncology knowledge base. JCO Precis Oncol 2017;2017.

49. Slamon DJ, Clark GM, Wong SG, et al. Human breast cancer: correlation of relapse and survival with amplification of the HER-2/neu oncogene. Science 1987;235(4785):177–82.

50. Slamon DJ, Godolphin W, Jones LA, et al. Studies of the HER-2/neu proto-oncogene in human breast and ovarian cancer. Science 1989;244(4905): 707–12.

51. Available at: https://www.fda.gov/medical-devices/vitro-diagnostics/list-cleared-or-approved-companion-diagnostic-devices-vitro-and-imaging-tools. Accessed November 12, 2020.

52. Ross DS, Zehir A, Cheng DT, et al. Next-generation assessment of human epidermal growth factor receptor 2 (ERBB2) amplification status: clinical validation in the context of a hybrid capture-based, comprehensive solid tumor genomic profiling assay. J Mol Diagn 2017;19(2):244–54.

53. Available at: https://www.accessdata.fda.gov/scripts/cder/daf/index.cfm. Accessed November 12, 2020.

54. Piccart-Gebhart MJ, Procter M, Leyland-Jones B, et al. Trastuzumab after adjuvant chemotherapy in HER2-positive breast cancer. N Engl J Med 2005; 353(16):1659–72.

55. Romond EH, Perez EA, Bryant J, et al. Trastuzumab plus adjuvant chemotherapy for operable HER2-positive breast cancer. N Engl J Med 2005; 353(16):1673–84.

56. Slamon D, Eiermann W, Robert N, et al. Adjuvant trastuzumab in HER2-positive breast cancer. N Engl J Med 2011;365(14):1273–83.

57. Perez EA, Romond EH, Suman VJ, et al. Trastuzumab plus adjuvant chemotherapy for human epidermal growth factor receptor 2-positive breast cancer: planned joint analysis of overall survival from NSABP B-31 and NCCTG N9831. J Clin Oncol 2014;32(33):3744–52.

58. von Minckwitz G, Procter M, de Azambuja E, et al. Adjuvant pertuzumab and trastuzumab in early HER2-positive breast cancer. N Engl J Med 2017; 377(2):122–31.

59. von Minckwitz G, Huang CS, Mano MS, et al. Trastuzumab emtansine for residual invasive HER2-positive breast cancer. N Engl J Med 2019; 380(7):617–28.

60. Chan A, Delaloge S, Holmes FA, et al. Neratinib after trastuzumab-based adjuvant therapy in patients with HER2-positive breast cancer (ExteNET): a multicentre, randomised, double-blind, placebo-controlled, phase 3 trial. Lancet Oncol 2016; 17(3):367–77.

61. Alberti L, Carniti C, Miranda C, et al. RET and NTRK1 proto-oncogenes in human diseases. J Cell Physiol 2003;195(2):168–86.

62. Ross DS, Liu B, Schram AM, et al. Enrichment of kinase fusions in ESR1 wild-type, metastatic breast cancer revealed by a systematic analysis of 4854 patients. Ann Oncol 2020;31(8):991–1000.

63. Amatu A, Sartore-Bianchi A, Siena S. NTRK gene fusions as novel targets of cancer therapy across multiple tumour types. ESMO Open 2016;1(2): e000023.

64. Drilon A, Laetsch TW, Kummar S, et al. Efficacy of larotrectinib in TRK fusion-positive cancers in adults and children. N Engl J Med 2018;378(8): 731–9.

65. Shukla N, Roberts SS, Baki MO, et al. Successful targeted therapy of refractory pediatric ETV6-NTRK3 fusion-positive secretory breast carcinoma. JCO Precis Oncol 2017;2017. PO.17.00034.

66. Bader AG, Kang S, Zhao L, et al. Oncogenic PI3K deregulates transcription and translation. Nat Rev Cancer 2005;5(12):921–9.

67. Zardavas D, Te Marvelde L, Milne RL, et al. Tumor PIK3CA genotype and prognosis in early-stage breast cancer: a pooled analysis of individual patient data. J Clin Oncol 2018;36(10):981–90.

68. Razavi P, Chang MT, Xu G, et al. The genomic landscape of endocrine-resistant advanced breast cancers. Cancer Cell 2018;34(3):427–38.e6.

69. Andre F, Ciruelos E, Rubovszky G, et al. Alpelisib for PIK3CA-mutated, hormone receptor-positive advanced breast cancer. N Engl J Med 2019; 380(20):1929–40.

70. Bose R, Kavuri SM, Searleman AC, et al. Activating HER2 mutations in HER2 gene amplification negative breast cancer. Cancer Discov 2013;3(2):224–37.

71. Gaibar M, Beltran L, Romero-Lorca A, et al. Somatic mutations in HER2 and implications for current treatment paradigms in HER2-positive breast cancer. J Oncol 2020;2020:6375956.

72. Kurozumi S, Alsaleem M, Monteiro CJ, et al. Targetable ERBB2 mutation status is an independent marker of adverse prognosis in estrogen receptor positive, ERBB2 non-amplified primary lobular breast carcinoma: a retrospective in silico analysis of public datasets. Breast Cancer Res 2020;22(1):85.

73. Petrelli F, Tomasello G, Barni S, et al. Clinical and pathological characterization of HER2 mutations in human breast cancer: a systematic review of the literature. Breast Cancer Res Treat 2017;166(2):339–49.

74. Subramanian J, Katta A, Masood A, et al. Emergence of ERBB2 mutation as a biomarker and an actionable target in solid cancers. Oncologist 2019;24(12):e1303–14.

75. Hyman DM, Piha-Paul SA, Won H, et al. HER kinase inhibition in patients with HER2- and HER3-mutant cancers. Nature 2018;554(7691):189–94.

76. Exman P, Barroso-Sousa R, Tolaney SM. Evidence to date: talazoparib in the treatment of breast cancer. Onco Targets Ther 2019;12:5177–87.

77. Oza AM, Tinker AV, Oaknin A, et al. Antitumor activity and safety of the PARP inhibitor rucaparib in patients with high-grade ovarian carcinoma and a germline or somatic BRCA1 or BRCA2 mutation: integrated analysis of data from Study 10 and ARIEL2. Gynecol Oncol 2017;147(2):267–75.

78. Balasubramaniam S, Beaver JA, Horton S, et al. FDA approval summary: rucaparib for the treatment of patients with deleterious BRCA mutation-associated advanced ovarian cancer. Clin Cancer Res 2017;23(23):7165–70.

79. Bleeker FE, Felicioni L, Buttitta F, et al. AKT1(E17K) in human solid tumours. Oncogene 2008;27(42):5648–50.

80. Kim MS, Jeong EG, Yoo NJ, et al. Mutational analysis of oncogenic AKT E17K mutation in common solid cancers and acute leukaemias. Br J Cancer 2008;98(9):1533–5.

81. Rudolph M, Anzeneder T, Schulz A, et al. AKT1 (E17K) mutation profiling in breast cancer: prevalence, concurrent oncogenic alterations, and blood-based detection. BMC Cancer 2016;16:622.

82. Bazzichetto C, Conciatori F, Pallocca M, et al. PTEN as a prognostic/predictive biomarker in cancer: an unfulfilled promise? Cancers (Basel) 2019;11(4):435.

83. Hyman DM, Smyth LM, Donoghue MTA, et al. AKT inhibition in solid tumors with AKT1 mutations. J Clin Oncol 2017;35(20):2251–9.

84. Early Breast Cancer Trialists' Collaborative Group. Effects of chemotherapy and hormonal therapy for early breast cancer on recurrence and 15-year survival: an overview of the randomised trials. Lancet 2005;365(9472):1687–717.

85. Mouridsen H, Gershanovich M, Sun Y, et al. Phase III study of letrozole versus tamoxifen as first-line therapy of advanced breast cancer in postmenopausal women: analysis of survival and update of efficacy from the International Letrozole Breast Cancer Group. J Clin Oncol 2003;21(11):2101–9.

86. Toy W, Shen Y, Won H, et al. ESR1 ligand-binding domain mutations in hormone-resistant breast cancer. Nat Genet 2013;45(12):1439–45.

87. Robinson DR, Wu YM, Vats P, et al. Activating ESR1 mutations in hormone-resistant metastatic breast cancer. Nat Genet 2013;45(12):1446–51.

88. Fribbens C, O'Leary B, Kilburn L, et al. Plasma ESR1 mutations and the treatment of estrogen receptor-positive advanced breast cancer. J Clin Oncol 2016;34(25):2961–8.

89. Chandarlapaty S, Chen D, He W, et al. Prevalence of ESR1 mutations in cell-free DNA and outcomes in metastatic breast cancer: a secondary analysis of the BOLERO-2 clinical trial. JAMA Oncol 2016;2(10):1310–5.

90. Razavi P, Dickler MN, Shah PD, et al. Alterations in PTEN and ESR1 promote clinical resistance to alpelisib plus aromatase inhibitors. Nat Cancer 2020;1(4):382–93.

91. Turner N, Pearson A, Sharpe R, et al. FGFR1 amplification drives endocrine therapy resistance and is a therapeutic target in breast cancer. Cancer Res 2010;70(5):2085–94.

92. Hickey TE, Irvine CM, Dvinge H, et al. Expression of androgen receptor splice variants in clinical breast cancers. Oncotarget 2015;6(42):44728–44.

93. Nik-Zainal S, Davies H, Staaf J, et al. Landscape of somatic mutations in 560 breast cancer whole-genome sequences. Nature 2016;534(7605):47–54.

94. Lord CJ, Ashworth A. BRCAness revisited. Nat Rev Cancer 2016;16(2):110–20.

95. Vonderheide RH, Domchek SM, Clark AS. Immunotherapy for breast cancer: what are we missing? Clin Cancer Res 2017;23(11):2640–6.

96. Schmid P, Adams S, Rugo HS, et al. Atezolizumab and Nab-Paclitaxel in advanced triple-negative breast cancer. N Engl J Med 2018;379(22):2108–21.

97. Cortes-Ciriano I, Lee S, Park WY, et al. A molecular portrait of microsatellite instability across multiple cancers. Nat Commun 2017;8:15180.

98. Le DT, Uram JN, Wang H, et al. PD-1 blockade in tumors with mismatch-repair deficiency. N Engl J Med 2015;372(26):2509–20.

99. Garcia-Murillas I, Schiavon G, Weigelt B, et al. Mutation tracking in circulating tumor DNA predicts relapse in early breast cancer. Sci Transl Med 2015;7(302):302ra133.

100. Chu D, Paoletti C, Gersch C, et al. ESR1 mutations in circulating plasma tumor DNA from metastatic breast cancer patients. Clin Cancer Res 2016;22(4):993–9.

101. O'Leary B, Hrebien S, Morden JP, et al. Early circulating tumor DNA dynamics and clonal selection with palbociclib and fulvestrant for breast cancer. Nat Commun 2018;9(1):896.

Molecular Alterations in Pediatric Solid Tumors

Jonathan C. Slack, MD, Alanna J. Church, MD*

KEYWORDS

• Pediatric pathology • Molecular • Solid tumors • Soft tissue and bone tumors

Key Points

- Extracranial pediatric solid tumors exclude hematologic malignancies and central nervous system tumors.
- Pediatric solid tumors typically have a simpler molecular signature than their adult counterparts, with many harboring a single genetic alteration, often a gene fusion.
- Clinically significant molecular alterations in pediatric solid tumors are diagnostic, prognostic, or predictive of response to targeted therapy.
- Next-generation sequencing panels are increasingly being used in the evaluation of pediatric solid tumors and allow simultaneous assessment of a wide variety of gene fusions, sequence variants, and copy number alterations.
- Children with cancer have a high probability of having a germline cancer predisposition syndrome.

ABSTRACT

Pediatric tumors can be divided into hematologic malignancies, central nervous system tumors, and extracranial solid tumors of bone, soft tissue, or other organ systems. Molecular alterations that impact diagnosis, prognosis, treatment, and familial cancer risk have been described in many pediatric solid tumors. In addition to providing a concise summary of clinically relevant molecular alterations in extracranial pediatric solid tumors, this review discusses conventional and next-generation sequencing–based molecular techniques, relevant tumor predisposition syndromes, and the increasing integration of molecular data into the practice of diagnostic pathology for children with solid tumors.

OVERVIEW

Malignant tumors in infancy, childhood, and adolescence can be divided into 3 broad groups: hematologic (leukemias, lymphomas, other), central nervous system tumors (brain and spinal cord), and extracranial solid tumors. Although most extracranial pediatric solid tumors (PSTs) are rare individually; together, they account for nearly 40% of all childhood cancers.[1,2] PSTs can be further subdivided into mesenchyme-derived

Declarations of interest: Dr Church is a consultant for Bayer Oncology and has received speaker fees from Bio-Rad Laboratories.
Department of Pathology, Boston Children's Hospital, Harvard Medical School, 300 Longwood Avenue, Boston, MA 02115, USA
* Corresponding author.
E-mail address: Alanna.Church@childrens.harvard.edu

Surgical Pathology 14 (2021) 473–492
https://doi.org/10.1016/j.path.2021.05.010
1875-9181/21/© 2021 Elsevier Inc. All rights reserved.

tumors that occur primarily in bone and soft tissue and predominantly epithelial tumors that occur in other organs.

In adulthood, the vast majority of solid tumors are carcinomas of epithelial origin.[3] Carcinogenesis often follows via a well-characterized stepwise progression: from mature normal tissue to low-grade dysplasia, then high-grade dysplasia, and ultimately invasion of the basement membrane and cancer. In contrast, pediatric tumors almost never arise from a dysplastic precursor. Carcinomas are rare in childhood, with most PSTs differentiating toward mesenchymal or primitive stem cell populations ('-blastomas').[1,2,4,5] The histologic appearance of PSTs often includes sheets of monomorphic cells with minimal cytoplasm and lack obvious morphologic evidence of differentiation, colloquially referred to as small round blue cell tumors. The histomorphologic diagnosis can be extremely challenging, often requiring extensive ancillary testing, including histochemistry, immunoperoxidase, and molecular methods, to be diagnosed accurately.[6]

Owing to an increasing availability of molecular techniques including next-generation sequencing (NGS), there has been significant progress in the understanding of molecular alterations in PSTs in recent years. Relative to their adult counterparts, pediatric tumors typically have fewer molecular alterations, with many being characterized by a single recurrent gene fusion or sequence variant that is highly specific, or even pathognomonic, for a given entity.[7] Molecular testing can support specific diagnoses, prognostication, and risk stratification, and can identify options for targeted therapy. In some cases, molecular testing can identify a germline (familial) cancer predisposition syndrome.

We provide a review of clinically actionable alterations in PSTs, including those that impact the diagnosis, prognosis, treatment, and familial risk of cancer. The somatic and germline alterations presented meet the criteria for clinically actionable alterations in cancer and germline variants, respectively.[8,9]

CATEGORIZATION OF PEDIATRIC EXTRACRANIAL SOLID TUMORS

There are several ways to categorize pediatric extracranial solid tumors (PSTs), which essentially represent a collection of rare tumors. For the following description of molecular alterations, we have subdivided PSTs into 2 major groups: tumors of bone and soft tissue and those arising from other organs.

Most PSTs arising in bone and soft tissue are sarcomas that exhibit mesenchymal differentiation, although many also include evidence of epithelial differentiation morphologically and with an expression of cytokeratin, for example, biphasic synovial sarcoma and pseudomyogenic hemangioendothelioma. In contrast, PSTs arising in other organ systems may demonstrate a far broader range of differentiation, including undifferentiated (blastemal), epithelial (carcinomas), or mesenchymal/stromal (sarcomatous). Nowhere is this more evident than in PSTs arising from embryonic progenitor cells (-blastomas). The prototypical example of complex differentiation is triphasic a Wilms tumor (also known as nephroblastoma) in which blastemal, epithelial, and stromal elements occur in the same tumor.

According to epidemiologic data, the most common mesenchymal PSTs are rhabdomyosarcomas, fibroblastic or myofibroblastic tumors, Ewing sarcomas, osteosarcomas, and vascular tumors.[10,11] Common organ-based PSTs include neuroblastoma, Wilms tumor (nephroblastoma), retinoblastoma, and hepatoblastoma (by descending order of prevalence).[2,10,12] Of note, many of the mesenchymal tumors can occur as organ-based tumors.

Key Points

- PSTs can be subdivided into 2 major groups:
  - Bone and soft tissue tumors
  - Other organ systems
- Most PSTs arising in bone and soft tissue are mesenchymal, but in other tissues may demonstrate a broad variety of differentiation.

MOLECULAR ALTERATIONS IN PEDIATRIC BONE AND SOFT TISSUE TUMORS

Key molecular alterations in pediatric bone and soft tissue tumors are summarized in **Table 1**. Many of these alterations are included in the National Comprehensive Cancer Network guidelines for the diagnosis, prognosis, and selection of targeted therapies.[13]

DIAGNOSTIC

Fusions are the most common type of molecular alteration in bone and soft tissue PSTs. Notable rearrangements include *TP53* alterations in osteosarcoma and pathognomonic fusions such as *SS18* (synovial sarcoma), *CIC-DUX4*, and *BCOR-CCNB3*.

Table 1
Key molecular alterations in pediatric bone and soft tissue tumors

Tumor	Gene(s)	Alteration	Significance
Adipocytic			
Lipoblastoma[14,15]	*PLAG1*	Fusions	Dx
Myxoid/round cell liposarcoma[16]	*FUS-DDIT3*	Fusions	Dx
Fibroblastic/myofibroblastic			
Fibrous hamartoma of infancy[17]	*EGFR* exon 20	Sequence variants	Dx, Tx
Nodular fasciitis[18]	*MYH9-USP6*	Fusions	Dx
Cranial fasciitis[19]	*MYH9-USP6, USP6*	Fusions	Dx
	CTNNB1	Sequence variants	Dx
Myofibroma[20–23]	*RELA,*	Fusions	
	PDGFRB, NOTCH3	Sequence variants	Dx
Solitary fibrous tumor[24]	*NAB2-STAT6*	Fusion	Dx
Desmoid fibromatosis[25]	*CTNNB1, APC*	Sequence variants	Dx, Fam
Gardner fibroma[26]	*APC*	Sequence variants	Dx, Fam
Dermatofibrosarcoma protuberans[27,28] and giant cell fibroblastoma	*COL1A1-PDGFB*	Fusions	Dx, Tx
Inflammatory myofibroblastic tumor[29–32]	*RANBP2-ALK, ALK, NTRK3, ROS, RET*	Fusions	Dx, Prog, Tx
Low-grade fibromyxoid sarcoma[33]	*FUS-CREB3L1/2*	Fusions	Dx
Sclerosing epithelioid fibrosarcoma[33–35]	*FUS-CREB3L2, YAP1 KMT2A*	Fusions	Dx
Infantile/congenital fibrosarcoma[36–39]	*NTRK3, RET, BRAF*	Fusions	Dx, Tx
Primitive myxoid mesenchymal tumor of infancy, undifferentiated round cell sarcoma[40–42]	*BCOR*	Internal tandem duplication	Dx
Vascular			
Spindle cell hemangioma[43]	*IDH1, IDH2*	Sequence variants	Dx
Pseudomyogenic hemangioendothelioma[44]	*SERPINE1-FOSB*	Fusions	Dx, Tx
Epithelioid hemangioendothelioma[45]	*WWTR1-CAMTA1*	Fusions	Dx
Bone			
Aneurysmal bone cyst[46–48]	*USP6*	Fusions	Dx
Giant cell tumor of bone[49]	*H3F3A*	Sequence variants	Dx

(continued on next page)

Table 1
(continued)

Tumor	Gene(s)	Alteration	Significance
Osteosarcoma[50,51]	TP53	Sequence variants or fusions	Dx
Cartilage			
Chondroblastoma[49]	H3F3B	Sequence variants	Dx
Mesenchymal chondrosarcoma[52]	HEY1-NCOA2	Fusions	Dx
Myogenic			
Alveolar rhabdomyosarcoma[53–56]	PAX3/PAX7-FOXO1	Fusions	Dx, Prog
Embryonal rhabdomyosarcoma[56]	FGFR4 KRAS, NRAS, HRAS, TP53	Copy gains, sequence variants Sequence variants Sequence variants	Dx Dx, Fam Dx, Fam
Spindle cell/sclerosing rhabdomyosarcoma[57–59]	VGLL2, NCOA2 MYOD1	Fusions Sequence variant	Dx, Prog
Peripheral nerve sheath			
Malignant peripheral nerve sheath tumor[60–62]	TP53,SUZ12, EED,CDKN2A H3K27me3 NF1	Sequence variants, deletion Epigenetic methylation Sequence variants	Dx Dx, Prog Dx, Fam
Other			
Ewing sarcoma[13,63,64]	EWSR1-FLI1, EWSR1-ERG STAG2	Fusions Sequence variants	Dx Prog
CIC-rearranged sarcoma[64–66]	CIC-DUX4, CIC-NUTM1, other CIC	Fusions	Dx
BCOR-rearranged sarcoma[64,67,68]	BCOR-CCNB3, BCOR	Fusions	Dx
Synovial sarcoma[63,69,70]	SS18-SSX1/2/4	Fusions	Dx
Angiomatoid fibrous histiocytoma[71–74]	EWSR1-CREB1, EWSR1-CREM, EWSR1/FUS-ATF1	Fusions	Dx
Desmoplastic small round cell tumor[63,75]	EWSR1-WT1	Fusions	Dx
Alveolar soft part sarcoma[63]	ASPCR1-TFE3	Fusions	Dx
Ossifying fibromyxoid tumor[76,77]	PHF1	Fusions	Dx

Abbreviations: Dx, diagnostic; Fam, familial cancer risk; Prog, prognostic; Tx, treatment.

PROGNOSTIC

Few alterations are prognostic for this group of tumors. In alveolar rhabdomyosarcoma, *PAX3-FOXO1* and *PAX7-FOXO1* fusion-positive cases are associated with a poor prognosis, with *PAX3-FOXO1* associated with a lower overall survival than with *PAX7* gene fusions.[53–55] Identification of *RANBP2* as the fusion partner for *ALK* in inflammatory myofibroblastic tumors allows for a more accurate diagnosis and prognostication, because these tumors have an unusual (epithelioid) morphology and are associated with a worse

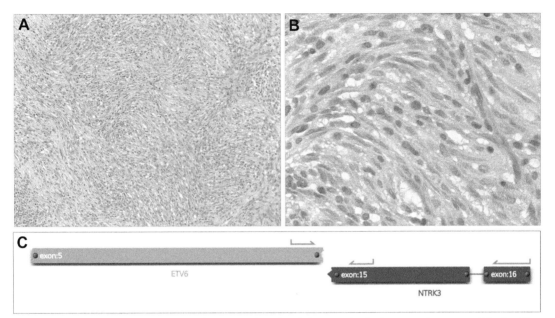

Fig. 1. A soft tissue mass in the thigh of a 6-month-old girl shows a fascicular growth pattern (*A*) of uniform cellular population of spindle to oval cells with mild nuclear atypia (*B*). This tumor was associated with the *ETV6-NTRK3* fusion (*C*), which supports the pathologic diagnosis of infantile fibrosarcoma (red *arrows* = primers with polymerase chain reaction direction; red dots = breakpoints). Oncogenic fusions involving the *NTRK* family genes are associated with response to new targeted kinase inhibitors.

prognosis.[29] Inactivating *STAG2* alterations may be associated with aggressive disease in patients with Ewing sarcoma.[63] *MYOD1* mutations in spindle cell or sclerosing rhabdomyosarcoma are associated with a poor prognosis.[57,58]

TREATMENT

The identification of gene fusions allows for targeted therapy.[63,78,79] Notable examples include those involving *NTRK* and *ALK*, each treated with targeted kinase inhibition (**Fig. 1**). Clinical trials and case reports including children show significant responses to targeted treatment.[63,80]

Key Points

- Many pediatric bone and soft tissue tumors are defined by recurrent gene fusions. Other abnormalities are less common.

- Prognostic associations are rare, and include *FOXO1* fusions in alveolar rhabdomyosarcoma, which are associated with aggressive disease.

- Kinase gene fusions are increasingly recognized in this group of tumors, and are associated with response to targeted inhibition.

MOLECULAR ALTERATIONS IN ORGAN-BASED SOLID TUMORS

Key molecular alterations in nonbone and soft tissue PSTs are summarized in **Table 2**.

DIAGNOSTIC

Most PSTs have at least 1 diagnostically significant sequence variation. Recurrent gene fusions occur in many of tumors listed elsewhere in this article. Other, less common molecular alterations in this group include microRNA cluster alterations (undifferentiated embryonal sarcoma), internal tandem duplications (clear cell sarcoma of kidney), and gene amplifications (neuroblastoma).

PROGNOSTIC

Molecular subtyping can aid in prognostication for many of the most common PSTs, including papillary thyroid carcinoma, Wilms tumor, and neuroblastoma. Notably, *MYCN* amplification in neuroblastoma is associated with decreased overall survival, and its detection is used clinically for risk stratification with intensification of treatment (**Fig. 2**).

Table 2
Recurrent molecular alterations in organ-based PSTs

Tumor	Gene(s)	Alteration	Significance
Salivary gland			
Mucoepidermoid carcinoma[81]	*MECT1-MAML2*	Fusions	Dx
Pleomorphic adenoma[82,83]	*PLAG1, HMGA2*	Fusions	Dx
Acinic cell carcinoma[84,85]	*HTN3-MSANTD3*	Fusions	Dx
Thyroid			
Conventional PTC[86,87]	*BRAF, RAS, DICER1, TP53, AKT1, TERT RET, NTRK1/2/3, ALK*	Sequence variants Fusions	Dx, Prog, Tx, Fam Dx, Prog, Tx
Cribriform-morular variant PTC[86,88,89]	*APC* *CTNNB1*	Sequence variants Sequence variants	Dx, Fam Dx
Diffuse-sclerosing variant PTC[90,91]	*RET*	Fusions	Dx, Tx
Follicular thyroid carcinoma[86,87,91,92]	*PPARG* *RAS, PIK3CA*	Fusions Sequence variants	Dx, Tx Dx, Tx
Medullary thyroid carcinoma[86,87,93,94]	*RET, ALK*	Fusions, sequence variants	Dx, Tx, Fam
Noninvasive follicular thyroid PTC[87,92]	*NRAS, KRAS*	Sequence variants	Dx
Lung			
Pleuropulmonary blastoma[95–97]	*DICER1*	Sequence variants	Dx, Fam
Pulmonary blastoma[98]	*CTNNB1*	Sequence variants	Dx
Gastrointestinal			
Gastrointestinal stromal tumor[99–101]	*KIT, SDHA/B/C/D, PDGFRA*	Sequence variants	Dx, Tx, Fam
Hepatobiliary			
Hepatoblastoma[102]	*CTNNB1*	Sequence variants	Dx
Fibrolamellar carcinoma[103]	*DNAJB1-PRKACA*	Fusions	Dx
Undifferentiated embryonal sarcoma of liver[104,105]	*C19 MC* *MALAT1*	miRNA cluster alt. Fusion	Dx
Mesenchymal hamartoma of infancy[104]	*MALAT1*	Fusions	Dx
Pancreatoblastoma[106]	*APC* *CTNNB1*	Sequence variants Sequence variants	Dx, Fam Dx
Adrenal and kidney			
Adrenocortical carcinoma[107]	*TP53*	sequence variants	Dx, Fam
Neuroblastoma[6,108–115]	*MYCN* *ALK, PHOX2B* *ATRX chr7/17* *chr11q*	Amplification Mutation, amplification Sequence variants Copy gain Copy loss	Prog Prog, Tx, Fam Prog Prog Prog
Wilms tumor[116–119]	*WT1, DIS3L2, TP53, WTX chr11*	Sequence variants, deletion Deletion, methylation	Dx, Fam Dx, Fam
	chr1q 1p/16q	Copy gain LOH	Prog Prog

(continued on next page)

Table 2
(continued)

Tumor	Gene(s)	Alteration	Significance
Clear cell sarcoma of kidney[42,120,121]	BCOR	Tandem duplication	Dx
	YWHAE	Fusions	
Congenital mesoblastic nephroma[38,80,122,123]	ETV6-NTRK3, NTRK3	Fusions	Dx, Tx
Translocation-associated renal cell carcinoma[124,125]	TFE3, TFEB	Fusions	Dx
Metanephric adenoma[126]	BRAF	Sequence variants	Dx
Malignant rhabdoid tumor[127–129]	SMARCB1, SMARCA4	Sequence variants	Dx, Tx, Fam
Pediatric cystic nephroma,[130,131] cystic partially differentiating nephroblastoma, and DICER1-associated renal sarcoma	DICER1	Sequence variants	Dx, Fam
Gonad			
Juvenile granulosa cell tumor[132]	AKT1	Tandem duplication	Dx
Sertoli–Leydig cell tumor[133]	DICER1	Sequence variants	Dx, Fam
Other			
Paraganglioma/ pheochromocytoma[134,135]	SDHA/B/C/D	Sequence variants	Dx, Fam
Retinoblastoma[136]	RB1	Sequence variants, deletion, LOH	Dx, Fam
Spitz tumor[137–139]	ROS1, NTRK1/2/3, ALK, MET, RET BRAF, BAP1, NRAS, HRAS	Fusions Variants	Dx, Tx, Fam

Abbreviations: Dxdiagnostic; Fam, familial cancer risk; LOH, loss of heterozygosity; Prog, prognostic; PTC, papillary thyroid carcinoma; Tx, treatment.

TREATMENT

Targeted therapies are increasingly available for many of these tumors, including targeted kinase inhibition in papillary and follicular thyroid carcinoma, gastrointestinal stromal tumor, congenital mesoblastic nephroma, and Spitz tumors.[63,80,137,140]

- Molecular prognostication is increasingly being used. For example, *MYCN* amplification is associated with a poor prognosis in neuroblastoma and is routinely used in risk stratification.

- Targeted therapies options can be identified in pediatric tumors, including thyroid carcinomas, gastrointestinal stromal tumors, congenital mesoblastic nephroma, and Spitz tumors.

- Tumor predisposition syndromes are particularly prevalent in this group of tumors.

Key Points

- Recurrent sequence variants have been identified in most PSTs that occur outside of bone and soft tissue.

- In contrast with pediatric bone and soft tissue tumors, gene fusions are less common, although sequence variants and copy number alterations are more significant clinically.

DIFFERENCES FROM ADULT SOLID TUMORS

As demonstrated in **Tables 1 and 2**, PSTs encompass a heterogeneous group of tumors, many of which are individually rare or exclusive to childhood, such that a comparison between these

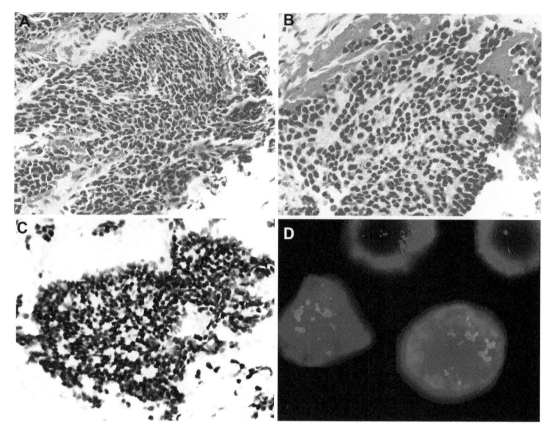

Fig. 2. An adrenal mass of a 2-year-old girl shows a Schwannian stroma-poor neuroblastic tumor composed of round cells with relatively uniform nuclei, evenly distributed chromatin, and scant cytoplasm (*A* and *B*). Neuropil is noted focally (*B*). PHOX2B immunostain is diffusely expressed in tumor cell nuclei (*C*). *MYCN* amplification, detected by fluorescence in situ hybridization with a pink probe (*D*), is associated with a poor prognosis in patients with neuroblastoma.

tumors and their adult counterparts is challenging. Despite this heterogeneity, there are several notable differences between solid tumors in pediatric patients and those occurring in adulthood, including the following.

- *Tissue of origin:* In adulthood, the majority of solid tumors are carcinomas of epithelial origin, which in childhood are exceedingly rare.[4] Conversely, mesenchymal-derived tumors of bone and soft tissue are proportionally far more common in children and infants.[1,2,4,10]
- Clinical characteristics
  - *Limited understanding of clinical associations*: The evidence-based clinical significance of molecular alterations depends on the available literature describing the diagnostic, prognostic, and therapeutic associations with respect to the specific tumor type.[8,9] Because pediatric tumors are rare, there are often limited data, such that potential associations are often extrapolated

from adult datasets. Therapeutic associations are particularly difficult because children have not been included in many clinical trials. New legislation supports the increasing inclusion of children in trials going forward,[5,141] and pediatric cancer groups continue to participate in multi-institutional trials.[78,142,143]
  - *Different anatomic distribution*: Although not relevant when discussing organ-specific PSTs, soft tissue and bone PSTs are more likely to occur on the head and neck, and less likely to occur on the extremities, than in adults.[10,63]
  - *Different prognosis*: PSTs have a generally favorable clinical course when compared with their adult counterparts.[10,144] For example, the overall 5-year relative survival in soft tissue sarcomas (all types) decreases from 75% in pediatric patients (0–19 years of age) to 56% in elderly patients (≥7+ years of age).[10] Unfortunately, survivors of

childhood cancer face significant late long-term side effects of radiation and cytotoxic chemotherapy, including growth delays and secondary cancers.[145–147]

o *Association with germline tumor predisposition*: As described elsewhere in this article, children with cancer are more likely than adults with cancer to have a tumor predisposition syndrome.[148–150] An accurate diagnosis and molecular characterization in this setting can support a germline diagnosis, which may benefit the patient and their family.

- *Molecular alterations:* Roughly 95% of mutations in adult solid tumors are single-base substitutions that accumulate over time. The overwhelming majority of these acquired somatic mutations do not substantially contribute to the neoplastic process, so-called passenger mutations, whereas those that contribute to oncogenesis are designated as drivers. Although each driver mutation typically confers a small selective growth advantage, as these mutations accumulate, oncogenesis proceeds through a stepwise progression, from normal tissue to a precursor with low-grade dysplasia, then high-grade dysplasia, and ultimately invasive carcinoma.[7,151]

Conversely, PSTs are typically associated with a single catastrophic molecular event, rather than a gradual progression over years owing to the accumulation of multiple point mutations. This event is often a gene rearrangement connecting 2 previously noncontiguous genes, which results in an oncogenic fusion. These fusions typically represent the only known driver for that tumor and are present in every neoplastic cell.

The advantages associated with the simpler genetics of PSTs include often looking for just 1 genetic change to support a specific diagnosis. Data about the efficacy of targeted therapies in children are evolving, but some investigators theorize that pediatric tumors with a single dominant molecular abnormality may be more vulnerable to targeted inhibition than an adult tumor with multiple stochastic alterations and subclones. Indeed, many pediatric tumors have demonstrated remarkable responses to precision or targeted therapy.[79,152,153]

Data about the clinical significance of tumor mutational burden (TMB) are still emerging; however, there is increasing evidence that a high TMB is associated with an improved response to immune checkpoint inhibition.[154–156] Thresholds of TMB, measured in mutations per megabase, predicting response to immunotherapy are under

investigation. It is possible that different thresholds may be appropriate for predicting response to immunotherapy in children, given that TMB tends to be lower for childhood tumors.[7] The evaluation of the TMB has also proved helpful in identifying patients with cancer predisposition syndromes including POLE deficiency, Lynch syndrome, and congenital mismatch repair deficiency.[157,158]

PSTs represent a collection of rare tumors, each with its own characteristic genetic profile. The incorporation of molecular diagnostics into the care of children with cancer may serve as a model for care of adult patients with rare tumors.[144]

Key Points

- PSTs represent a unique group of rare tumors, largely different from adult tumors. Mesenchymal tumors are relatively more common and carcinomas far rarer.

- Owing to their rarity, our understanding of PSTs is incomplete. Research is ongoing and new legislation supports the inclusion of children in future clinical trials.

- Pediatric tumors typically lack precursor lesions, have relatively simple genetic profiles, and are often associated with oncogenic gene fusions.

- Children with cancer have had significant responses to targeted therapies.

TUMOR PREDISPOSITION SYNDROMES IN PEDIATRIC SOLID TUMORS

Children with cancer have a high prior probability of having a germline cancer predisposition, with more than 10% having an identifiable syndrome.[148–150] A notable example is DICER1 tumor predisposition syndrome, first associated with pleuropulmonary blastoma and now with a several tumor types distributed throughout the body (**Fig. 3**).[95,130,133,159] Bone and soft tissue PSTs occur less commonly in the context of a tumor predisposition syndrome, with the notable exceptions of Gardner fibroma and desmoid fibromatosis, where a subset of *APC* sequence variants are associated with familial adenomatous polyposis.[25,26] How to identify, prioritize, and report potential germline variants is an important consideration for any laboratory or medical practice. If possible, access to genetic counseling is recommended. A list of selected tumor predisposition syndromes relevant to PSTs is provided in **Table 3**. For a more comprehensive review of the topic the following references are recommended.[178–180]

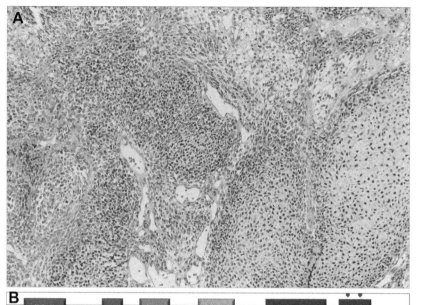

Fig. 3. Pleuropulmonary blastoma (PPB) in the lung of a 3-year-old boy. (*A*) Histology shows an arrangement of light and dark areas, as well as differentiation into cartilage (*right*). PPBs are associated with *DICER1* syndrome in approximately 70% of cases. DICER1-associated tumors including PPBs typically have 2 alterations in the *DICER1* gene: 1 loss-of-function variant and 1 hotspot variant in the RNaseIIb domain at one of the metal-binding sites (*red arrows*) (*B*).

MOLECULAR TECHNIQUES

Molecular techniques are rapidly evolving. The selection of which molecular techniques to incorporate into a clinical practice is complex. Considerations include clinical usefulness, efficient use of scant tissue, assay availability, cost, and reimbursement. An overview of some conventional molecular and NGS techniques are provided elsewhere in this article.

CONVENTIONAL MOLECULAR TECHNIQUES

Conventional molecular techniques remain a mainstay of clinical practice (**Table 4**). Targeted analyses including fluorescence in situ hybridization and single gene assays are cost effective, if limited in scope.

USE OF NEXT-GENERATION SEQUENCING–BASED MOLECULAR ASSAYS IN PEDIATRIC SOLID TUMORS

NGS refers to a variety of platforms that use massively parallel, high-throughput sequencing to provide simultaneous reads of million or billions of RNA and/or DNA strands.[181] Many NGS-based molecular assays have been developed in recent years for use in solid tumors that allow the simultaneous assessment of some or all of the following: sequence variants, insertions and/or deletions, copy number alterations, and gene fusions. Owing to its ability to interrogate multiple genes and alteration types simultaneously, NGS is an efficient tool for the evaluation of PSTs, which are essentially a collection of rare tumors with overlapping morphologies, in which tumor tissue is limited.[78,182]

A comparison of different available platforms is beyond the scope of this article. However, because many are designed for use in adult laboratories, we recommend that any group evaluating PSTs using NGS consider the following points.

CLINICS CARE POINTS

- How well are the molecular alterations in PSTs covered by the assay?
  - Many are specific to pediatric patients and not routinely included on many adult-based assays.
- How much priority is given to fusions on the assay?
  - Coverage of introns takes up a lot of sequencing space on a DNA panel, such

Table 3
Select pediatric tumor predisposition syndromes

Syndrome	Gene(s)	Associated Tumor(s)
DICER1 tumor predisposition syndrome[95,97,130,131,133,159–165]	DICER1	Thyroid carcinoma, pleuropulmonary blastoma, pediatric cystic nephroma, ovarian sex cord stromal tumor, pituitary or pineal blastoma, ciliary body medulloepithelioma, nasal chondromesenchymal hamartoma, DICER1-associated CNS sarcoma
Familial adenomatous polyposis[26,166]	APC	gastrointestinal tract polyposis and/or carcinoma, thyroid carcinoma, desmoid tumor, Gardner fibroma, hepatoblastoma, pancreatoblastoma, juvenile nasopharyngeal angiofibroma, CNS tumors
Noonan syndrome[167]	PTPN11, SOS1, RAF1, RIT1, KRAS	Juvenile myelomonocytic leukemia, neuroblastoma, rhabdomyosarcoma
Familial Wilms tumor[119,168–170]	WT1, BUB1B, DIS3L2	Wilms tumor
Multiple endocrine neoplasia, type II[135,171,172]	RET	Pheochromocytoma, parathyroid adenoma, medullary thyroid carcinoma, neuroma, ganglioneuroma
Familial retinoblastoma[136,173]	RB1	Retinoblastoma, pineoblastoma, osteosarcoma, melanoma
Familial paranglioma-pheochromocytoma syndrome[134,135]	SDHA/B/C/D	Paraganglioma, pheochromocytoma, GIST, renal cell carcinoma
Li–Fraumeni syndrome[174,175]	TP53	Adrenocortical carcinomas, breast cancer, central nervous system tumors, osteosarcomas, soft tissue sarcomas, and others
Constitutional mismatch repair deficiency syndrome[157,176,177]	MLH1, MSH2, MSH6, PMS2, EPCAM, MSH3	Malignant brain tumors, gastrointestinal adenomas and carcinomas, hematologic malignancies (T-NHL, T-ALL, AML), and others

Abbreviations: AML, acute myelogenous leukemia; CNS, central nervous system; GIST, gastrointestinal stromal tumor; T-ALL, T-cell acute lymphoblastic leukemia; T-NHL, T-cell non-Hodgkin lymphoma.

that rare pediatric fusions may not be prioritized. The addition of RNA-based fusion detection may be considered.
- How are fusions reported?
  - For some PSTs, the specific fusion partner is of diagnostic, prognostic, or predictive significance.
- How much priority is given to variants that are rare in adults but important in pediatric patients (eg, DICER1 and MYOD1)?
  - NGS-based molecular assays designed specifically for use in pediatric patients typically prioritize these variants.
- How are germline or potential germline variants handled?
  - Each institution or laboratory must determine how to address the identification of incidental findings of potential germline significance, in accordance with their local laws and practice.

Table 4
Conventional molecular techniques used in clinical evaluation of PSTs, with key advantages and limitations

Technique	Advantages	Limitations
Karyotype	Evaluates the whole genome in an unbiased analysis Good for discovery of novel alterations	Requires fresh tissue May be confounded by overgrowth of non-neoplastic cells Unable to detect small changes including some fusions and copy number alterations (eg, *DNAJB1-PRKACA* fusion) Unable to identify sequence variants
Fluorescence in situ hybridization	Widely available Works well with formalin-fixed, paraffin-embedded tissue Break apart fluorescence in situ hybridization is efficient at screening for known fusions	If it becomes necessary to evaluate multiple targets, the costs and use of tissue can increase substantially Typically does not identify the fusion partner (which may be diagnostically important, as in *EWSR1-WT1* to support a diagnosis of desmoplastic small round cell tumor)
Single gene assays	Typically designed for a thorough analysis of a single gene, for example, *KIT* in GIST, *ETV6-NRTK3* reverse transcriptase polymerase chain reaction High sensitivity and specificity for targeted alterations	Relatively costly for evaluation of a single target Limited scope, only identifying alterations in 1 gene
Microarray	The gold standard for copy number alterations and loss of heterozygosity Still routinely used for prognostication in Wilms tumor and neuroblastoma	Does not assess broadly for sequence variants or gene fusions

Abbreviation: GIST, gastrointestinal stromal tumor.

EMERGING CONCEPTS

The traditional practice of surgical pathology has been to use diagnostic categories that are based on the histomorphology and clinical characteristics of each tumor. As molecular techniques are increasingly integrated into clinical practice, the genomic associations are being incorporated into diagnostic categorization. This shift toward molecularly defined diagnoses has already been evident in both hematologic malignancies and central nervous system tumors.[183,184] New diagnostic entities are emerging in sarcomas and PSTs, including the addition of *CIC*-rearranged tumors as a unique entity in the recent World Health Organization classification, which had previously been included in the description of Ewing or Ewing-like sarcoma.[185] Two notable PSTs defined by their genetics are *NTRK*- and *RET*-rearranged mesenchymal tumors, which are morphologically indistinguishable from one another, yet associated with response to unique targeted therapies.[36,37,80] This paradigm shift of molecular integration is exemplified by the "integrated pathology report," which incorporates histomorphology, immunohistochemistry, clinical features, and molecular data.[186,187] The increasing integration of molecular alterations may support a more accurate diagnosis, allow better prognostication, and identify promising targets for precision therapies.

SUMMARY

We provide a review of the clinically actionable molecular alterations in PSTs occurring outside of the central nervous system. These entities include molecular alterations with diagnostic or prognostic significance, those that predict response to targeted therapies, or those that are associated with a tumor predisposition. PSTs have unique clinical, epidemiologic, and molecular features in comparison with their adult counterparts, notably simpler genetic signatures, and a greater proportion of gene fusions. The unique features of PSTs require careful consideration as the practice of pathology transitions from conventional molecular techniques to NGS-based assays, many of which have been designed for adult cancers. A thoughtful approach to the integration of molecular techniques supports the best of care for our young patients with cancer.

FUNDING

No financial support.

ACKNOWLEDGMENTS

The authors thank Drs Alyaa Al-Ibraheemi, Adrian Dubuc, and Sara Vargas for generously contributing images of their cases.

REFERENCES

1. Allen-Rhoades W, Whittle SB, Rainusso N. Pediatric solid tumors of infancy: an overview. Pediatr Rev 2018;39(2):57–67.
2. Allen-Rhoades W, Whittle SB, Rainusso N. Pediatric solid tumors in children and adolescents: an overview. Pediatr Rev 2018;39(9):444–53.
3. Centers for Disease Control and Prevention. United States Cancer Statistics: Highlights from 2017 Incidence. USCS Data Brief, no. 17. Atlanta, GA: Centers for Disease Control and Prevention, US Department of Health and Human Services; 2020. Available at: https://www.cdc.gov/cancer/uscs/about/data-briefs/no17-USCS-highlights-2017-incidence.htm. Accessed June 18, 2021.
4. Vargas SO. Childhood carcinoma. Surg Pathol Clin 2010;3(3):689–710.
5. U.S. Cancer Statistics Working Group. U.S. Cancer Statistics Data Visualizations Tool, based on 2020 submission data (1999–2018): U.S. Department of Health and Human Services, Centers for Disease Control and Prevention and National Cancer Institute; www.cdc.gov/cancer/dataviz, June 2021. Available at: https://www.cdc.gov/cancer/uscs/dataviz/index.htm. Accessed June 18, 2021.
6. Parham DM. Modern diagnosis of small cell malignancies of children. Surg Pathol Clin 2010;3(3):515–51.
7. Vogelstein B, Papadopoulos N, Velculescu VE, et al. Cancer genome landscapes. Science 2013;339(6127):1546–58.
8. Li MM, Datto M, Duncavage EJ, et al. Standards and guidelines for the interpretation and reporting of sequence variants in cancer: a joint consensus recommendation of the association for molecular pathology, American Society of Clinical Oncology, and College of American Pathologists. J Mol Diagn 2017;19(1):4–23.
9. Richards S, Aziz N, Bale S, et al. Standards and guidelines for the interpretation of sequence variants: a joint consensus recommendation of the American College of Medical Genetics and Genomics and the Association for Molecular Pathology. Genet Med 2015;17(5):405–24.
10. Ferrari A, Sultan I, Huang TT, et al. Soft tissue sarcoma across the age spectrum: a population-based study from the Surveillance Epidemiology and End Results database. Pediatr Blood Cancer 2011;57(6):943–9.
11. Coffin CM, Dehner LP. Fibroblastic-myofibroblastic tumors in children and adolescents: a clinicopathologic study of 108 examples in 103 patients. Pediatr Pathol 1991;11(4):569–88.
12. Scotting PJ, Walker DA, Perilongo G. Childhood solid tumours: a developmental disorder. Nat Rev Cancer 2005;5(6):481–8.
13. von Mehren M, Randall RL, Benjamin RS, et al. Soft tissue sarcoma, version 2.2018, NCCN clinical practice guidelines in oncology. J Natl Compr Canc Netw 2018;16(5):536–63.
14. Hibbard MK, Kozakewich HP, Dal Cin P, et al. PLAG1 fusion oncogenes in lipoblastoma. Cancer Res 2000;60(17):4869–72.
15. Lopez-Nunez O, Alaggio R, Ranganathan S, et al. New molecular insights into the pathogenesis of lipoblastomas: clinicopathologic, immunohistochemical, and molecular analysis in pediatric cases. Hum Pathol 2020;104:30–41.
16. Knight JC, Renwick PJ, Dal Cin P, et al. Translocation t(12;16)(q13;p11) in myxoid liposarcoma and round cell liposarcoma: molecular and cytogenetic analysis. Cancer Res 1995;55(1):24–7.
17. Park JY, Cohen C, Lopez D, et al. EGFR Exon 20 insertion/duplication mutations characterize fibrous hamartoma of infancy. Am J Surg Pathol 2016;40(12):1713–8.
18. Erickson-Johnson MR, Chou MM, Evers BR, et al. Nodular fasciitis: a novel model of transient neoplasia induced by MYH9-USP6 gene fusion. Lab Invest 2011;91(10):1427–33.
19. Paulson VA, Stojanov IA, Wasman JK, et al. Recurrent and novel USP6 fusions in cranial fasciitis

identified by targeted RNA sequencing. Mod Pathol 2020;33(5):775–80.

20. Agaimy A, Bieg M, Michal M, et al. Recurrent Somatic PDGFRB mutations in sporadic infantile/solitary adult myofibromas but not in angioleiomyomas and myopericytomas. Am J Surg Pathol 2017;41(2):195–203.

21. Antonescu CR, Sung YS, Zhang L, et al. Recurrent SRF-RELA fusions define a novel subset of cellular myofibroma/myopericytoma: a potential diagnostic pitfall with sarcomas with myogenic differentiation. Am J Surg Pathol 2017;41(5):677–84.

22. Cheung YH, Gayden T, Campeau PM, et al. A recurrent PDGFRB mutation causes familial infantile myofibromatosis. Am J Hum Genet 2013; 92(6):996–1000.

23. Koo SC, Janeway KA, Harris MH, et al. A distinctive genomic and immunohistochemical profile for NOTCH3 and PDGFRB in myofibroma with diagnostic and therapeutic implications. Int J Surg Pathol 2020;28(2):128–37.

24. Chmielecki J, Crago AM, Rosenberg M, et al. Whole-exome sequencing identifies a recurrent NAB2-STAT6 fusion in solitary fibrous tumors. Nat Genet 2013;45(2):131–2.

25. Alman BA, Li C, Pajerski ME, et al. Increased beta-catenin protein and somatic APC mutations in sporadic aggressive fibromatoses (desmoid tumors). Am J Pathol 1997;151(2):329–34.

26. Coffin CM, Hornick JL, Zhou H, et al. Gardner fibroma: a clinicopathologic and immunohistochemical analysis of 45 patients with 57 fibromas. Am J Surg Pathol 2007;31(3):410–6.

27. Patel KU, Szabo SS, Hernandez VS, et al. Dermatofibrosarcoma protuberans COL1A1-PDGFB fusion is identified in virtually all dermatofibrosarcoma protuberans cases when investigated by newly developed multiplex reverse transcription polymerase chain reaction and fluorescence in situ hybridization assays. Hum Pathol 2008;39(2):184–93.

28. Stacchiotti S, Pantaleo MA, Negri T, et al. Efficacy and biological activity of imatinib in metastatic dermatofibrosarcoma protuberans (DFSP). Clin Cancer Res 2016;22(4):837–46.

29. Marino-Enriquez A, Wang WL, Roy A, et al. Epithelioid inflammatory myofibroblastic sarcoma: an aggressive intra-abdominal variant of inflammatory myofibroblastic tumor with nuclear membrane or perinuclear ALK. Am J Surg Pathol 2011;35(1):135–44.

30. Lovly CM, Gupta A, Lipson D, et al. Inflammatory myofibroblastic tumors harbor multiple potentially actionable kinase fusions. Cancer Discov 2014; 4(8):889–95.

31. Lee JC, Li CF, Huang HY, et al. ALK oncoproteins in atypical inflammatory myofibroblastic tumours: novel RRBP1-ALK fusions in epithelioid inflammatory myofibroblastic sarcoma. J Pathol 2017;241(3):316–23.

32. Lopez-Nunez O, John I, Panasiti RN, et al. Infantile inflammatory myofibroblastic tumors: clinicopathological and molecular characterization of 12 cases. Mod Pathol 2020;33(4):576–90.

33. Guillou L, Benhattar J, Gengler C, et al. Translocation-positive low-grade fibromyxoid sarcoma: clinicopathologic and molecular analysis of a series expanding the morphologic spectrum and suggesting potential relationship to sclerosing epithelioid fibrosarcoma: a study from the French Sarcoma Group. Am J Surg Pathol 2007;31(9):1387–402.

34. Kao YC, Lee JC, Zhang L, et al. Recurrent YAP1 and KMT2A Gene Rearrangements in a Subset of MUC4-negative Sclerosing Epithelioid Fibrosarcoma. Am J Surg Pathol 2020;44(3):368–77.

35. Puls F, Agaimy A, Flucke U, et al. Recurrent fusions between YAP1 and KMT2A in morphologically distinct neoplasms within the spectrum of low-grade fibromyxoid sarcoma and sclerosing epithelioid fibrosarcoma. Am J Surg Pathol 2020;44(5):594–606.

36. Davis JL, Lockwood CM, Albert CM, et al. Infantile NTRK-associated mesenchymal tumors. Pediatr Dev Pathol 2018;21(1):68–78.

37. Davis JL, Vargas SO, Rudzinski ER, et al. Recurrent RET gene fusions in paediatric spindle mesenchymal neoplasms. Histopathology 2020;76(7):1032–41.

38. Church AJ, Calicchio ML, Nardi V, et al. Recurrent EML4-NTRK3 fusions in infantile fibrosarcoma and congenital mesoblastic nephroma suggest a revised testing strategy. Mod Pathol 2018;31(3):463–73.

39. Antonescu CR, Dickson BC, Swanson D, et al. Spindle cell tumors with RET gene fusions exhibit a morphologic spectrum akin to tumors with NTRK gene fusions. Am J Surg Pathol 2019; 43(10):1384–91.

40. Antonescu CR, Kao YC, Xu B, et al. Undifferentiated round cell sarcoma with BCOR internal tandem duplications (ITD) or YWHAE fusions: a clinicopathologic and molecular study. Mod Pathol 2020;33(9):1669–77.

41. Kao YC, Sung YS, Zhang L, et al. Recurrent BCOR internal tandem duplication and YWHAE-NUTM2B fusions in soft tissue undifferentiated round cell sarcoma of infancy: overlapping genetic features with clear cell sarcoma of kidney. Am J Surg Pathol 2016;40(8):1009–20.

42. Santiago T, Clay MR, Allen SJ, et al. Recurrent BCOR internal tandem duplication and BCOR or BCL6 expression distinguish primitive myxoid mesenchymal tumor of infancy from congenital

infantile fibrosarcoma. Mod Pathol 2017;30(6): 884–91.

43. Kurek KC, Pansuriya TC, van Ruler MA, et al. R132C IDH1 mutations are found in spindle cell hemangiomas and not in other vascular tumors or malformations. Am J Pathol 2013;182(5):1494–500.

44. Walther C, Tayebwa J, Lilljebjorn H, et al. A novel SERPINE1-FOSB fusion gene results in transcriptional up-regulation of FOSB in pseudomyogenic haemangioendothelioma. J Pathol 2014;232(5): 534–40.

45. Errani C, Zhang L, Sung YS, et al. A novel WWTR1-CAMTA1 gene fusion is a consistent abnormality in epithelioid hemangioendothelioma of different anatomic sites. Genes Chromosomes Cancer 2011;50(8):644–53.

46. Oliveira AM, Perez-Atayde AR, Inwards CY, et al. USP6 and CDH11 oncogenes identify the neoplastic cell in primary aneurysmal bone cysts and are absent in so-called secondary aneurysmal bone cysts. Am J Pathol 2004;165(5):1773–80.

47. Guseva NV, Jaber O, Tanas MR, et al. Anchored multiplex PCR for targeted next-generation sequencing reveals recurrent and novel USP6 fusions and upregulation of USP6 expression in aneurysmal bone cyst. Genes Chromosomes Cancer 2017;56(4):266–77.

48. Oliveira AM, Hsi BL, Weremowicz S, et al. USP6 (Tre2) fusion oncogenes in aneurysmal bone cyst. Cancer Res 2004;64(6):1920–3.

49. Cleven AH, Hocker S, Briaire-de Bruijn I, et al. Mutation analysis of H3F3A and H3F3B as a diagnostic tool for giant cell tumor of bone and chondroblastoma. Am J Surg Pathol 2015;39(11): 1576–83.

50. Chen X, Bahrami A, Pappo A, et al. Recurrent somatic structural variations contribute to tumorigenesis in pediatric osteosarcoma. Cell Rep 2014; 7(1):104–12.

51. Perry JA, Kiezun A, Tonzi P, et al. Complementary genomic approaches highlight the PI3K/mTOR pathway as a common vulnerability in osteosarcoma. Proc Natl Acad Sci U S A 2014;111(51): E5564–73.

52. Wang L, Motoi T, Khanin R, et al. Identification of a novel, recurrent HEY1-NCOA2 fusion in mesenchymal chondrosarcoma based on a genome-wide screen of exon-level expression data. Genes Chromosomes Cancer 2012;51(2):127–39.

53. Sorensen PH, Lynch JC, Qualman SJ, et al. PAX3-FKHR and PAX7-FKHR gene fusions are prognostic indicators in alveolar rhabdomyosarcoma: a report from the children's oncology group. J Clin Oncol 2002;20(11):2672–9.

54. Rudzinski ER, Anderson JR, Chi YY, et al. Histology, fusion status, and outcome in metastatic rhabdomyosarcoma: a report from the Children's

Oncology Group. Pediatr Blood Cancer 2017; 64(12).

55. Gallego S, Zanetti I, Orbach D, et al. Fusion status in patients with lymph node-positive (N1) alveolar rhabdomyosarcoma is a powerful predictor of prognosis: experience of the European Paediatric Soft Tissue Sarcoma Study Group (EpSSG). Cancer 2018;124(15):3201–9.

56. Shern JF, Chen L, Chmielecki J, et al. Comprehensive genomic analysis of rhabdomyosarcoma reveals a landscape of alterations affecting a common genetic axis in fusion-positive and fusion-negative tumors. Cancer Discov 2014;4(2): 216–31.

57. Agaram NP, LaQuaglia MP, Alaggio R, et al. MYOD1-mutant spindle cell and sclerosing rhabdomyosarcoma: an aggressive subtype irrespective of age. A reappraisal for molecular classification and risk stratification. Mod Pathol 2019;32(1):27–36.

58. Rekhi B, Upadhyay P, Ramteke MP, et al. MYOD1 (L122R) mutations are associated with spindle cell and sclerosing rhabdomyosarcomas with aggressive clinical outcomes. Mod Pathol 2016; 29(12):1532–40.

59. Alaggio R, Zhang L, Sung YS, et al. A molecular study of pediatric spindle and sclerosing rhabdomyosarcoma: identification of novel and recurrent VGLL2-related fusions in infantile cases. Am J Surg Pathol 2016;40(2):224–35.

60. Lee W, Teckie S, Wiesner T, et al. PRC2 is recurrently inactivated through EED or SUZ12 loss in malignant peripheral nerve sheath tumors. Nat Genet 2014;46(11):1227–32.

61. Mito JK, Qian X, Doyle LA, et al. Role of Histone H3K27 trimethylation loss as a marker for malignant peripheral nerve sheath tumor in fine-needle aspiration and small biopsy specimens. Am J Clin Pathol 2017;148(2):179–89.

62. Brohl AS, Kahen E, Yoder SJ, et al. The genomic landscape of malignant peripheral nerve sheath tumors: diverse drivers of Ras pathway activation. Sci Rep 2017;7(1):14992.

63. Crompton BD, Stewart C, Taylor-Weiner A, et al. The genomic landscape of pediatric Ewing sarcoma. Cancer Discov 2014;4(11):1326–41.

64. Machado I, Navarro L, Pellin A, et al. Defining Ewing and Ewing-like small round cell tumors (SRCT): the need for molecular techniques in their categorization and differential diagnosis. A study of 200 cases. Ann Diagn Pathol 2016;22:25–32.

65. Antonescu CR, Owosho AA, Zhang L, et al. Sarcomas with CIC-rearrangements are a distinct pathologic entity with aggressive outcome: a clinicopathologic and molecular study of 115 cases. Am J Surg Pathol 2017;41(7):941–9.

66. Yoshimoto T, Tanaka M, Homme M, et al. CIC-DUX4 induces small round cell sarcomas distinct from Ewing sarcoma. Cancer Res 2017;77(11):2927–37.

67. Peters TL, Kumar V, Polikepahad S, et al. BCOR-CCNB3 fusions are frequent in undifferentiated sarcomas of male children. Mod Pathol 2015;28(4):575–86.

68. Pierron G, Tirode F, Lucchesi C, et al. A new subtype of bone sarcoma defined by BCOR-CCNB3 gene fusion. Nat Genet 2012;44(4):461–6.

69. Clark J, Rocques PJ, Crew AJ, et al. Identification of novel genes, SYT and SSX, involved in the t(X;18)(p11.2;q11.2) translocation found in human synovial sarcoma. Nat Genet 1994;7(4):502–8.

70. McBride MJ, Pulice JL, Beird HC, et al. The SS18-SSX Fusion Oncoprotein Hijacks BAF Complex Targeting and Function to Drive Synovial Sarcoma. Cancer Cell 2018;33(6):1128–41.e1127.

71. Yoshida A, Wakai S, Ryo E, et al. Expanding the phenotypic spectrum of mesenchymal tumors harboring the EWSR1-CREM fusion. Am J Surg Pathol 2019;43(12):1622–30.

72. Hallor KH, Mertens F, Jin Y, et al. Fusion of the EWSR1 and ATF1 genes without expression of the MITF-M transcript in angiomatoid fibrous histiocytoma. Genes Chromosomes Cancer 2005;44(1):97–102.

73. Rossi S, Szuhai K, Ijszenga M, et al. EWSR1-CREB1 and EWSR1-ATF1 fusion genes in angiomatoid fibrous histiocytoma. Clin Cancer Res 2007;13(24):7322–8.

74. Waters BL, Panagopoulos I, Allen EF. Genetic characterization of angiomatoid fibrous histiocytoma identifies fusion of the FUS and ATF-1 genes induced by a chromosomal translocation involving bands 12q13 and 16p11. Cancer Genet Cytogenet 2000;121(2):109–16.

75. Benjamin LE, Fredericks WJ, Barr FG, et al. Fusion of the EWS1 and WT1 genes as a result of the t(11;22)(p13;q12) translocation in desmoplastic small round cell tumors. Med Pediatr Oncol 1996;27(5):434–9.

76. Antonescu CR, Sung YS, Chen CL, et al. Novel ZC3H7B-BCOR, MEAF6-PHF1, and EPC1-PHF1 fusions in ossifying fibromyxoid tumors–molecular characterization shows genetic overlap with endometrial stromal sarcoma. Genes Chromosomes Cancer 2014;53(2):183–93.

77. Gebre-Medhin S, Nord KH, Moller E, et al. Recurrent rearrangement of the PHF1 gene in ossifying fibromyxoid tumors. Am J Pathol 2012;181(3):1069–77.

78. Forrest SJ, Geoerger B, Janeway KA. Precision medicine in pediatric oncology. Curr Opin Pediatr 2018;30(1):17–24.

79. Burdach SEG, Westhoff MA, Steinhauser MF, et al. Precision medicine in pediatric oncology. Mol Cell Pediatr 2018;5(1):6.

80. Hong DS, DuBois SG, Kummar S, et al. Larotrectinib in patients with TRK fusion-positive solid tumours: a pooled analysis of three phase 1/2 clinical trials. Lancet Oncol 2020;21(4):531–40.

81. Okabe M, Miyabe S, Nagatsuka H, et al. MECT1-MAML2 fusion transcript defines a favorable subset of mucoepidermoid carcinoma. Clin Cancer Res 2006;12(13):3902–7.

82. Martins C, Fonseca I, Roque L, et al. PLAG1 gene alterations in salivary gland pleomorphic adenoma and carcinoma ex-pleomorphic adenoma: a combined study using chromosome banding, in situ hybridization and immunocytochemistry. Mod Pathol 2005;18(8):1048–55.

83. Katabi N, Ghossein R, Ho A, et al. Consistent PLAG1 and HMGA2 abnormalities distinguish carcinoma ex-pleomorphic adenoma from its de novo counterparts. Hum Pathol 2015;46(1):26–33.

84. Haller F, Skalova A, Ihrler S, et al. Nuclear NR4A3 immunostaining is a specific and sensitive novel marker for acinic cell carcinoma of the salivary glands. Am J Surg Pathol 2019;43(9):1264–72.

85. Andreasen S, Varma S, Barasch N, et al. The HTN3-MSANTD3 fusion gene defines a subset of acinic cell carcinoma of the salivary gland. Am J Surg Pathol 2019;43(4):489–96.

86. Paulson VA, Rudzinski ER, Hawkins DS. Thyroid Cancer in the Pediatric Population. Genes (Basel) 2019;10(9):723.

87. Haddad RI, Nasr C, Bischoff L, et al. NCCN guidelines insights: thyroid carcinoma, version 2.2018. J Natl Compr Canc Netw 2018;16(12):1429–40.

88. Lam AK, Saremi N. Cribriform-morular variant of papillary thyroid carcinoma: a distinctive type of thyroid cancer. Endocr Relat Cancer 2017;24(4):R109–21.

89. Xu B, Yoshimoto K, Miyauchi A, et al. Cribriform-morular variant of papillary thyroid carcinoma: a pathological and molecular genetic study with evidence of frequent somatic mutations in exon 3 of the beta-catenin gene. J Pathol 2003;199(1):58–67.

90. Joung JY, Kim TH, Jeong DJ, et al. Diffuse sclerosing variant of papillary thyroid carcinoma: major genetic alterations and prognostic implications. Histopathology 2016;69(1):45–53.

91. Mostoufi-Moab S, Labourier E, Sullivan L, et al. Molecular testing for oncogenic gene alterations in pediatric thyroid lesions. Thyroid 2018;28(1):60–7.

92. Hung YP, Fletcher CDM, Hornick JL. Evaluation of Pan-TRK immunohistochemistry in infantile fibrosarcoma, lipofibromatosis-like neural tumor, and histologic mimics. Histopathology 2018;73(4):634–44.

93. Vanden Borre P, Schrock AB, Anderson PM, et al. Pediatric, adolescent, and young adult thyroid carcinoma harbors frequent and diverse targetable genomic alterations, including kinase fusions. Oncologist 2017;22(3):255–63.

94. Hillier K, Hughes A, Shamberger RC, et al. A novel ALK fusion in pediatric medullary thyroid carcinoma. Thyroid 2019;29(11):1704–7.

95. Messinger YH, Stewart DR, Priest JR, et al. Pleuropulmonary blastoma: a report on 350 central pathology-confirmed pleuropulmonary blastoma cases by the International Pleuropulmonary Blastoma Registry. Cancer 2015;121(2):276–85.

96. Priest JR, Watterson J, Strong L, et al. Pleuropulmonary blastoma: a marker for familial disease. J Pediatr 1996;128(2):220–4.

97. Pugh TJ, Yu W, Yang J, et al. Exome sequencing of pleuropulmonary blastoma reveals frequent biallelic loss of TP53 and two hits in DICER1 resulting in retention of 5p-derived miRNA hairpin loop sequences. Oncogene 2014;33(45):5295–302.

98. Nakatani Y, Miyagi Y, Takemura T, et al. Aberrant nuclear/cytoplasmic localization and gene mutation of beta-catenin in classic pulmonary blastoma: beta-catenin immunostaining is useful for distinguishing between classic pulmonary blastoma and a blastomatoid variant of carcinosarcoma. Am J Surg Pathol 2004;28(7):921–7.

99. Agaram NP, Laquaglia MP, Ustun B, et al. Molecular characterization of pediatric gastrointestinal stromal tumors. Clin Cancer Res 2008;14(10):3204–15.

100. Joensuu H, Rutkowski P, Nishida T, et al. KIT and PDGFRA mutations and the risk of GI stromal tumor recurrence. J Clin Oncol 2015;33(6):634–42.

101. Postow MA, Robson ME. Inherited gastrointestinal stromal tumor syndromes: mutations, clinical features, and therapeutic implications. Clin Sarcoma Res 2012;2(1):16.

102. Lopez-Terrada D, Gunaratne PH, Adesina AM, et al. Histologic subtypes of hepatoblastoma are characterized by differential canonical Wnt and Notch pathway activation in DLK+ precursors. Hum Pathol 2009;40(6):783–94.

103. Honeyman JN, Simon EP, Robine N, et al. Detection of a recurrent DNAJB1-PRKACA chimeric transcript in fibrolamellar hepatocellular carcinoma. Science 2014;343(6174):1010–4.

104. Mathews J, Duncavage EJ, Pfeifer JD. Characterization of translocations in mesenchymal hamartoma and undifferentiated embryonal sarcoma of the liver. Exp Mol Pathol 2013;95(3):319–24.

105. Setty BA, Jinesh GG, Arnold M, et al. The genomic landscape of undifferentiated embryonal sarcoma of the liver is typified by C19MC structural rearrangement and overexpression combined with TP53 mutation or loss. Plos Genet 2020;16(4):e1008642.

106. Isobe T, Seki M, Yoshida K, et al. Integrated molecular characterization of the lethal pediatric cancer pancreatoblastoma. Cancer Res 2018;78(4):865–76.

107. Wasserman JD, Novokmet A, Eichler-Jonsson C, et al. Prevalence and functional consequence of TP53 mutations in pediatric adrenocortical carcinoma: a children's oncology group study. J Clin Oncol 2015;33(6):602–9.

108. Goto S, Umehara S, Gerbing RB, et al. Histopathology (International Neuroblastoma Pathology Classification) and MYCN status in patients with peripheral neuroblastic tumors: a report from the Children's Cancer Group. Cancer 2001;92(10):2699–708.

109. Barr EK, Applebaum MA. Genetic predisposition to neuroblastoma. Children (Basel) 2018;5(9):119.

110. Bown N, Cotterill S, Lastowska M, et al. Gain of chromosome arm 17q and adverse outcome in patients with neuroblastoma. N Engl J Med 1999;340(25):1954–61.

111. Bresler SC, Weiser DA, Huwe PJ, et al. ALK mutations confer differential oncogenic activation and sensitivity to ALK inhibition therapy in neuroblastoma. Cancer Cell 2014;26(5):682–94.

112. Pinto NR, Applebaum MA, Volchenboum SL, et al. Advances in risk classification and treatment strategies for neuroblastoma. J Clin Oncol 2015;33(27):3008–17.

113. Trochet D, Bourdeaut F, Janoueix-Lerosey I, et al. Germline mutations of the paired-like homeobox 2B (PHOX2B) gene in neuroblastoma. Am J Hum Genet 2004;74(4):761–4.

114. Twist CJ, Schmidt ML, Naranjo A, et al. Maintaining outstanding outcomes using response- and biology-based therapy for intermediate-risk neuroblastoma: a report from the children's oncology group study ANBL0531. J Clin Oncol 2019;37(34):3243–55.

115. Valentijn LJ, Koster J, Zwijnenburg DA, et al. TERT rearrangements are frequent in neuroblastoma and identify aggressive tumors. Nat Genet 2015;47(12):1411–4.

116. Gadd S, Huff V, Walz AL, et al. A Children's Oncology Group and TARGET initiative exploring the genetic landscape of Wilms tumor. Nat Genet 2017;49(10):1487–94.

117. Gratias EJ, Dome JS, Jennings LJ, et al. Association of chromosome 1q gain with inferior survival in favorable-histology Wilms tumor: a report from the children's oncology group. J Clin Oncol 2016;34(26):3189–94.

118. Grundy PE, Breslow NE, Li S, et al. Loss of heterozygosity for chromosomes 1p and 16q is an adverse prognostic factor in favorable-histology

Wilms tumor: a report from the National Wilms Tumor Study Group. J Clin Oncol 2005;23(29): 7312–21.

119. Lipska-Ziętkiewicz BS. WT1 Disorder. 2020 Apr 30 [Updated 2021 Apr 29]. In: Adam MP, Ardinger HH, Pagon RA, et al., editors. GeneReviews® [Internet]. Seattle (WA): University of Washington, Seattle; 1993-2021. Available at: https://www.ncbi.nlm.nih.gov/books/NBK556455/

120. Roy A, Kumar V, Zorman B, et al. Recurrent internal tandem duplications of BCOR in clear cell sarcoma of the kidney. Nat Commun 2015;6:8891.

121. Wong MK, Ng CCY, Kuick CH, et al. Clear cell sarcomas of the kidney are characterised by BCOR gene abnormalities, including exon 15 internal tandem duplications and BCOR-CCNB3 gene fusion. Histopathology 2018;72(2):320–9.

122. Anderson J, Gibson S, Sebire NJ. Expression of ETV6-NTRK in classical, cellular and mixed subtypes of congenital mesoblastic nephroma. Histopathology 2006;48(6):748–53.

123. Drilon A, Laetsch TW, Kummar S, et al. Efficacy of Larotrectinib in TRK fusion-positive cancers in adults and children. N Engl J Med 2018;378(8): 731–9.

124. Argani P. MiT family translocation renal cell carcinoma. Semin Diagn Pathol 2015;32(2):103–13.

125. Armah HB, Parwani AV. Xp11.2 translocation renal cell carcinoma. Arch Pathol Lab Med 2010; 134(1):124–9.

126. Marsden L, Jennings LJ, Gadd S, et al. BRAF exon 15 mutations in pediatric renal stromal tumors: prevalence in metanephric stromal tumors. Hum Pathol 2017;60:32–6.

127. Pawel BR. SMARCB1-deficient tumors of childhood: a practical guide. Pediatr Dev Pathol 2018; 21(1):6–28.

128. Biegel JA, Kalpana G, Knudsen ES, et al. The role of INI1 and the SWI/SNF complex in the development of rhabdoid tumors: meeting summary from the workshop on childhood atypical teratoid/rhabdoid tumors. Cancer Res 2002;62(1):323–8.

129. Eaton KW, Tooke LS, Wainwright LM, et al. Spectrum of SMARCB1/INI1 mutations in familial and sporadic rhabdoid tumors. Pediatr Blood Cancer 2011;56(1):7–15.

130. Li Y, Pawel BR, Hill DA, et al. Pediatric cystic nephroma is morphologically, immunohistochemically, and genetically distinct from adult cystic nephroma. Am J Surg Pathol 2017;41(4):472–81.

131. Doros LA, Rossi CT, Yang J, et al. DICER1 mutations in childhood cystic nephroma and its relationship to DICER1-renal sarcoma. Mod Pathol 2014; 27(9):1267–80.

132. Auguste A, Bessiere L, Todeschini AL, et al. Molecular analyses of juvenile granulosa cell tumors bearing AKT1 mutations provide insights into tumor biology and therapeutic leads. Hum Mol Genet 2015;24(23):6687–98.

133. Schultz KAP, Harris AK, Finch M, et al. DICER1-related Sertoli-Leydig cell tumor and gynandroblastoma: clinical and genetic findings from the International Ovarian and Testicular Stromal Tumor Registry. Gynecol Oncol 2017;147(3):521–7.

134. Wong MY, Andrews KA, Challis BG, et al. Clinical practice guidance: surveillance for phaeochromocytoma and paraganglioma in paediatric succinate dehydrogenase gene mutation carriers. Clin Endocrinol (Oxf) 2019;90(4):499–505.

135. Else T, Greenberg S, Fishbein L. Hereditary Paraganglioma-Pheochromocytoma Syndromes. 2008 May 21 [Updated 2018 Oct 4]. In: Adam MP, Ardinger HH, Pagon RA, et al., editors. GeneReviews® [Internet]. Seattle (WA): University of Washington, Seattle; 1993-2021. Available at: https://www.ncbi.nlm.nih.gov/books/NBK1548/

136. McEvoy JD, Dyer MA. Genetic and epigenetic discoveries in human retinoblastoma. Crit Rev Oncog 2015;20(3–4):217–25.

137. Wiesner T, Kutzner H, Cerroni L, et al. Genomic aberrations in spitzoid melanocytic tumours and their implications for diagnosis, prognosis and therapy. Pathology 2016;48(2):113–31.

138. Bartenstein DW, Fisher JM, Stamoulis C, et al. Clinical features and outcomes of spitzoid proliferations in children and adolescents. Br J Dermatol 2019;181(2):366–72.

139. Wiesner T, He J, Yelensky R, et al. Kinase fusions are frequent in Spitz tumours and spitzoid melanomas. Nat Commun 2014;5:3116.

140. Picarsic JL, Buryk MA, Ozolek J, et al. Molecular characterization of sporadic pediatric thyroid carcinoma with the DNA/RNA ThyroSeq v2 next-generation sequencing assay. Pediatr Dev Pathol 2016;19(2):115–22.

141. President Signs STAR Act for Kids' Cancers. Cancer Discov 2018;8(7):785–6.

142. Harris MH, DuBois SG, Glade Bender JL, et al. Multicenter feasibility study of tumor molecular profiling to inform therapeutic decisions in advanced pediatric solid tumors: the individualized cancer therapy (iCat) study. JAMA Oncol 2016;2(5):608–15.

143. ClinicalTrials.gov. Targeted therapy directed by genetic testing in treating pediatric patients with relapsed or refractory advanced solid tumors, non-Hodgkin lymphomas, or histiocytic disorders (The Pediatric MATCH Screening Trial). Bethesda, Maryland: Medicine USNLo; 2017. Available at: https://clinicaltrials.gov/ct2/show/NCT03155620. Accessed June 18, 2021.

144. Gatta G, van der Zwan JM, Casali PG, et al. Rare cancers are not so rare: the rare cancer burden in Europe. Eur J Cancer 2011;47(17):2493–511.

145. Landier W, Skinner R, Wallace WH, et al. Surveillance for Late Effects in Childhood Cancer Survivors. J Clin Oncol 2018;36(21):2216–22.

146. Michel G, Mulder RL, van der Pal HJH, et al. Evidence-based recommendations for the organization of long-term follow-up care for childhood and adolescent cancer survivors: a report from the PanCareSurFup Guidelines Working Group. J Cancer Surviv 2019;13(5):759–72.

147. Armstrong GT, Liu Q, Yasui Y, et al. Late mortality among 5-year survivors of childhood cancer: a summary from the Childhood Cancer Survivor Study. J Clin Oncol 2009;27(14):2328–38.

148. Parsons DW, Roy A, Yang Y, et al. Diagnostic yield of clinical tumor and germline whole-exome sequencing for children with solid tumors. JAMA Oncol 2016;2(5):616–24.

149. Zhang J, Walsh MF, Wu G, et al. Germline mutations in predisposition genes in pediatric cancer. N Engl J Med 2015;373(24):2336–46.

150. Ripperger T, Bielack SS, Borkhardt A, et al. Childhood cancer predisposition syndromes-A concise review and recommendations by the Cancer Predisposition Working Group of the Society for Pediatric Oncology and Hematology. Am J Med Genet A 2017;173(4):1017–37.

151. Bozic I, Antal T, Ohtsuki H, et al. Accumulation of driver and passenger mutations during tumor progression. Proc Natl Acad Sci U S A 2010;107(43):18545–50.

152. Lee JA. Solid tumors in children and adolescents. J Korean Med Sci 2018;33(41):e269.

153. Hudson MM, Link MP, Simone JV. Milestones in the curability of pediatric cancers. J Clin Oncol 2014;32(23):2391–7.

154. Chalmers ZR, Connelly CF, Fabrizio D, et al. Analysis of 100,000 human cancer genomes reveals the landscape of tumor mutational burden. Genome Med 2017;9(1):34.

155. Samstein RM, Lee CH, Shoushtari AN, et al. Tumor mutational load predicts survival after immunotherapy across multiple cancer types. Nat Genet 2019;51(2):202–6.

156. Cristescu R, Mogg R, Ayers M, et al. Pan-tumor genomic biomarkers for PD-1 checkpoint blockade-based immunotherapy. Science 2018;362(6411):eaar3593.

157. Shlien A, Campbell BB, de Borja R, et al. Combined hereditary and somatic mutations of replication error repair genes result in rapid onset of ultra-hypermutated cancers. Nat Genet 2015;47(3):257–62.

158. Koch L. Cancer genomics: the driving force of cancer evolution. Nat Rev Genet 2017;18(12):703.

159. Kamihara J, Paulson V, Breen MA, et al. DICER1-associated central nervous system sarcoma in children: comprehensive clinicopathologic and genetic analysis of a newly described rare tumor. Mod Pathol 2020;33(10):1910–21.

160. de Kock L, Priest JR, Foulkes WD, et al. An update on the central nervous system manifestations of DICER1 syndrome. Acta Neuropathol 2019;139(4):689–701.

161. de Kock L, Sabbaghian N, Druker H, et al. Germline and somatic DICER1 mutations in pineoblastoma. Acta Neuropathol 2014;128(4):583–95.

162. de Kock L, Sabbaghian N, Plourde F, et al. Pituitary blastoma: a pathognomonic feature of germ-line DICER1 mutations. Acta Neuropathol 2014;128(1):111–22.

163. Foulkes WD, Priest JR, Duchaine TF. DICER1: mutations, microRNAs and mechanisms. Nat Rev Cancer 2014;14(10):662–72.

164. Koelsche C, Mynarek M, Schrimpf D, et al. Primary intracranial spindle cell sarcoma with rhabdomyosarcoma-like features share a highly distinct methylation profile and DICER1 mutations. Acta Neuropathol 2018;136(2):327–37.

165. Wu MK, Vujanic GM, Fahiminiya S, et al. Anaplastic sarcomas of the kidney are characterized by DICER1 mutations. Mod Pathol 2018;31(1):169–78.

166. Jasperson KW, Patel SG, Ahnen DJ. APC-Associated Polyposis Conditions. 1998 Dec 18 [Updated 2017 Feb 2]. In: Adam MP, Ardinger HH, Pagon RA, et al., editors. GeneReviews® [Internet]. Seattle (WA): University of Washington, Seattle; 1993-2021. Available at: https://www.ncbi.nlm.nih.gov/books/NBK1345/.

167. Allanson JE, Roberts AE. Noonan Syndrome. 2001 Nov 15 [Updated 2019 Aug 8]. In: Adam MP, Ardinger HH, Pagon RA, et al., editors. GeneReviews® [Internet]. Seattle (WA): University of Washington, Seattle; 1993-2021. Available at: https://www.ncbi.nlm.nih.gov/books/NBK1124/.

168. Dome JS, Huff V. Wilms Tumor Predisposition. 2003 Dec 19 [Updated 2016 Oct 20]. In: Adam MP, Ardinger HH, Pagon RA, et al., editors. GeneReviews® [Internet]. Seattle (WA): University of Washington, Seattle; 1993-2021. Available at: https://www.ncbi.nlm.nih.gov/books/NBK1294/.

169. Ehrlich PF, Chi YY, Chintagumpala MM, et al. Results of treatment for patients with multicentric or bilaterally predisposed unilateral Wilms tumor (AREN0534): a report from the Children's Oncology Group. Cancer 2020;126(15):3516–25.

170. Astuti D, Morris MR, Cooper WN, et al. Germline mutations in DIS3L2 cause the Perlman syndrome of overgrowth and Wilms tumor susceptibility. Nat Genet 2012;44(3):277–84.

171. Eng C. Multiple Endocrine Neoplasia Type 2. 1999 Sep 27 [Updated 2019 Aug 15]. In: Adam MP, Ardinger HH, Pagon RA, et al., editors. GeneReviews® [Internet]. Seattle (WA): University of

Washington, Seattle; 1993-2021. Available at: https://www.ncbi.nlm.nih.gov/books/NBK1257/.

172. Wells SA Jr, Asa SL, Dralle H, et al. Revised American Thyroid Association guidelines for the management of medullary thyroid carcinoma. Thyroid 2015;25(6):567–610.

173. Rodriguez-Galindo C, Orbach DB, VanderVeen D. Retinoblastoma. Pediatr Clin North Am 2015; 62(1):201–23.

174. Kratz CP, Achatz MI, Brugieres L, et al. Cancer screening recommendations for individuals with Li-Fraumeni syndrome. Clin Cancer Res 2017; 23(11):e38–45.

175. Schneider K, Zelley K, Nichols KE, et al. Li-Fraumeni Syndrome. 1999 Jan 19 [Updated 2019 Nov 21]. In: Adam MP, Ardinger HH, Pagon RA, et al., editors. GeneReviews® [Internet]. Seattle (WA): University of Washington, Seattle; 1993-2021. Available at: https://www.ncbi.nlm.nih.gov/books/NBK1311/.

176. Bakry D, Aronson M, Durno C, et al. Genetic and clinical determinants of constitutional mismatch repair deficiency syndrome: report from the constitutional mismatch repair deficiency consortium. Eur J Cancer 2014;50(5):987–96.

177. Tabori U, Hansford JR, Achatz MI, et al. Clinical management and tumor surveillance recommendations of inherited mismatch repair deficiency in childhood. Clin Cancer Res 2017;23(11):e32–7.

178. Coury SA, Schneider KA, Schienda J, et al. Recognizing and managing children with a pediatric cancer predisposition syndrome: a guide for the pediatrician. Pediatr Ann 2018;47(5):e204–16.

179. Scollon S, Anglin AK, Thomas M, et al. A comprehensive review of pediatric tumors and associated cancer predisposition syndromes. J Genet Couns 2017;26(3):387–434.

180. Kesserwan C, Friedman Ross L, Bradbury AR, et al. The advantages and challenges of testing children for heritable predisposition to cancer. Am Soc Clin Oncol Educ Book 2016;35:251–69.

181. Groisberg R, Roszik J, Conley A, et al. The role of next-generation sequencing in sarcomas: evolution from light microscope to molecular microscope. Curr Oncol Rep 2017;19(12):78.

182. Pinches RS, Clinton CM, Ward A, et al. Making the most of small samples: optimization of tissue allocation of pediatric solid tumors for clinical and research use. Pediatr Blood Cancer 2020;67(9): e28326.

183. Louis DN, Perry A, Reifenberger G, et al. The 2016 World Health Organization classification of tumors of the central nervous system: a summary. Acta Neuropathol 2016;131(6):803–20.

184. Leonard JP, Martin P, Roboz GJ. Practical implications of the 2016 revision of the World Health Organization classification of lymphoid and myeloid neoplasms and acute leukemia. J Clin Oncol 2017;35(23):2708–15.

185. Kallen ME, Hornick JL. The 2020 WHO classification: what's new in soft tissue tumor pathology? Am J Surg Pathol 2020;45(1):e1–23.

186. Lee SC. Diffuse gliomas for nonneuropathologists: the new integrated molecular diagnostics. Arch Pathol Lab Med 2018;142(7):804–14.

187. Feldman AZ, Jennings LJ, Wadhwani NR, et al. The essentials of molecular testing in CNS tumors: what to order and how to integrate results. Curr Neurol Neurosci Rep 2020;20(7):23.

Molecular Pathology of Thyroid Tumors
Old Problems and New Concepts

Juan C. Hernandez-Prera, MD

KEYWORDS

- RAS mutation • NIFTP • Hürthel cell carcinoma • Hyalinizing trabecular tumor • GLIS1
- Secretory carcinoma • ETV6-NTRK3 • Sclerosing mucoepidermoid carcinoma with eosinophilia

Key points

- RAS mutant thyroid nodules predominately, if not exclusively, exhibit follicular architecture and consist of a broad spectrum of histopathological diagnoses ranging from adenomatous/hyperplastic nodules to high-risk thyroid cancers.

- Hürthel cell neoplasms are a distinctive group of thyroid tumors molecularly characterized by near genome haploidization and mitochondrial DNA mutations.

- Hyalinizing trabecular tumor and secretory carcinoma of thyroid have recurrent GLIS1 rearrangement and ETV6-NTRK3 fusion, respectively.

- Sclerosing mucoepidermoid carcinoma with eosinophilia does not harbor mutations seen in follicular cell–derived thyroid tumors and salivary gland mucoepidermoid carcinoma.

- Immunohistochemistry for BRAFV600E (clone VE1) and pan-TRK (clone EPR17341) is emerging as a rapid, accessible, and inexpensive technique to identify targetable alterations.

ABSTRACT

The molecular signatures of many thyroid tumors have been uncovered. These discoveries have translated into clinical practice and are changing diagnostic and tumor classification paradigms. Here, the findings of recent studies are presented with special emphasis on how molecular insights are impacting the understating of RAS mutant thyroid nodules, Hürthel cell neoplasms, and unusual thyroid tumors, such as hyalinizing trabecular tumor, secretory carcinoma of the thyroid, and sclerosing mucoepidermoid carcinoma with eosinophilia. In addition, the utility of detecting actionable molecular alterations by immunohistochemistry in advanced and aggressive thyroid cancer is also discussed.

OVERVIEW

During the last few decades, there have been tremendous advances in understanding the molecular mechanisms of thyroid tumors. These discoveries have translated into clinical practice and are changing diagnostic and treatment paradigms. A remarkable milestone was the molecular characterization of papillary thyroid carcinoma (PTC) by The Cancer Genome Atlas (TCGA), which included a comprehensive analysis of 496 primary tumors and observed the PTC is characterized by highly prevalent mutually exclusive somatic alterations in *BRAFV600E*, point mutations in the *RAS* gene family, and fusions in tyrosine kinase receptors genes, such as *RET*.[1] The mutually exclusive occurrence of *BRAFV600E* and *RAS* mutations in PTC correlated with biological and morphologic

Department of Pathology, Moffitt Cancer Center, 12902 Magnolia Drive, Tampa, Florida 33612, USA
E-mail address: juan.hernandez-prera@moffitt.org

Surgical Pathology 14 (2021) 493–506
https://doi.org/10.1016/j.path.2021.05.011
1875-9181/21/© 2021 Elsevier Inc. All rights reserved.

differences. This binary obversion set the framework to categorize other genetic alterations and, in general, follicularcell derived -thyroid tumors, such as *BRAFV600E*-like and *RAS*-like.[1] Despite these important advances, some recognized dilemmas remain unsolved, and novel concepts emerged. This review focuses on 4 important topics that highlight application of molecular pathology in thyroid tumors.

THE *RAS* MUTANT THYROID NODULE

Follicular cell–derived thyroid nodules are commonly encountered in clinical practice. It is estimated that between 2% and 6% of the population has a palpable thyroid nodule, and the prevalence increases up to 68% when high-frequency ultrasound technology is used as a screening tool in individuals presenting for routine health examinations.[2,3] Identifying a thyroid nodule raises the concern for cancer; fortunately, only around 5% to 10% of all thyroid nodules are malignant.[4] The most accurate and cost-effective method for evaluating thyroid nodules, when clinically indicated, is fine-needle aspiration (FNA).[5] With the purpose of standardizing FNA reports and guiding appropriate management, in 2009, the Bethesda System for Reporting Thyroid Cytopathology introduced a widely accepted reporting schema that established 6 diagnostic categories associated with estimated risks of malignancy.[6] This system is not without flaws, as some, up to 25% to 30% of the FNAs, render an indeterminate cytology result that provides a variable range of risk of malignancy (atypia/follicular lesion of undetermined significance [Bethesda III], 6% to 18%; follicular neoplasm/suspicious for follicular neoplasm [Bethesda IV], 10% to 40%; and suspicious for malignancy [Bethesda V], 45%–60%).[7,8] To this end, the use of commercially available oncogene panels to evaluate cytology specimens with indeterminate results has become a common tool to supplement preoperative risk assessment.[9] By identifying specific mutations or gene fusions in thyroid nodules, these panels provide additional information that may influence the decision of proceeding to surveillance, diagnostic surgery, or therapeutic thyroidectomy.[10] The most common molecular events identified in thyroid nodules with indeterminate cytology are point mutations in the *RAS* gene family.[11]

The *RAS* gene family includes 3 highly homologous genes: *H-RAS*, *K-RAS*, *N-RAS*. The *RAS* genes encode highly related proteins with GTPases activity that are located at the inner surface of the cell membrane. RAS protein cycles between inactive (GDP-bound) and active (GTP-bound) forms, and when activated, the RAS protein triggers several downstream effectors, including the MAPK and the PI3K-AKT-mTOR pathways.[12–14] Once an activating mutation occurs, the *RAS* gene encodes a protein resistant to the hydrolysis of GTPase, which converts GTP into GDP, which results in permanently active GTP-bound forms and activation of downstream signaling pathways.[15] The association of RAS mutations and thyroid tumorigenesis dates back to the late 1980s when it was first described in thyroid cancer, predominately in follicular thyroid carcinoma.[16,17] Subsequently, all 3 mutant isoforms of the *RAS* gene were reported as driving molecular event in both benign and malignant thyroid tumors, and *N-RAS* seems to be the most affected isoform by an amino acid substitution at position 61 from a glutamine to an arginine (*NRAS Q61R*).[17–22]

The presence of a *RAS* mutation in a thyroid nodule does not confirm the malignant biology of the lesion, as this alteration can be harbored by a broad spectrum of histopathological diagnosis, ranging from adenomatous/hyperplastic nodules (AHN) to high-risk thyroid cancers (**Fig. 1**).[22,23] Two main problems derive from the occurrence of these molecular alterations in different thyroid tumors. First, the true prevalence of *RAS* mutations is difficult to estimate because the frequency of histologic tumor types varies significantly among reports.[24] Second, the positive predictive value (PPV) of a *RAS* mutation in thyroid nodules with indeterminate cytology when interpreted alone is difficult to establish. In a recent systematic literature review and meta-analysis, Nabhan and colleagues[25] demonstrated marked variation in the PPV of *RAS* mutations across 23 studies, ranging from 0% to 100%, 28% to 100%, and 0% to 100% in Bethesda III, IV, and V nodules, respectively. This significant heterogeneity limits the clinical application of *RAS* mutation as stand-alone marker of malignancy. Most resected *RAS* mutant tumors discovered by molecular testing of FNA specimens are either benign or low-risk tumors.[26–28] Therefore, it has been argued that an isolated *RAS* mutation in nodules with indeterminate cytology and no clinical and radiological concern for malignancy merits conservative surgical management or even observation.[26,28]

A different scenario may apply when other mutations coexist with *RAS*, particularity mutations in the promoter of the *telomerase reverse transcriptase* (*TERT*) gene. The *TERT* gene encodes the catalytic protein subunit of telomerase, which is responsible for maintaining chromosomal integrity and genome stability by adding tandem repeats of TTAGGG sequence to the end of

Fig. 1. Four RAS mutant thyroid nodules showing follicular architecture but with different histopathological diagnosis: (*A*) AHN (hematoxilin-eosin stain, 2 x 10 magnification); (*B*) follicular adenoma; (*C*) NIFTP (hematoxilin-eosin stain, 2 x 10 magnification); (*D*) follicular carcinoma (hematoxilin-eosin stain, 20 x 10 magnification). All the images taken at 40 × 10 magnification.

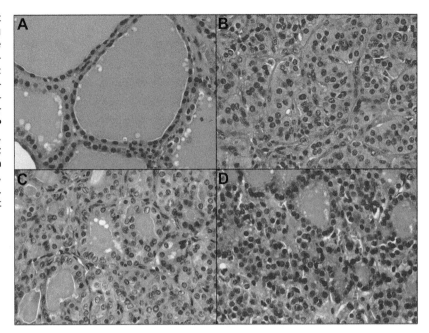

chromosomes.[29] *TERT* activation is naturally silent in most somatic differentiated cells, and when critical telomere length is reached, cells enter replicative senescence.[30] In many cancer types, *TERT* is transcriptionally activated via promoter mutation, and there are 2 common hotspots for mutations in thyroid cancer, C228T and C250T, with the former being more common. *TERT* promoter mutations have strongly been associated with aggressive behavior in well-differentiated thyroid cancer and progression to poorly and/or undifferentiated (anaplastic) thyroid cancer.[31] This association leads to the incorporation of *TERT* promoter mutation analysis in oncogene panels performed on cytology specimens.[32,33] Therefore, a *RAS* mutant thyroid nodule with a coexisting *TERT* promoter mutation is surgically excised with concern for a cancer with more aggressive phenotype. However, current clinical guidelines still do not routinely incorporate *TERT* status in the postoperative risk stratification assessment of thyroid cancer and recognize that mutations should be interpreted in the context of other clinicopathologic risk factors.[5] Other genes that can be comutated with *RAS* and appear to increase the risk of malignancy are *TP53* and *EIF1AX*.[26]

Most *RAS* mutant tumors predominately, if not exclusively, exhibit follicular architecture.[34] This might be one of the sources for the heterogenous performance of an isolated *RAS* mutation as a marker of malignancy.[23] Oncogene panels provide objective evidence of a *RAS* mutation, which contrast with the well-documented subjectivity

and interobserver variability of the histologic diagnosis of follicular pattern lesions of the thyroid. To this end, it is important to recognize that 1 study has shown that up to 50% or more of *RAS* mutant tumors could be reclassified as noninvasive follicular thyroid neoplasm with papillary-like nuclear features (NIFTP).[35] The terminology NIFTP was originally coined to rename a subset of tumors diagnosed as follicular variant of PTC (FVPTC).[36] This change emerged from the observation that tumors regarded as FVPTC lacking an invasive growth pattern have a highly indolent behavior without metastatic potential.[37–39] This difference has been further supported by the high rate of *RAS* mutations in noninvasive FVPTC in contrast to higher incidence of *BRAFV600E* mutations in infiltrative tumors.[40] These clinical, morphologic, and molecular differences led to the change in nomenclature with the purpose of reducing the psychological and clinical consequences associated with the term "cancer."[36]

The original criteria of NIFTP included an encapsulated/well-demarcated follicular pattern with less than 1% of papillae formation, tumor cells showing nuclear atypia diagnostic of PTC, absence of capsular and vascular invasion, absence of ≥30% of solid growth, absence of tumor necrosis, and absence of increased mitotic activity (defined as ≥3 mitoses per 10 high-power fields).[36] The criteria of NIFTP were subsequently revised to become more rigid criteria and included 0% papillae and lack of *BRAFV600E*-like or high-risk mutations (**Table 1**).[41] This

Table 1
Common mutations or gene fusion involved in thyroid tumorigenesis

BRAF-like Group	RAS-like Group	High-Risk Mutation Group
BRAFV600E	RAS family	TERT
NTRK3 fusions	of genes	promoter
RET fusions	(NRAS,	TP53
BRAF fusions	HRAS,	
	KRAS)	
	EIF1AX	
	BRAFK601E	
	PTEN	
	IDH2	
	DICER1	
	PPARG fusions	
	THADA fusions	

amendment was based on the observation that when the cutoff of 1% papilla was applied to noninvasive tumors the rate of lymph node metastasis was 3% and a BRAFV600E mutation was present in 10% of those cases.[42] These new criteria should not convey the message that molecular testing is required to establish a diagnosis of NIFTP. However, if a tumor with possible NIFTP features has been tested preoperatively by an oncogene panel and shows BRAFV600E-like mutation, the diagnosis of NIFTP should not be rendered. In many of these cases, extensive sampling and thorough microscopic evaluation might identify invasion or true papillae. Moreover, if a noninvasive tumor exhibits widespread and unequivocal nuclear features of PTC, a positive result for BRAFV600E immunohistochemistry (IHC) will weigh against the diagnosis of NIFTP.[43] It is important to remember that some NIFTP can harbor a BRAFK601E mutation but, unlike BRAFV600E, this alteration does not exclude its diagnosis.[44]

A problem that arises with these stricter criteria is how to designate tumors with a known preoperative RAS-like mutation that would have been classified as NIFTP, if the less than 1% papillae threshold would have not been changed. The original NIFTP study included only RAS-like mutant tumors and showed 0% risk of nodal metastasis in their cohort.[36] This observation was recently confirmed by another study that showed that encapsulated FVPTC enriched with NRASQ61 R mutations have 0% risk of nodal metastasis even if very few (<1%) true papillae are present.[45] Moreover, the recommendation that a diagnosis of NIFTP should be avoided in the presence of high-risk mutations, such a TERT promoter or

TP53, is more cautionary and requires further investigation with follow-up.[46,47]

An intriguing fact about RAS mutant tumors is that despite having a clonal molecular abnormality, many of them have the morphologic appearance of AHN, which is conceptually considered a nonneoplastic process.[22] Differentiating between an AHN from an adenoma by light microscopy might be arbitrary in some cases; however, a nodule showing poor encapsulation, variable microfollicular and macrofollicular architecture, and occurring in the background of a goitrous thyroid gland would be diagnosed as AHN by most pathologists. The observation that AHNs might be true clonal proliferations dates back to the mid-1990s, and recent study has shown that additional mutually exclusive mutations in SPOP, ZNF148, and EZH1 are identified in 24.3% of thyroid nodules diagnosed as AHN.[48,49] The presence of driving mutations in nonneoplastic-appearing nodules suggests that the tumorigenesis events start very early and support an adenoma-carcinoma sequence in thyroid oncogenesis.[50] With respect to RAS mutant tumors, this proposed sequence from an AHN to a high-risk cancer appears to correlate with the expression of genes involved in cell cycle and apoptosis, the PI3K pathway, and angiogenesis.[22] In addition, this concept allows for the existence of the intermediate category that would lie between benign and malignant thyroid neoplasms, hypothetically NIFTP.[22]

HÜRTHEL CELL NEOPLASMS

Oncocytes are cells with abundant granular eosinophilic cytoplasms typically showing round nuclei and prominent nucleoli and lacking nuclear features of PTC. Their cytoplasmic characteristics are secondary to the presence of abundant mitochondria, which stain intensively with eosin.[51] In the thyroid, these cells have historically been designated as Hürthel cells.[52] Consequently, noninvasive oncocytic follicular lesions are designated as Hürthel cell adenoma (HCA), whereas cases with capsular and/or vascular invasion are called Hürthel cell carcinoma (HCC) (Fig. 2). The classification of oncocytic follicular pattern lesions of the thyroid has been encumbered by multiple assumptions and misconceptions. First, there has been lack of agreement on what percentage of a neoplasm must be composed of Hürthel cells to be included within this group of tumors.[53] Second, it is not clear in classification schemes if Hürthel cell lesions represent a distinct entity or a variant of follicular adenoma/carcinoma.[54] Third, extensive oncocytic cytoplasmic changes can be

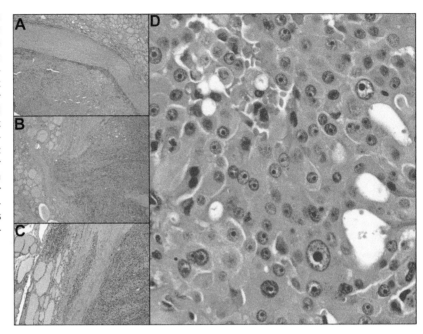

Fig. 2. HCC showing (*A*) a well-formed thick capsule; (*B*) capsular invasion; (*C*) focus of vascular invasion; and (*D*) composed of tumor cells with abundant eosinophilic granular cytoplasm with round nuclei and prominent nucleoli. *Data from* Cerami E, Gao J, Dogrusoz U, et al. The cBio Cancer Genomics Portal: An Open Platform for Exploring Multidimensional Cancer Genomics Data: Figure 1. Cancer Discov. 2012;2(5):401-404.

present in other thyroid tumor and nonneoplastic lesions.[52] Fourth, many clinicians have the belief that all oncocytic lesions of the thyroid are malignant regardless of the presence or absence of invasion.[55] To this end, molecular profiling of Hürthel cell lesions has helped in clarifying these conundrums.

The early attempts to elucidate the molecular characteristics of Hürthel cell lesions reported high prevalence of alterations in mitochondrial DNA (mtDNA) genes and nuclear DNA (nDNA) genes coding for mitochondrial proteins.[56–59] The alterations in mtDNA tend to be disruptive mutations in genes coding subunits of the complex I of the electron transport chain (*ND1, ND2, ND4,* and *ND5*).[57,60] In addition, mutations in *NDUFA13* (*GRIM-19*), an nDNA gene that encodes for proteins also involved in the mitochondrial electron transport, were reported in 16% of Hürthel cell tumors.[59] Consequently, there is impairment of oxidative phosphorylation, which induces an accumulation of dysfunctional mitochondrial as a feedback mechanism.[61] These initial observations explained the characteristic oncocytic phenotype of Hürthel cell tumors; however, the role of mitochondrial abnormalities in their tumorigenesis was not well understood.[61] Numerical chromosomal aberrations are a dominant feature that was also described in Hürthel cell neoplasms, and early reports found an association between recurrence in HCC and gains of certain chromosomes, in particular, chromosome 7.[62–64] It was also reported that HCC is characterized by near

haploidization.[65,66] Moreover, mutations in the most common thyroid oncogenes, *BRAFV600E* and *RAS* family of genes, are absent or infrequent in Hürthel cell tumors, respectively.[62,65,67]

Two recent articles providing a compressive and integrative genomic characterization of HCC support prior observations and expand the understating of these tumors.[68,69] Collectively, they confirmed that mtDNA mutations in complex I of the electron transport chain are enriched in HCC and that extensive chromosomal losses is a hallmark of these tumors with a common near-haploid state that leads to widespread loss of heterozygosity.[68,69] Gopal and colleagues[69] conducted a phylogenic analysis of tumor samples from the same patients obtained at different moments (ie, primary, recurrence, distant metastasis) and showed both abnormalities are early clonal events maintained during tumor progression and proposed them as drivers of tumorigenesis, albeit not understanding their coevolution. Ganly and colleagues[68] show that whole chromosomal duplication of chromosome 7 is a feature that correlates with tumor aggressiveness and identified multiple gene rearrangements, of which *TMEM233_PRKAB1* appears to be a functional gene fusion. Both investigator teams also described multiple somatic recurrent mutations in nDNA, but they differ from the mutational profile described by TCGA.[1] Both teams of investigators also interrogated TERT promoter variants relevant to thyroid cancer (C228T and C250T) and overall found that 22% to 32% of HCC have them and it appears that they cluster with aggressive tumors. Alternative mechanisms to stabilizing the length of the telomere, including amplifications of the TERT gene and DAXX or ATRX mutations, were seen in a minority of cases.[68,69]

Even though most studies focus on HCC, altogether, these molecular discoveries are strong evidence to support that Hürthel cell lesions are distinctive type thyroid neoplasms. The application of this finding has translated in clinical practice in the detection of DNA copy number alterations (CAN) by the newest versions of ThyroSeq V3.[70,71] This approach improves the testing ability to identify HCCs; however, CAN is not specific for malignancy.[70,71] It is anticipated that the emerging understating molecular characteristics of HCC will provide new tools for their diagnosis and prognostication in near future.

MOLECULAR ALTERATION IN UNUSUAL THYROID TUMORS

The discovery of recurrent molecular alteration in rare thyroid tumors has help to define their clinicopathological characteristics as distinct entities.

HYALINIZING TRABECULAR TUMOR

HTT was originally described as hyalinizing trabecular adenoma (HTA) in 1987 by Carney and colleagues [72] and subsequently by Bronner and colleagues[73] as paraganglioma-like adenoma of the thyroid.HTT has elicited multiple controversies, and the 2 major points of contention have been its designation as a benign or malignant tumor and its relationship, if any, with PTC.[74,75] Most reported cases of HTT have a benign clinical course after surgical resection; however, cases with lymph node metastases are rarely reported except for 1 case with distant metastasis.[74,76]

Histologically, HTT is a well-circumscribed cellular proliferation predominately composed of wide trabeculae or exhibiting a nested growth, which confers a Zellballen appearance (**Fig. 3**). Microcystic formation can be identified, and with the trabeculae, there is variable and distinctive stromal hyalinization. The tumor cells are polygonal or elongated and tend to be perpendicularly oriented toward the intertrabecular stroma. The cytoplasm is clear to eosinophilic with occasional yellow pigmented coarse granules. The nuclei are round and show membrane irregularities, grooves, and inclusions, reminiscent of nuclear features of PTC. Calcification of the intertrabecular stroma can also produce structures suggestive of psammoma bodies.[74]

There is no doubt that HTT has some morphologic overlap with PTC, and the controversy over whether these 2 tumors were related was further encouraged by studies reporting *RET/PTC1* rearrangements in 40% to 75% of HTT.[75,77] The results of these publications were challenged because of the lack of rigorous inclusion criteria and possible technical flaws leading to false

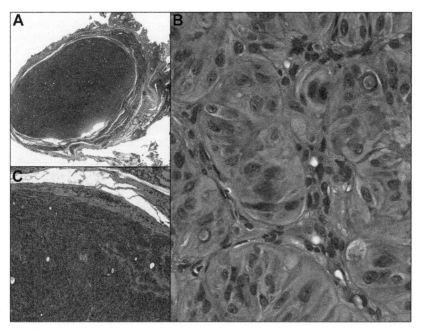

Fig. 3. Hyalinizing trabecular tumor characterized by (*A*) a well-circumscribed cellular proliferation (hematoxilin-eosin stain, Whole slide scan); and (*B*) tumor cells with eosinophilic round to oval nuclei with occasional grooves and inclusions (hematoxilin-eosin stain, 4 x 10 magnification). (*C*) Arranged in trabeculae with stromal hyalinization (hematoxilin-eosin stain, 20 x 10 magnification).

positive molecular results.[78,79] One could also argue that the reported metastatic cases of HTT probably represented true PTC that were misclassed because of the morphologic overlap.

Recently, recurrent GLIS-rearrangements have been recognized as the underlining molecular event in HTT. Using RNA-Seq technology, Nikiforova and colleagues[80] identified an in-frame fusion between exon 2 of the PAX8 gene and exon 3 of the GLIS3 gene in the index cases. The fusion is a consequence of an interchromosomal rearrangement between chromosome 2q14.1 (PAX8) and chromosome 9p24.2 (GLIS3). The investigators further confirm the presence of the PAX8–GLIS3 fusion in 10 additional cases and described an alternative PAX8–GLIS1 fusion in 1 case. None of the GLIS-rearrangement tumors harbor RET/PTC1 rearrangements or mutations in BRAFV600E or RAS family of genes. Moreover, 3 cases originally diagnosed as HTT and negative for fusion were reclassified as other tumor types (Follicular adenoma [FA] with spindle cells, HCA, PTC solid variant).[80] These observations have independently been validated by another group that further demonstrated the oncogenic properties of the PAX8–GLIS3 fusion in a xenograft model.[81]

The discovery of GLIS-rearrangements in HTT is an important hallmark that confirms the distinctiveness of this neoplasm. In addition, it also provides insight into its peculiar morphology, as fusion-positive tumors show upregulation of extracellular matrix-related genes, including collagen genes, which hypothetically lead to excessive accumulation of collagen IV deposition.[80] Importantly, available follow-up in 9 fusion-positive HTT did not report recurrences, which probably support classifying these lesions as benign and justify the original designation of HTA.

SECRETORY CARCINOMA OF THE THYROID

Secretory carcinoma (SC) is a distinctive entity characterized by recurrent ETV6-NTRK3 gene fusions.[82,83] This tumor was initially recognized in the breast, and it is regarded in that organ as a triple-negative carcinoma with a favorable prognosis predominately occurring in younger women.[84,85] SC received major attention in 2010 when Skalova and colleagues[83,86] coined the term mammary analogue secretory carcinoma (MASC) to describe a unique salivary gland adenocarcinoma with pathologic and molecular features analogous to the tumor arising in the breast. Histologically, most MASC are characterized by an infiltrative lobulated growth and fibrous septa with microcystic/cribriform, solid, tubular/glandular, follicular, and papillary-cystic structures and

intraluminal secretions.[86] The tumor cells have eosinophilic granular to vacuolated–appearing cytoplasm and typically round to oval nuclei with hyperchromatic to vesicular nuclei with inconspicuous to small nucleoli, and strong diffuse immunoreactivity for S100 protein and mammaglobin, and absence of DOG1staining is characteristic.[86–88] Similar to tumors in the breast, MASC usually exhibits an indolent behavior, although up to 25% of cases may have locoregional lymph nodes metastasis and rarely metastasize distantly. Since the initial description, additional publications have confirm the observations by Skalova and colleagues,[83,86] and interestingly, SC has been reported to occur in unusual locations, including 11 cases presenting as primary thyroid tumors (Fig. 4).[89–95]

Desai and colleagues[95] recently summarized the clinical characteristics of thyroid SCs based on the published cases and reported an apparent strong female predominance with mean age of 59 years (range, 36–74) at presentation. Most SC of the thyroid present at an advance tumor state with up to 50% cases having lymph node metastasis. Distant metastatic disease has been reported in 3 patients who subsequently died of disease.[90,91,95] Based on limited cases, SC of the thyroid appears to have a more aggressive clinical behavior compared with tumors in the breast and salivary glands. In addition, the diagnosis of SC of the thyroid is challenging, as it shares morphologic and molecular features with PTC. IHC can aid in this distinction because all reported cases have been consistently negative for TTF-1 and thyroglobulin; however, PAX 8 can be misleading, as it can show variable positivity. In addition, the strong and diffuse immunoreactivity for S100 protein is not typically seen in all thyroid SC, whereas mammaglobin appears to be a more reliable marker.[95] In breast and salivary glands, ETV6-NTRK3 gene fusion is strong diagnostic evidence of SC. This is not the case in the thyroid, as NTRK fusions have been described in a subset of thyroid cancers.[96] NTRK-rearranged PTC share morphologic features and commonly exhibit a multinodular growth with mixed follicular and papillary architecture and scattered glomeruloid structures (Fig. 5).[96,97]

SCLEROSING MUCOEPIDERMOID CARCINOMA WITH EOSINOPHILIA

SMECE is a distinct and rare thyroid neoplasm frequently arising in a background of chronic lymphocytic thyroiditis (Fig. 6). This neoplasm is arranged in infiltrative small nests, narrow strands, and anastomosing cords embedded in an

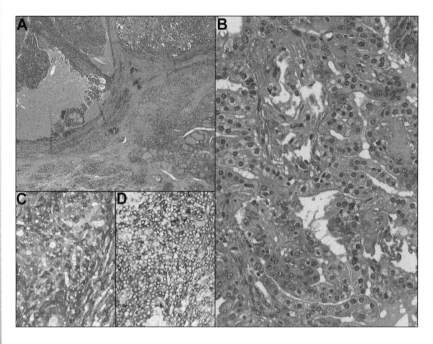

Fig. 4. SC of the thyroid showing (*A*) an infiltrative lobulated growth with microcystic/cribriform, and papillary-cystic architecture (hematoxilin-eosin stain, 4 x 10 magnification). (*B*) Tumor cells have eosinophilic to vacuolated–appearing cytoplasm and round nuclei with inconspicuous to nucleoli (hematoxilin-eosin stain, 10 x 10 magnification). (*C*) Strong diffuse immunoreactivity for S100 protein (S100 immunohistochemistry 10 x 10 magnification) and (*D*) mammaglobin S100 immunohistochemistry 10 x 10 magnification

.

eosinophil-rich dense fibrohyaline stroma. The tumor cells show squamous differentiation characterized by cohesive growth with intercellular bridges and variable degrees of true keratinization, including the formation of keratin pearl. Admixed with the squamous cell, there are neoplastic cells exhibiting glandular differentiation consisting of mucous-secreting cells and pools of mucin.[98]

Immunohistochemically, the tumor cells are characterized by strong p63 reactivity, variable positivity for TTF-1, and negativity for thyroglobulin.[99–101] Local recurrence and distant metastases are seen in approximately one-third of patients which warrants closer follow-up.[100,102]

The enigmatic pathologic features of SMECE have elicited many questions regarding its cell of

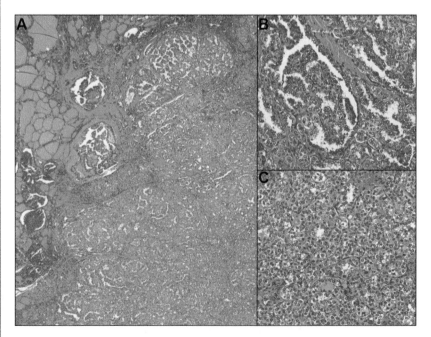

Fig. 5. ETV6-NTRK fusion positive PTC exhibiting (*A*) multinodular growth with mixed [hematoxilin-eosin stain, 4 x 10 magnification] (*B*) papillary architecture with glomeruloid structures (hematoxilin-eosin stain, 4 x 10 magnification), and (*C*) follicular architecture (hematoxilin-eosin stain, 10 x 10 magnification).

Fig. 6. SMECE arising in (*A*) a background of chronic lymphocytic thyroiditis (hematoxilin-eosin stain, 4 x 10 magnification); (*B*) tumor cells show squamous differentiation including keratin pearls(hematoxilin-eosin stain, 4 x 10 magnification); and (*C*) glandular differentiation consisting of mucous-secreting cells (hematoxilin-eosin stain, 10 x 10 magnification).

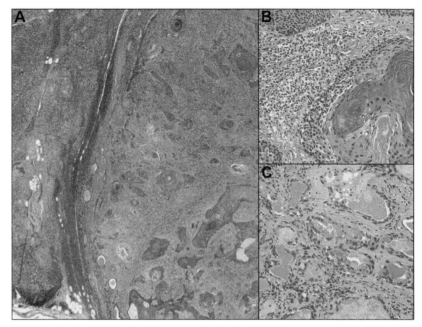

origin, and molecular interrogation of this tumor has help to exclude some hypotheses. Using next-generation sequencing targeting, Shah and colleagues[102] reported that none of 8 SMECEs harbored known and common mutations or gene fusion involved in thyroid tumorigenesis, and in addition, none of them had significant expression of thyroid follicular cell-specific *mRNA*, including *TG*, *NIS*, and *TTF1*. The cases were also tested for *MAML2* gene rearrangements by fluorescence in situ hybridization, and all of them were negative. Altogether, these findings argue against the possibility that SMECE represents a metaplastic variant of follicular cell-derived thyroid cancer or ectopic salivary gland carcinoma.

DETERMINING ACTIONABLE MOLECULAR ALTERATIONS BY IMMUNOHISTOCHEMISTRY

The treatment options based on actionable mutations for patients with advanced and aggressive thyroid cancer are expanding to include BRAFV600E mutant inhibitors, such as dabrafenib, and *NTRK* inhibitors, such as larotrectinib and entrectinib.[103] This supports the role of molecular testing in this setting, and IHC using formalin-fixed paraffin-embedded tissue is emerging as a rapid, accessible, and inexpensive technique to identify these alterations (**Fig. 7**). The monoclonal antibody clone VE1 to assess *BRAFV600E* mutations developed by Capper and colleagues[104] is the most studied and available clone. Multiple

studies have assessed the performance of this clone by comparing it with other molecular techniques, such as DNA direct sequencing and polymerase chain reaction (PCR)-based methods. In a recent meta-analysis that included 23 studies focusing on surgical resections, Parker and colleagues[105] reported a pooled sensitivity and specificity of 99% (95% confidence interval [CI]: 0.98–1.00) and 84% (95% CI, 0.72–0.91), respectively. The investigators noted that the studies that used direct sequencing as the comparing method showed slightly more false positive results (6.3%) in contrast to studies using PCR techniques (2.8%) and also reported that there is variability in the scoring criteria used among studies.[105] The original interpretation criteria introduced by Capper and colleagues[104] define a positive staining as unambiguous cytoplasmic staining of any intensity (weak, moderate, strong) for VE1 in a substantial fraction of viable tumor cells, whereas faint diffuse staining, any type of isolated nuclear staining, weak staining of single interspersed cells, or staining of inflammatory cells is considered negative. The intensity of the staining is reduced in areas adjected to tumor necrosis and impaired by temporary cryofixation, which may lead to false negative results in small biopsies and tissue samples subjected to frozen section evaluation. Adequate tissue fixation for 12 to 24 hours within 2 hours of tissue collection with 10% neutral buffered formalin appears to provide the best results.[106] Moreover, it has been shown that other preanalytical conditions of the staining

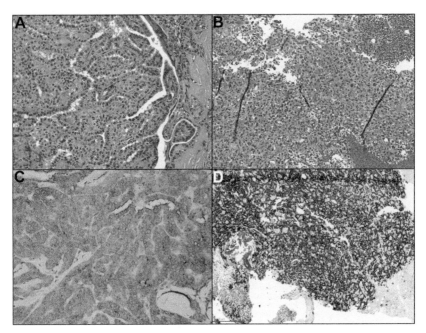

Fig. 7. (*A*) PTC showing immunoreactivity (hematoxilin-eosin stain, 4 x 10 magnification) for (*C*) BRAFV600E (clone VE1) [BRAFV600E immunohistochemistry 10 x 10 magnification]; and (*B*) anaplastic thyroid carcinoma with a confirmed *TMP-NTRK1* fusion showing immunoreactivity for (hematoxilin-eosin stain, 4 x 10 magnification) (*D*) pan-TRK (clone EPR17341) [pan-TRK immunohistochemistry 10 x 10 magnification]. (Figures B & D are *Courtesy of* Jaclyn F. Hechtman, MD, New York, with permission.)

protocol, such as antigen retrieval, are tumor specific. Zhang and colleagues[107] reported that for PTC the optimal retrieval time using EDTA is 64 minutes compared with 32 minutes for colorectal cancer.

The *NTRK* family of proto-oncogenes includes *NTRK1*, *NTRK2*, and *NTRK3*, which encode Trk A, Trk B, and Trk C proteins, respectively. The monoclonal antibody clone EPR17341 is a pan-Trk marker that reacts with a conserved proprietary peptide in C-terminus of TrkA-C. Lately, few studies have assessed the utility of clone EPR17341 as a screening tool for the detection of *NTRK1-3* fusions in solid tumors irrespective of tumor histology, and these studies have reported a sensitivity and specificity of 75% to 95.2% and 95.9% to 100%, respectively.[108,109] However, the sensitivity of the identification of *NTRK3* fusions is lower compared with *NTRK1* and *-2*, and tumor histology and organ-specific variations exist.[109,110]Cytoplasmic reactivity of various intensities above the background in at least 1% is the most common positive staining pattern seen in *NTRK* fusion-positive tumors.[110] Interestingly, additional staining patterns (perinuclear, membranous, nuclear) can be observed and correlate with the subcellular localization of the protein encoded by the fusion partner gene.[108] The utility of pan-Trk IHC in thyroid tumors is limited, and based on current available information, the overall sensitivity and specificity for detecting *NTRK* fusions are 81.8% and 100%, respectively, with a PPV of 100%. These data are promising but require further studies.

CLINICS CARE POINTS

- *RAS* mutations are the most common molecular alterations in thyroid nodules with indeterminate cytology results.

- The presence of a *RAS* mutation in a thyroid nodule does not confirm the diagnosis of malignancy.

- *GLIS1* rearrangements are the underlying molecular alterations in hyalinizing trabecular tumor.

- Secretory carcinoma of thyroid and a subset of papillary thyroid carcinomas are molecularly characterized by recurrent *ETV6-NTRK3* fusions.

- BRAFV600E (clone VE1) and pan-TRK (clone EPR17341) immunohistochemistry are clinical useful to identify targetable alterations in thyroid cancer.

DISCLOSURE

The author has nothing to disclose.

ACKNOWLEDGMENTS

The author would like to give special thanks to Dr Jaclyn F. Hechtman (Department of Pathology, Memorial Sloan Kettering Cancer Center, New York) for providing **Fig. 7**B & D.

REFERENCES

1. Integrated genomic characterization of papillary thyroid carcinoma. Cell 2014;159(3):676–90.
2. Dean DS, Gharib H. Epidemiology of thyroid nodules. Best Pract Res Clin Endocrinol Metab 2008; 22(6):901–11.
3. Guth S, Theune U, Aberle J, et al. Very high prevalence of thyroid nodules detected by high frequency (13 MHz) ultrasound examination. Eur J Clin Invest 2009;39(8):699–706.
4. Mazzaferri EL. Management of a solitary thyroid nodule. N Engl J Med 1993;328(8):553–9.
5. Haugen BR, Alexander EK, Bible KC, et al. 2015 American Thyroid Association Management Guidelines for adult patients with thyroid nodules and differentiated thyroid cancer: the American Thyroid Association Guidelines Task Force on Thyroid Nodules and Differentiated Thyroid Cancer. Thyroid 2016;26(1):1–133.
6. Cibas ES, Ali SZ. The Bethesda system for reporting thyroid cytopathology. Am J Clin Pathol 2009; 132(5):658–65.
7. Cibas ES, Ali SZ. The 2017 Bethesda system for reporting thyroid cytopathology. Thyroid 2017;27(11): 1341–6.
8. Bongiovanni M, Spitale A, Faquin WC, et al. The Bethesda system for reporting thyroid cytopathology: a meta-analysis. Acta Cytol 2012;56(4):333–9.
9. Roth MY, Witt RL, Steward DL. Molecular testing for thyroid nodules: review and current state. Cancer 2018;124(5):888–98.
10. Nikiforov YE. Role of molecular markers in thyroid nodule management: then and now. Endocr Pract 2017;23(8):979–88.
11. Valderrabano P, Khazai L, Leon ME, et al. Evaluation of ThyroSeq v2 performance in thyroid nodules with indeterminate cytology. Endocr Relat Cancer 2017;24(3):127–36.
12. Karnoub AE, Weinberg RA. Ras oncogenes: split personalities. Nat Rev Mol Cell Biol 2008;9(7): 517–31.
13. Wood KW, Sarnecki C, Roberts TM, et al. ras mediates nerve growth factor receptor modulation of three signal-transducing protein kinases: MAP kinase, Raf-1, and RSK. Cell 1992;68(6):1041–50.
14. Rodriguez-Viciana P, Warne PH, Dhand R, et al. Phosphatidylinositol-3-OH kinase as a direct target of Ras. Nature 1994;370(6490):527–32.
15. McGrath JP, Capon DJ, Goeddel DV, et al. Comparative biochemical properties of normal and activated human ras p21 protein. Nature 1984; 310(5979):644–9.
16. Suarez H, Du Villard J, Caillou BA, et al. Detection of activated ras oncogenes in human thyroid carcinomas. Oncogene 1988;2(4):403.
17. Lemoine NR, Mayall ES, Wyllie FS, et al. Activated ras oncogenes in human thyroid cancers. Cancer Res 1988;48(16):4459–63.
18. Vasko V, Ferrand M, Di Cristofaro J, et al. Specific pattern of RAS oncogene mutations in follicular thyroid tumors. J Clin Endocrinol Metab 2003;88(6): 2745–52.
19. Lemoine N, Mayall E, Wyllie F, et al. High frequency of ras oncogene activation in all stages of human thyroid tumorigenesis. Oncogene 1989;4(2): 159–64.
20. Gire V, Wynford-Thomas D. RAS oncogene activation induces proliferation in normal human thyroid epithelial cells without loss of differentiation. Oncogene 2000;19:737.
21. Miller KA, Yeager N, Baker K, et al. Oncogenic Kras requires simultaneous PI3K signaling to induce ERK activation and transform thyroid epithelial cells in vivo. Cancer Res 2009;69(8):3689–94.
22. Hernandez-Prera JC, Valderrabano P, Creed JH, et al. Molecular determinants of thyroid nodules with indeterminate cytology and RAS mutations. Thyroid 2021;31(1):36–49.
23. Marcadis AR, Valderrabano P, Ho AS, et al. Interinstitutional variation in predictive value of the ThyroSeq v2 genomic classifier for cytologically indeterminate thyroid nodules. Surgery 2019; 165(1):17–24.
24. Howell GM, Hodak SP, Yip L. RAS mutations in thyroid cancer. Oncologist 2013;18(8):926–32.
25. Nabhan F, Porter K, Lupo MA, et al. Heterogeneity in positive predictive value of RAS mutations in cytologically indeterminate thyroid nodules. Thyroid 2018;28(6):729–38.
26. Guan H, Toraldo G, Cerda S, et al. Utilities of RAS mutations in preoperative fine needle biopsies for decision making for thyroid nodule management: results from a single-center prospective cohort. Thyroid 2020;30(4):536–47.
27. Valderrabano P, Khazai L, Thompson ZJ, et al. Impact of oncogene panel results on surgical management of cytologically indeterminate thyroid nodules. Head Neck 2018;40(8):1812–23.
28. Medici M, Kwong N, Angell TE, et al. The variable phenotype and low-risk nature of RAS-positive thyroid nodules. BMC Med 2015;13:184.
29. Blasco MA. Telomeres and human disease: ageing, cancer and beyond. Nat Rev Genet 2005;6(8): 611–22.
30. Bell RJ, Rube HT, Xavier-Magalhães A, et al. Understanding TERT promoter mutations: a common path to immortality. Mol Cancer Res 2016;14(4): 315–23.
31. Liu X, Bishop J, Shan Y, et al. Highly prevalent TERT promoter mutations in aggressive thyroid cancers. Endocr Relat Cancer 2013;20(4):603–10.

32. Liu R, Xing M. Diagnostic and prognostic TERT promoter mutations in thyroid fine-needle aspiration biopsy. Endocr Relat Cancer 2014;21(5): 825–30.

33. Nikiforov YE, Carty SE, Chiosea SI, et al. Highly accurate diagnosis of cancer in thyroid nodules with follicular neoplasm/suspicious for a follicular neoplasm cytology by ThyroSeq v2 next-generation sequencing assay. Cancer 2014; 120(23):3627–34.

34. Gupta N, Dasyam AK, Carty SE, et al. RAS mutations in thyroid FNA specimens are highly predictive of predominantly low-risk follicular-pattern cancers. J Clin Endocrinol Metab 2013;98(5): E914–22.

35. Paulson VA, Shivdasani P, Angell TE, et al. Noninvasive follicular thyroid neoplasm with papillary-like nuclear features accounts for more than half of "carcinomas" harboring RAS mutations. Thyroid 2017;27(4):506–11.

36. Nikiforov YE, Seethala RR, Tallini G, et al. Nomenclature revision for encapsulated follicular variant of papillary thyroid carcinoma: a paradigm shift to reduce overtreatment of indolent tumors. JAMA Oncol 2016;2(8):1023–9.

37. Liu J, Singh B, Tallini G, et al. Follicular variant of papillary thyroid carcinoma: a clinicopathologic study of a problematic entity. Cancer 2006;107(6): 1255–64.

38. Rivera M, Tuttle RM, Patel S, et al. Encapsulated papillary thyroid carcinoma: a clinico-pathologic study of 106 cases with emphasis on its morphologic subtypes (histologic growth pattern). Thyroid 2009;19(2):119–27.

39. Piana S, Frasoldati A, Di Felice E, et al. Encapsulated well-differentiated follicular-patterned thyroid carcinomas do not play a significant role in the fatality rates from thyroid carcinoma. Am J Surg Pathol 2010;34(6):868–72.

40. Rivera M, Ricarte-Filho J, Knauf J, et al. Molecular genotyping of papillary thyroid carcinoma follicular variant according to its histological subtypes (encapsulated vs infiltrative) reveals distinct BRAF and RAS mutation patterns. Mod Pathol 2010; 23(9):1191–200.

41. Nikiforov YE, Baloch ZW, Hodak SP, et al. Change in diagnostic criteria for noninvasive follicular thyroid neoplasm with papillarylike nuclear features. JAMA Oncol 2018;4(8):1125–6.

42. Cho U, Mete O, Kim MH, et al. Molecular correlates and rate of lymph node metastasis of non-invasive follicular thyroid neoplasm with papillary-like nuclear features and invasive follicular variant papillary thyroid carcinoma: the impact of rigid criteria to distinguish non-invasive follicular thyroid neoplasm with papillary-like nuclear features. Mod Pathol 2017;30(6):810–25.

43. Johnson DN, Sadow PM. Exploration of BRAFV600E as a diagnostic adjuvant in the non-invasive follicular thyroid neoplasm with papillary-like nuclear features (NIFTP). Hum Pathol 2018; 82:32–8.

44. Afkhami M, Karunamurthy A, Chiosea S, et al. Histopathologic and clinical characterization of thyroid tumors carrying the BRAF(K601E) mutation. Thyroid 2016;26(2):242–7.

45. Xu B, Serrette R, Tuttle RM, et al. How many papillae in conventional papillary carcinoma? A clinical evidence-based pathology study of 235 unifocal encapsulated papillary thyroid carcinomas, with emphasis on the diagnosis of noninvasive follicular thyroid neoplasm with papillary-like nuclear features. Thyroid 2019;29(12):1792–803.

46. Guerrero D, Valderrabano P, Tarasova V, et al. Clinical significance of TERT promoter and TP53 mutations in thyroid nodules with indeterminate cytology. Paper presented at: LABORATORY INVESTIGATION. 2020.

47. Jiang XS, Harrison GP, Datto MB. Young investigator challenge: molecular testing in noninvasive follicular thyroid neoplasm with papillary-like nuclear features. Cancer Cytopathol 2016;124(12): 893–900.

48. Apel RL, Ezzat S, Bapat BV, et al. Clonality of thyroid nodules in sporadic goiter. Diagn Mol Pathol 1995;4(2):113–21.

49. Ye L, Zhou X, Huang F, et al. The genetic landscape of benign thyroid nodules revealed by whole exome and transcriptome sequencing. Nat Commun 2017;8(1):15533.

50. Xing M. Molecular pathogenesis and mechanisms of thyroid cancer. Nat Rev Cancer 2013;13(3): 184–99.

51. Tallini G. Oncocytic tumours. Virchows Arch 1998; 433(1):5–12.

52. Mete O, Asa SL. Oncocytes, oxyphils, Hürthle, and Askanazy cells: morphological and molecular features of oncocytic thyroid nodules. Endocr Pathol 2010;21(1):16–24.

53. Lloyd R, Osamura R, Klöppel G, et al. WHO classification of tumours of endocrine organs. 4th edn. Lyon: France International Agency for Research on Cancer (IARC); 2017.

54. DeLellis RA. Pathology and genetics of tumours of endocrine organs, 8. Lyon: IARC; 2004.

55. Thompson NW, Dunn EL, Batsakis JG, et al. Hürthle cell lesions of the thyroid gland. Surg Gynecol Obstet 1974;139(4):555–60.

56. Tallini G, Ladanyi M, Rosai J, et al. Analysis of nuclear and mitochondrial DNA alterations in thyroid and renal oncocytic tumors. Cytogenet Cell Genet 1994;66(4):253–9.

57. Máximo V, Soares P, Lima J, et al. Mitochondrial DNA somatic mutations (point mutations and large

deletions) and mitochondrial DNA variants in human thyroid pathology: a study with emphasis on Hürthle cell tumors. Am J Pathol 2002;160(5): 1857–65.

58. Máximo V, Sobrinho-Simões M. Mitochondrial DNA 'common' deletion in Hürthle cell lesions of the thyroid. J Pathol 2000;192(4):561–2.

59. Máximo V, Botelho T, Capela J, et al. Somatic and germline mutation in GRIM-19, a dual function gene involved in mitochondrial metabolism and cell death, is linked to mitochondrion-rich (Hürthle cell) tumours of the thyroid. Br J Cancer 2005; 92(10):1892–8.

60. Gasparre G, Porcelli AM, Bonora E, et al. Disruptive mitochondrial DNA mutations in complex I subunits are markers of oncocytic phenotype in thyroid tumors. Proc Natl Acad Sci U S A 2007;104(21):9001–6.

61. Máximo V, Lima J, Prazeres H, et al. The biology and the genetics of Hurthle cell tumors of the thyroid. Endocr Relat Cancer 2012;19(4):R131–47.

62. Tallini G, Hsueh A, Liu S, et al. Frequent chromosomal DNA unbalance in thyroid oncocytic (Hürthle cell) neoplasms detected by comparative genomic hybridization. Lab Invest 1999;79(5):547–55.

63. Wada N, Duh Q-Y, Miura D, et al. Chromosomal aberrations by comparative genomic hybridization in Hürthle cell thyroid carcinomas are associated with tumor recurrence. J Clin Endocrinol Metab 2002;87(10):4595–601.

64. Erickson LA, Jalal SM, Goellner JR, et al. Analysis of Hurthle cell neoplasms of the thyroid by interphase fluorescence in situ hybridization. Am J Surg Pathol 2001;25(7):911–7.

65. Corver WE, Ruano D, Weijers K, et al. Genome haploidisation with chromosome 7 retention in oncocytic follicular thyroid carcinoma. PLoS One 2012;7(6):e38287.

66. Corver WE, van Wezel T, Molenaar K, et al. Near-haploidization significantly associates with oncocytic adrenocortical, thyroid, and parathyroid tumors but not with mitochondrial DNA mutations. Genes Chromosomes Cancer 2014;53(10):833–44.

67. Ganly I, Ricarte Filho J, Eng S, et al. Genomic dissection of Hurthle cell carcinoma reveals a unique class of thyroid malignancy. J Clin Endocrinol Metab 2013;98(5):E962–72.

68. Ganly I, Makarov V, Deraje S, et al. Integrated genomic analysis of Hürthle cell cancer reveals oncogenic drivers, recurrent mitochondrial mutations, and unique chromosomal landscapes. Cancer Cell 2018;34(2):256–70.e5.

69. Gopal RK, Kübler K, Calvo SE, et al. Widespread chromosomal losses and mitochondrial DNA alterations as genetic drivers in Hürthle cell carcinoma. Cancer Cell 2018;34(2):242–55.e5.

70. Nikiforova MN, Mercurio S, Wald AI, et al. Analytical performance of the ThyroSeq v3 genomic classifier for cancer diagnosis in thyroid nodules. Cancer 2018;124(8):1682–90.

71. Steward DL, Carty SE, Sippel RS, et al. Performance of a multigene genomic classifier in thyroid nodules with indeterminate cytology: a prospective blinded multicenter study. JAMA Oncol 2019;5(2):204–12.

72. Carney JA, Ryan J, Goellner JR. Hyalinizing trabecular adenoma of the thyroid gland. Am J Surg Pathol 1987;11(8):583–91.

73. Bronner M. PLAT: paraganglioma-like adenomas of the thyroid. Surg Pathol 1988;1:383–9.

74. Carney JA, Hirokawa M, Lloyd RV, et al. Hyalinizing trabecular tumors of the thyroid gland are almost all benign. Am J Surg Pathol 2008;32(12):1877–89.

75. Cheung CC, Boerner SL, MacMillan CM, et al. Hyalinizing trabecular tumor of the thyroid: a variant of papillary carcinoma proved by molecular genetics. Am J Surg Pathol 2000;24(12):1622–6.

76. McCluggage WG, Sloan JM. Hyalinizing trabecular carcinoma of thyroid gland. Histopathology 1996; 28(4):357–62.

77. Papotti M, Volante M, Giuliano A, et al. RET/PTC activation in hyalinizing trabecular tumors of the thyroid. Am J Surg Pathol 2000;24(12):1615–21.

78. LiVolsi VA. Hyalinizing trabecular tumor of the thyroid: adenoma, carcinoma, or neoplasm of uncertain malignant potential? Am J Surg Pathol 2000; 24(12):1683–4.

79. Lloyd RV. Hyalinizing trabecular tumors of the thyroid: a variant of papillary carcinoma? Adv Anat Pathol 2002;9(1):7–11.

80. Nikiforova MN, Nikitski AV, Panebianco F, et al. GLIS rearrangement is a genomic hallmark of hyalinizing trabecular tumor of the thyroid gland. Thyroid 2019;29(2):161–73.

81. Marchiò C, Da Cruz Paula A, Gularte-Merida R, et al. PAX8-GLIS3 gene fusion is a pathognomonic genetic alteration of hyalinizing trabecular tumors of the thyroid. Mod Pathol 2019;32(12):1734–43.

82. Tognon C, Knezevich SR, Huntsman D, et al. Expression of the ETV6-NTRK3 gene fusion as a primary event in human secretory breast carcinoma. Cancer Cell 2002;2(5):367–76.

83. Skalova A, Vanecek T, Sima R, et al. Mammary analogue secretory carcinoma of salivary glands, containing the ETV6-NTRK3 fusion gene: a hitherto undescribed salivary gland tumor entity. Am J Surg Pathol 2010;34(5):599–608.

84. McDivitt RW, Stewart FW. Breast carcinoma in children. JAMA 1966;195(5):388–90.

85. Vasudev P, Onuma K. Secretory breast carcinoma: unique, triple-negative carcinoma with a favorable prognosis and characteristic molecular expression. Arch Pathol Lab Med 2011;135(12):1606–10.

86. Skalova A, Bell D, Bishop JA, et al. Secretory carcinoma. In: El-Naggar AK, Chan JKC, Grandis JR, et al, editors. World Health Organization

classification of tumours: pathology and genetics of head and neck tumours. 4th ed. Lyon: IARC Press; 2017. p. 177–8.

87. Bishop JA, Yonescu R, Batista D, et al. Utility of mammaglobin immunohistochemistry as a proxy marker for the ETV6-NTRK3 translocation in the diagnosis of salivary mammary analogue secretory carcinoma. Hum Pathol 2013;44(10):1982–8.

88. Said-Al-Naief N, Carlos R, Vance GH, et al. Combined DOG1 and mammaglobin immunohistochemistry is comparable to ETV6-breakapart analysis for differentiating between papillary cystic variants of acinic cell carcinoma and mammary analogue secretory carcinoma. Int J Surg Pathol 2017;25(2):127–40.

89. Dogan S, Wang L, Ptashkin RN, et al. Mammary analog secretory carcinoma of the thyroid gland: a primary thyroid adenocarcinoma harboring ETV6-NTRK3 fusion. Mod Pathol 2016;29(9):985–95.

90. Reynolds S, Shaheen M, Olson G, et al. A case of primary mammary analog secretory carcinoma (MASC) of the thyroid masquerading as papillary thyroid carcinoma: potentially more than a one off. Head Neck Pathol 2016;10(3):405–13.

91. Dettloff J, Seethala RR, Stevens TM, et al. Mammary analog secretory carcinoma (MASC) involving the thyroid gland: a report of the first 3 cases. Head Neck Pathol 2017;11(2):124–30.

92. Wu EY, Lebastchi J, Marqusee E, et al. A case of primary secretory carcinoma of the thyroid with high-grade features. Histopathology 2017;71(4):665–9.

93. Asa SL, Mete O. An unusual salivary gland tumor mimicking papillary thyroid carcinoma: mammary analog secretory carcinoma. Front Endocrinol 2018;9:555.

94. Liao H, Khan A, Miron PM, et al. Mammary analogue secretory carcinoma of the thyroid mimicking locally advanced papillary thyroid carcinoma: a rare case report. Int J Surg Pathol 2018;26(5):459–63.

95. Desai MA, Mehrad M, Ely KA, et al. Secretory carcinoma of the thyroid gland: report of a highly aggressive case clinically mimicking undifferentiated carcinoma and review of the literature. Head Neck Pathol 2019;13(4):562–72.

96. Seethala RR, Chiosea SI, Liu CZ, et al. Clinical and morphologic features of ETV6-NTRK3 translocated papillary thyroid carcinoma in an adult population without radiation exposure. Am J Surg Pathol 2017;41(4):446–57.

97. Chu Y-H, Dias-Santagata D, Farahani AA, et al. Clinicopathologic and molecular characterization of NTRK-rearranged thyroid carcinoma (NRTC). Mod Pathol 2020;33(11):2186–97.

98. Chan JK, Albores-Saavedra J, Battifora H, et al. Sclerosing mucoepidermoid thyroid carcinoma with eosinophilia. A distinctive low-grade malignancy arising from the metaplastic follicles of Hashimoto's thyroiditis. Am J Surg Pathol 1991;15(5):438–48.

99. Hunt JL, LiVolsi VA, Barnes EL. p63 expression in sclerosing mucoepidermoid carcinomas with eosinophilia arising in the thyroid. Mod Pathol 2004;17(5):526–9.

100. Quiroga-Garza G, Lee JH, El-Naggar A, et al. Sclerosing mucoepidermoid carcinoma with eosinophilia of the thyroid: more aggressive than previously reported. Hum Pathol 2015;46(5):725–31.

101. Albores-Saavedra J, Gu X, Luna MA. Clear cells and thyroid transcription factor I reactivity in sclerosing mucoepidermoid carcinoma of the thyroid gland. Ann Diagn Pathol 2003;7(6):348–53.

102. Shah AA, La Fortune K, Miller C, et al. Thyroid sclerosing mucoepidermoid carcinoma with eosinophilia: a clinicopathologic and molecular analysis of a distinct entity. Mod Pathol 2017;30(3):329–39.

103. National Comprehensive Cancer Network. Thyroid cancer (version 2.2020). www.nccn.org/professionals/physician_gls/pdf/thyroid.pdf. [Accessed 25 November 2020].

104. Capper D, Preusser M, Habel A, et al. Assessment of BRAF V600E mutation status by immunohistochemistry with a mutation-specific monoclonal antibody. Acta Neuropathol 2011;122(1):11–9.

105. Parker KG, White MG, Cipriani NA. Comparison of molecular methods and BRAF immunohistochemistry (VE1 Clone) for the detection of BRAF V600E mutation in papillary thyroid carcinoma: a meta-analysis. Head Neck Pathol 2020;14(4):1067–79.

106. Dvorak K, Aggeler B, Palting J, et al. Immunohistochemistry with the anti-BRAF V600E (VE1) antibody: impact of pre-analytical conditions and concordance with DNA sequencing in colorectal and papillary thyroid carcinoma. Pathology 2014;46(6):509–17.

107. Zhang X, Wang L, Wang J, et al. Immunohistochemistry is a feasible method to screen BRAF V600E mutation in colorectal and papillary thyroid carcinoma. Exp Mol Pathol 2018;105(1):153–9.

108. Hechtman JF, Benayed R, Hyman DM, et al. Pan-Trk immunohistochemistry is an efficient and reliable screen for the detection of NTRK fusions. Am J Surg Pathol 2017;41(11):1547–51.

109. Gatalica Z, Xiu J, Swensen J, et al. Molecular characterization of cancers with NTRK gene fusions. Mod Pathol 2019;32(1):147–53.

110. Solomon JP, Linkov I, Rosado A, et al. NTRK fusion detection across multiple assays and 33,997 cases: diagnostic implications and pitfalls. Mod Pathol 2020;33(1):38–46.

Pan-Cancer Molecular Biomarkers
A Paradigm Shift in Diagnostic Pathology

Fei Dong, MD

KEYWORDS

• Molecular pathology • Next-generation sequencing • Targeted therapy • Cancer biomarkers

Key points

- Clinical-grade next-generation sequencing has enabled the accurate identification of pan-cancer biomarkers.
- Targetable molecular alterations are shared between cancers from multiple anatomic sites.
- Some molecular biomarkers predict response to therapy regardless of the histologic diagnosis.
- New approaches to clinical trial design and the regulatory environment contribute to the increasing availability of new molecularly targeted therapies.

SYNOPSIS

The rapid adoption of next-generation sequencing in clinical oncology has enabled the detection of molecular biomarkers shared between multiple tumor types. These pan-cancer biomarkers include sequence-altering mutations, copy number changes, gene rearrangements, and mutational signatures and have been demonstrated to predict response to targeted therapy. This article reviews issues surrounding current and emerging pan-cancer molecular biomarkers in clinical oncology: technological advances that enable the broad detection of cancer mutations across hundreds of genes, the spectrum of driver and passenger mutations derived from human cancer genomes, and implications for patient care now and in the near future.

OVERVIEW

Cancer is traditionally classified based on tissue of origin and the morphologic relatedness between neoplastic cells and normal anatomic structures. This system of classification is embedded within the vocabulary of surgical pathology. The broad differential diagnosis of malignant neoplasms, carcinoma, sarcoma, lymphoma, and so forth, reflects derivation from epithelial, mesenchymal, or hematopoietic cell lineages and forms the basis of all subsequent diagnostic analysis. Traditional pathologic classification is extremely powerful. The anatomic pathologic diagnosis represents the clinical gold standard for informing prognosis and treatment selection.[1]

Advances in molecular diagnostics have identified key genetic alterations that drive the biology of neoplastic disorders. Discoveries of BCR-ABL1 translocations in chronic myelogenous leukemia and EGFR mutations in lung adenocarcinoma have led to the development of small-molecule inhibitors to specifically target the vulnerabilities of tumor cells at a molecular level, ushering in a new era of precision medicine.[2,3] For surgical pathologists, much of the interest in molecular diagnostics has been focused on identifying disease-specific mutations that can assist with traditional classification. However, cancer genetics is complex, and oncogenic mutations are frequently nonspecific and shared across different cancer types. For

The author has no conflict of interest to disclose.
Department of Pathology, Brigham and Women's Hospital, 75 Francis Street, Boston, MA 02115, USA
E-mail address: fdong1@bwh.harvard.edu

Surgical Pathology 14 (2021) 507–516
https://doi.org/10.1016/j.path.2021.05.012
1875-9181/21/© 2021 Elsevier Inc. All rights reserved.

example, recurrent gene rearrangements involving *ALK* are present in anaplastic large-cell lymphoma, inflammatory myofibroblastic tumor, lung adenocarcinoma, and other cancers.[4–6] Targeting *ALK*-rearranged cancers with small-molecule inhibitors has been associated with therapeutic response in multiple cancer types.[7,8]

Several recent approvals of cancer therapies by the Food and Drug Administration (FDA) have been based on molecular biomarkers without consideration of primary tumor site. These approvals represent a paradigm shift in diagnostic pathology and medical oncology. Larotrectinib and entrectinib, tyrosine kinase inhibitors, have been approved for solid tumors with NTRK gene fusions.[9–11] Pembrolizumab, an immune checkpoint inhibitor, has been approved for solid tumors with microsatellite instability[12] as well as solid tumors with high-tumor mutational burden.[13] These therapeutic indications reflect an evolution in clinical practice in which advanced molecular testing, specifically next-generation sequencing, has become standard of care for patients with cancer, and molecular results are more informative than microscopic diagnosis for therapy selection in some situations.

THE EMERGENCE OF PAN-CANCER MOLECULAR BIOMARKERS HAS BEEN ENABLED BY TECHNOLOGICAL ADVANCES IN CLINICAL CANCER SEQUENCING

The concept of pan-cancer molecular biomarkers requires clinical-grade molecular testing platforms that are broadly applicable across multiple cancer types. Before the advent of next-generation sequencing, traditional molecular tests would analyze specific genetic hotspots for the presence of clinically actionable mutations. Lung adenocarcinomas would be specifically evaluated for the presence of *EGFR* L858R, whereas melanomas would be specifically tested for *BRAF* V600E mutation.[14,15] According to these testing strategies, pathologic diagnosis guides molecular test selection. Although a small proportion of lung adenocarcinomas harbor *BRAF* mutations, *BRAF* would not be evaluated in this context because of a lack clinical actionability at that time.

Pan-cancer analysis has been made possible by the widespread adoption of panel next-generation sequencing (**Fig. 1**). Instead of using separate targeted assays for each cancer type, molecular laboratories can now validate a single assay that tests all clinically relevant genes across multiple cancer types. Next-generation sequencing assays applied to targeted cancer genomes detect a variety of somatic mutations, including nucleotide substitutions, insertions and deletions, copy number alterations, and in some situations, structural variants, such as inversions and translocations.[16,17] Multiple laboratory-developed cancer panels have been validated for clinical testing,[18–21] and sequencing library preparation methods have been adapted to detect gene fusion events detectable from messenger RNA.[22] These technological innovations have allowed molecular laboratories to detect a broader range of mutations[23] and consolidate the testing of multiple cancer types

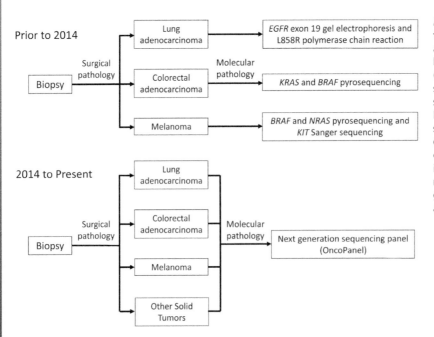

Fig. 1. Clinical molecular test selection at Brigham and Women's Hospital before (*top*) and after (*bottom*) next-generation sequencing.[21] Panel sequencing allows the molecular laboratory to streamline workflow, detect a broader spectrum of mutations, and rapidly initiate clinical testing as new indications for targeted therapies become available.

onto a single platform.[24,25] A College of American Pathologists survey in December 2014 showed that 72% of molecular laboratories had adopted or were planning to adopt next-generation sequencing within the following 2 years.[26] A nationally representative survey of medical oncologists showed that as of 2017, 76% of oncologists in the United States were using next-generation sequencing tests to guide treatment decisions for patients with advanced disease, determine eligibility for clinical trials, and prescribe off-label therapy.[27]

MANY TARGETABLE MUTATIONS ARE SHARED ACROSS TUMORS OF VARIOUS PRIMARY SITES

Large patient cohorts, such as The Cancer Genome Atlas and the International Cancer Genome Consortium, have provided insight into the genomic alterations that drive human cancer development.[28] Although understanding the full ramifications of cancer genomes remains complex, a reductionist perspective has argued that a typical cancer is defined by only 2 to 8 driver mutations, which involve a group of 125 cancer-associated genes in a handful of signaling pathways.[29] Frequently mutated pathways promote functions that are advantageous to tumor cells and have effects on cell survival, cell differentiation, and genome maintenance.

Although each cancer type has a unique distribution of mutations, many frequently mutated oncogenes in potentially targetable pathways are shared among multiple cancer types (Fig. 2). Based on these observations, the scientific field hypothesized that the efficacy of targeted therapies might be independent of tumor type as long as a targetable molecular alteration was present. An early test of this hypothesis was disappointing: BRAF small-molecule inhibitors vemurafenib and dabrafenib showed efficacy against melanomas with BRAF V600E mutation[30,31] but had little to no efficacy when used as monotherapy against colorectal cancers with the same mutation.[32,33] However, subsequent trials of another BRAF inhibitor encorafenib in combination with cetuximab, an anti-EGFR antibody therapy, showed benefit for patients with metastatic colorectal cancer after failing other therapeutic options.[34] Clinical benefit with combination targeted therapy has also been observed for patients with advanced lung cancers with BRAF V600E mutation.[35,36]

Similar treatment strategies have also been applied to other single-gene biomarkers, where standard-of-care therapies in 1 cancer type have been demonstrated to also be effective in another cancer with a lower frequency of the genetic alteration. For example, trastuzumab, a targeted antibody therapy against ERBB2 (HER2) that has long been used for ERBB2-amplified breast carcinomas, has also demonstrated efficacy against gastroesophageal,[37] colorectal,[38] and uterine serous carcinomas[39] with ERBB2 amplification. Mutation biomarkers that have been associated with at least 1 FDA-approved targeted therapy and have evidence of clinical significance in more than 1 tumor type are summarized in Table 1.

MOLECULAR BIOMARKERS BEYOND SINGLE MUTATIONS: MUTATIONAL SIGNATURES AND TUMOR MUTATIONAL BURDEN

Next-generation sequencing assays can provide more information than targetable mutational hotspots. In panels large enough to provide representative sampling of the cancer genome, patterns of somatic mutations emerge. Computational techniques by nonnegative matrix factorization have deconvoluted data from large cancer cohorts to derive several unique mutational signatures.[40] Mutational signatures reflect the underlying mechanisms of mutagenesis, such as spontaneous deamination of methylated cytosines in sporadic cancers associated with age,[41] dimerization of adjacent pyrimidine nucleic acids by ultraviolet radiation,[42] and the formation of DNA adducts by polycyclic aromatic hydrocarbons in tobacco smoke.[43]

The analysis of mutational signatures has clinical implications in some situations. Some mutational processes generate a high number of somatic mutations during the course of cancer development, and these mutations may be counted as tumor mutational burden, defined as the total number of somatic mutations divided by the genomic region covered by the sequencing panel. A higher number of somatic mutations may lead to the translation of novel peptides that can be processed into neoantigens, which may be able to elicit a response from the host immune system. Higher tumor mutational burden has been associated with favorable response to immune checkpoint inhibitor therapy for patients with melanoma,[44] non–small cell lung carcinoma,[45] and other cancer types.[46] Pembrolizumab has been recently approved for advanced solid tumors with high tumor mutational burden, defined as greater than 10 mutations per megabase, regardless of histologic diagnosis.[13]

Another mutational signature with direct clinical implications is microsatellite instability. In cancers with microsatellite instability, inactivation of at least

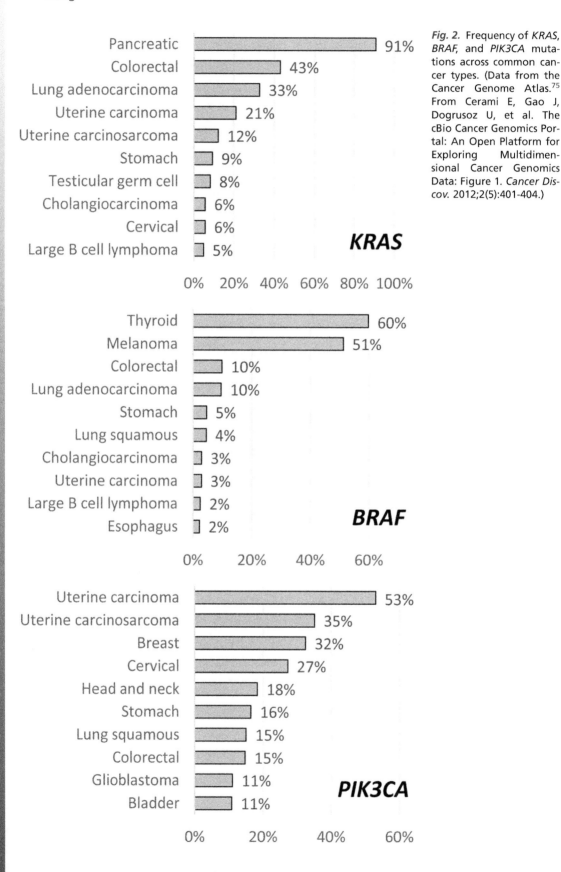

Fig. 2. Frequency of *KRAS*, *BRAF*, and *PIK3CA* mutations across common cancer types. (Data from the Cancer Genome Atlas.[75] From Cerami E, Gao J, Dogrusoz U, et al. The cBio Cancer Genomics Portal: An Open Platform for Exploring Multidimensional Cancer Genomics Data: Figure 1. *Cancer Discov.* 2012;2(5):401-404.)

Table 1
Mutational biomarkers with tumor-specific Food and Drug Administration–approved targeted therapies with evidence of clinical actionability in more than 1 cancer type

Gene	Alteration	Cancer Type	Indication	Level of Evidence
BRAF	V600E	Melanoma	Response to vemurafenib or dabrafenib with or without trametinib	FDA approval[30,76,77]
		Lung adenocarcinoma	Response to dabrafenib and trametinib	FDA approval[35,36]
		Colorectal adenocarcinoma	Response to encorafenib and cetuximab	FDA approval[34]
KRAS	Hotspot mutations	Colorectal adenocarcinoma	Lack of response to cetuximab and panitumumab	FDA label[78]
		Lung adenocarcinoma	Mutual exclusivity with other targetable oncogenic gene mutations	Practice guideline[79]
PIK3CA	Hotspot mutations	ER$^+$/HER2$^-$ breast carcinoma	Response to alpelisib	FDA approval[80]
	H1047R	Mixed	Response to PI3K pathway inhibitors	Clinical trial[81,82]
ERBB2	Amplification	Breast carcinoma	Response to trastuzumab	FDA approval[83,84]
		Gastric adenocarcinoma	Response to trastuzumab	FDA approval[37]
		Colorectal adenocarcinoma	Response to trastuzumab and lapatinib or trastuzumab and pertuzumab	Clinical trial[38,85]
		Uterine serous carcinoma	Response to trastuzumab	Clinical trial[39]
BRCA1 BRCA2	Deleterious mutation	Ovarian serous carcinoma	Response to olaparib, niraparib, or rucaparib	FDA approval[86]
		Breast carcinoma	Response to olaparib or talazoparib	FDA approval[87]
		Pancreatic adenocarcinoma	Response to olaparib	FDA approval[88]
		Prostatic adenocarcinoma	Response to rucaparib Response to olaparib	FDA approval Clinical trial[89]
ALK	Gene fusion	Lung adenocarcinoma	Response to crizotinib	FDA approval[8]
		Anaplastic large cell lymphoma	Response to crizotinib	Clinical trial[90]
		Inflammatory myofibroblastic tumor	Response to crizotinib	Clinical trial[7,90]
RET	Gene fusion	Lung adenocarcinoma Thyroid carcinoma	Response to selpercatinib	FDA approval
	Mutation	Medullary thyroid carcinoma		
FGFR2 or FGFR3	Mutation or gene fusion	Bladder cancer	Response to erdafitinib	FDA approval[91]
FGFR2	Gene fusion	Cholangiocarcinoma	Response to pemigatinib	FDA approval[92]

1 of 4 DNA mismatch repair proteins (MLH1, MSH2, MSH6, or PMS2) leads to a characteristic pattern of mutations. A hallmark feature is insertion and deletion mutations in tracts of repetitive DNA (microsatellites). Microsatellite instability was originally described as a shift in the size of the DNA repeat regions detectable by amplification and gel electrophoresis.[47,48] Microsatellite instability can also be inferred from next-generation sequencing data, either by evaluation of incidentally captured microsatellites[49–51] or by evaluation of mutations in short nucleotide repeats in coding regions.[52] These methods have been applied to solid tumors with relatively high rates of microsatellite instability, such as colorectal[53] and endometrial carcinomas,[54] as well as other solid tumors with lower frequencies of microsatellite instability, including upper gastrointestinal tract[55] and prostatic carcinomas.[56] Solid tumors with microsatellite instability have been associated with response to immune checkpoint inhibitor therapy.[57]

An emerging biomarker is a mutational signature in cancers with homologous recombination deficiency. Homologous recombination deficiency is most commonly associated with *BRCA1* or *BRCA2* loss-of-function mutations, but multiple genes play a role in the homologous recombination pathway.[58] Homologous recombination deficiency is associated with improved sensitivity to platinum chemotherapy[59] and is targetable with poly(ADP-ribose) polymerase (PARP) small-molecule inhibitors. A distinctive pattern of somatic mutations has been identified in solid tumors with BRCA1 or BRCA2 deficiency based on the pattern of nucleotide substitutions, deletion mutations, and loss of heterozygosity.[60–63] Genomic findings associated with homologous recombination deficiency have been aggregated in predictive scoring algorithms.[64] These mutational patterns have been postulated to be useful to guide prognosis[65] and predict sensitivity to PARP inhibitors for patients without detectable *BRCA1* or *BRCA2* alterations.[66,67]

NEW CLINICAL TRIAL DESIGN STRATEGIES IN THE VALIDATION OF PAN-CANCER BIOMARKERS

Although advanced molecular diagnostic testing is increasingly important in treatment selection, the clinical validation of new biomarkers does not depend on pathology alone. The availability of targeted therapies developed by pharmaceutical companies plays a major role in the clinical impact of diagnostic testing. Determining the efficacy of new therapies depends on carefully controlled clinical trials and approval by regulatory agencies.

The recent approvals of therapies based on pan-cancer biomarkers are the direct results of shifting trends in clinical trial design. Traditional clinical trials enroll patients based on cancer diagnosis or site of origin. The association between therapeutic response and molecular biomarkers may not be apparent until analysis is performed on molecular subgroups. Limitations of these methods were shown in early trials of EGFR small-molecular inhibitors in lung cancer, which did not demonstrate benefit compared with chemotherapy in a cohort of patients without *EGFR* mutation analysis.[68]

Basket trials directly test the core hypothesis of precision medicine: that therapy selection for patients with cancer should be predicated on molecular biomarkers representing direct targets or targetable phenotypes.[69] Centralized molecular testing, most commonly by next-generation sequencing, stratifies patients into 1 of several arms. Targeted therapy is provided based on molecular phenotype irrespective of the morphologic diagnosis, and patients are followed and evaluated for objective response. Basket trials have an advantage in enrolling patients with uncommon molecular alterations who may be candidates for targeted therapy. A search in PubMed for the term "basket trial" shows a steady increase in publications on this topic since 2015 (**Fig. 3**).

Last, the accelerated availability of targeted therapies associated with molecular biomarkers has been assisted by evolving trends in regulation. In 2012, the US Congress created the "breakthrough therapy" designation to expedite FDA approval for novel therapeutics with preliminary evidence of exceptional benefit. The rationale was to make effective therapies available in a more timely fashion and was in part supported by the success of molecularly targeted therapies.[70] The breakthrough therapy program, along with the accelerated approval track to expedite the availability of therapies that fulfill unmet medical needs, use surrogate endpoints, such as radiographic response, in lieu of primary endpoints, such as disease-specific or overall survival.

Despite the general excitement surrounding expedited drug approval, objective analysis has shown poor correlation between cancer drug approval based on a surrogate end point and subsequent demonstration of improved overall survival in randomized trials.[71,72] The accelerated approval of targeted therapies for tumor-agnostic indications remains controversial,[73,74] and it remains to be seen whether improvements in patient outcome can be demonstrated in randomized trials.

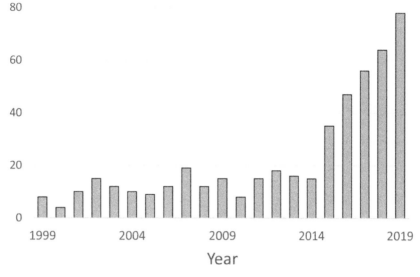

Fig. 3. Number of results on PubMed for the search term "basket trial," showing an increase in related publications since 2015.

SUMMARY

Surgical pathology has long been the standard for informing patient diagnosis and prognosis and directing therapeutic options. The integration of advanced molecular technologies into clinical practice has identified pan-cancer biomarkers that inform response to therapy irrespective of pathologic diagnosis. As of August 2020, the FDA has approved NTRK gene fusions, microsatellite instability, and tumor mutational burden as tumor-agnostic biomarkers linked to response to specific therapies for patients with advanced cancer, and the clinical, academic, pharmaceutical, and regulatory communities are clearly interested in promoting the availability of targeted therapies linked to molecular mechanisms. If current trends continue, there will be a continuing need to integrate results from advanced molecular diagnostic testing with surgical pathology to inform diagnosis and aid treatment decisions for patients with cancer.

CLINICS CARE POINTS

- Molecular diagnostics, including next-generation sequencing, is now routinely incorporated into the care of patients with advanced cancer.

- Advances in molecular diagnostic technology has enabled the clinical utilization of pan-cancer biomarkers.

- Evidence-based interpretation of molecular testing results can aid treatment decisions for patients with cancer.

REFERENCES

1. Abt AB, Abt LG, Olt GJ. The effect of interinstitution anatomic pathology consultation on patient care. Arch Pathol Lab Med 1995;119(6):514–7.

2. Kantarjian H, Sawyers C, Hochhaus A, et al. Hematologic and cytogenetic responses to imatinib mesylate in chronic myelogenous leukemia. N Engl J Med 2002;346(9):645–52.

3. Paez JG, Jänne PA, Lee JC, et al. EGFR mutations in lung cancer: correlation with clinical response to gefitinib therapy. Science 2004;304(5676):1497–500.

4. Morris S, Kirstein M, Valentine M, et al. Fusion of a kinase gene, ALK, to a nucleolar protein gene, NPM, in non-Hodgkin's lymphoma. Science 1994; 263(5151):1281–4.

5. Lawrence B, Perez-Atayde A, Hibbard MK, et al. TPM3-ALK and TPM4-ALK oncogenes in inflammatory myofibroblastic tumors. Am J Pathol 2000; 157(2):377–84.

6. Soda M, Choi YL, Enomoto M, et al. Identification of the transforming EML4–ALK fusion gene in non-small-cell lung cancer. Nature 2007;448(7153): 561–6.

7. Butrynski JE, D'Adamo DR, Hornick JL, et al. Crizotinib in ALK-rearranged inflammatory myofibroblastic tumor. N Engl J Med 2010;363(18):1727–33.

8. Shaw AT, Kim D-W, Nakagawa K, et al. Crizotinib versus chemotherapy in advanced ALK-positive lung cancer. N Engl J Med 2013;368(25):2385–94.

9. Hong DS, DuBois SG, Kummar S, et al. Larotrectinib in patients with TRK fusion-positive solid tumours: a pooled analysis of three phase 1/2 clinical trials. Lancet Oncol 2020;21(4):531–40.

10. Doebele RC, Drilon A, Paz-Ares L, et al. Entrectinib in patients with advanced or metastatic NTRK

fusion-positive solid tumours: integrated analysis of three phase 1–2 trials. Lancet Oncol 2020;21(2): 271–82.

11. Huang FW, Feng FY. A tumor-agnostic NTRK (TRK) inhibitor. Cell 2019;177(1):8.

12. Marcus L, Lemery SJ, Keegan P, et al. FDA approval summary: pembrolizumab for the treatment of microsatellite instability-high solid tumors. Clin Cancer Res 2019;25(13):3753–8.

13. Marabelle A, Fakih MG, Lopez J, et al. Association of tumour mutational burden with outcomes in patients with select advanced solid tumours treated with pembrolizumab in KEYNOTE-158. Ann Oncol 2019; 30:v477–8.

14. Ellison G, Zhu G, Moulis A, et al. EGFR mutation testing in lung cancer: a review of available methods and their use for analysis of tumour tissue and cytology samples. J Clin Pathol 2013;66(2):79–89.

15. Cheng L, Lopez-Beltran A, Massari F, et al. Molecular testing for BRAF mutations to inform melanoma treatment decisions: a move toward precision medicine. Mod Pathol 2018;31(1):24–38.

16. Metzker ML. Sequencing technologies — the next generation. Nat Rev Genet 2010;11(1):31–46.

17. Meyerson M, Gabriel S, Getz G. Advances in understanding cancer genomes through second-generation sequencing. Nat Rev Genet 2010; 11(10):685–96.

18. Frampton GM, Fichtenholtz A, Otto GA, et al. Development and validation of a clinical cancer genomic profiling test based on massively parallel DNA sequencing. Nat Biotechnol 2013;31(11):1023–31.

19. Pritchard CC, Salipante SJ, Koehler K, et al. Validation and implementation of targeted capture and sequencing for the detection of actionable mutation, copy number variation, and gene rearrangement in clinical cancer specimens. J Mol Diagn 2014; 16(1):56–67.

20. Cheng DT, Mitchell TN, Zehir A, et al. Memorial Sloan Kettering-integrated mutation profiling of actionable cancer targets (MSK-IMPACT): a hybridization capture-based next-generation sequencing clinical assay for solid tumor molecular oncology. J Mol Diagn 2015;17(3):251–64.

21. Garcia EP, Minkovsky A, Jia Y, et al. Validation of oncopanel a targeted next-generation sequencing assay for the detection of somatic variants in cancer. Arch Pathol Lab Med 2017;141(6):751–8.

22. Zheng Z, Liebers M, Zhelyazkova B, et al. Anchored multiplex PCR for targeted next-generation sequencing. Nat Med 2014;20(12):1479–84.

23. Costigan DC, Dong F. The extended spectrum of RAS-MAPK pathway mutations in colorectal cancer. Genes, Chromosom Cancer 2020;59(3):152–9.

24. Hyman DM, Solit DB, Arcila ME, et al. Precision medicine at Memorial Sloan Kettering Cancer Center: clinical next-generation sequencing enabling

next-generation targeted therapy trials. Drug Discov Today 2015;20(12):1422–8.

25. Sholl LM, Do K, Shivdasani P, et al. Institutional implementation of clinical tumor profiling on an unselected cancer population. JCI Insight 2016;1(19): e87062.

26. Nagarajan R, Bartley AN, Bridge JA, et al. A window into clinical next-generation sequencing-based oncology testing practices. Arch Pathol Lab Med 2017;141(12):1679–85.

27. Freedman AN, Klabunde CN, Wiant K, et al. Use of next-generation sequencing tests to guide cancer treatment: results from a nationally representative survey of oncologists in the United States. JCO Precis Oncol 2018;(2):1–13.

28. Campbell PJ, Getz G, Korbel JO, et al. Pan-cancer analysis of whole genomes. Nature 2020; 578(7793):82–93.

29. Vogelstein B, Papadopoulos N, Velculescu VE, et al. Cancer genome landscapes. Science 2013; 339(6127):1546–58.

30. Chapman PB, Hauschild A, Robert C, et al. Improved survival with vemurafenib in melanoma with BRAF V600E mutation. N Engl J Med 2011; 364(26):2507–16.

31. Hauschild A, Grob J-J, Demidov LV, et al. Dabrafenib in BRAF-mutated metastatic melanoma: a multicentre, open-label, phase 3 randomised controlled trial. Lancet 2012;380(9839):358–65.

32. Kopetz S, Desai J, Chan E, et al. Phase II pilot study of vemurafenib in patients with metastatic BRAF-mutated colorectal cancer. J Clin Oncol 2015; 33(34):4032–8.

33. Falchook GS, Long GV, Kurzrock R, et al. Dabrafenib in patients with melanoma, untreated brain metastases, and other solid tumours: a phase 1 dose-escalation trial. Lancet 2012;379(9829):1893–901.

34. Kopetz S, Grothey A, Yaeger R, et al. Encorafenib, binimetinib, and cetuximab in BRAF V600E-mutated colorectal cancer. N Engl J Med 2019; 381(17):1632–43.

35. Planchard D, Besse B, Groen HJM, et al. Dabrafenib plus trametinib in patients with previously treated BRAFV600E-mutant metastatic non-small cell lung cancer: an open-label, multicentre phase 2 trial. Lancet Oncol 2016;17(7):984–93.

36. Planchard D, Smit EF, Groen HJM, et al. Dabrafenib plus trametinib in patients with previously untreated BRAFV600E-mutant metastatic non-small-cell lung cancer: an open-label, phase 2 trial. Lancet Oncol 2017;18(10):1307–16.

37. Bang Y-J, Van Cutsem E, Feyereislova A, et al. Trastuzumab in combination with chemotherapy versus chemotherapy alone for treatment of HER2-positive advanced gastric or gastro-oesophageal junction cancer (ToGA): a phase 3, open-label, randomised controlled trial. Lancet 2010;376(9742):687–97.

38. Sartore-Bianchi A, Trusolino L, Martino C, et al. Dual-targeted therapy with trastuzumab and lapatinib in treatment-refractory, KRAS codon 12/13 wild-type, HER2-positive metastatic colorectal cancer (HERACLES): a proof-of-concept, multicentre, open-label, phase 2 trial. Lancet Oncol 2016;17(6):738–46.

39. Fader AN, Roque DM, Siegel E, et al. Randomized phase II trial of carboplatin-paclitaxel versus carboplatin-paclitaxel-trastuzumab in uterine serous carcinomas that overexpress human epidermal growth factor receptor 2/neu. J Clin Oncol 2018; 36(20):2044–51.

40. Alexandrov LB, Nik-Zainal S, Wedge DC, et al. Signatures of mutational processes in human cancer. Nature 2013;500:415–21.

41. Lindahl T. An N-glycosidase from Escherichia coli that releases free uracil from DNA containing deaminated cytosine residues. Proc Natl Acad Sci U S A 1974;71(9):3649–53.

42. Sinha RP, Häder D-P. UV-induced DNA damage and repair: a review. Photochem Photobiol Sci 2002;1(4): 225–36.

43. Seo K-Y, Jelinsky SA, Loechler EL. Factors that influence the mutagenic patterns of DNA adducts from chemical carcinogens. Mutat Res Mutat Res 2000; 463(3):215–46.

44. Van Allen EM, Miao D, Schilling B, et al. Genomic correlates of response to CTLA-4 blockade in metastatic melanoma. Science 2015;350(6257): 207–11.

45. Hellmann MD, Nathanson T, Rizvi H, et al. Genomic features of response to combination immunotherapy in patients with advanced non-small-cell lung cancer. Cancer Cell 2018;33(5):843–52.e4.

46. Samstein RM, Lee C-H, Shoushtari AN, et al. Tumor mutational load predicts survival after immunotherapy across multiple cancer types. Nat Genet 2019;51(2):202–6.

47. Aaltonen L, Peltomaki P, Leach F, et al. Clues to the pathogenesis of familial colorectal cancer. Science 1993;260(5109):812–6.

48. Thibodeau SN, Bren G, Schaid D. Microsatellite instability in cancer of the proximal colon. Science 1993;260(5109):816–9.

49. Niu B, Ye K, Zhang Q, et al. MSIsensor: microsatellite instability detection using paired tumor-normal sequence data. Bioinformatics 2014;30(7):1015–6.

50. Salipante SJ, Scroggins SM, Hampel HL, et al. Microsatellite instability detection by next generation sequencing. Clin Chem 2014;60(9):1192–9.

51. Huang MN, McPherson JR, Cutcutache I, et al. MSI-seq: software for assessing microsatellite instability from catalogs of somatic mutations. Sci Rep 2015; 5:13321.

52. Nowak JA, Yurgelun MB, Bruce JL, et al. Detection of mismatch repair deficiency and microsatellite instability in colorectal adenocarcinoma by targeted next-generation sequencing. J Mol Diagn 2017; 19(1):84–91.

53. Papke DJ, Nowak JA, Yurgelun MB, et al. Validation of a targeted next-generation sequencing approach to detect mismatch repair deficiency in colorectal adenocarcinoma. Mod Pathol 2018; 31(12):1882–90.

54. Dong F, Costigan DC, Howitt BE. Targeted next-generation sequencing in the detection of mismatch repair deficiency in endometrial cancers. Mod Pathol 2018;32(2):252–7.

55. Christakis AG, Papke DJ, Nowak JA, et al. Targeted cancer next-generation sequencing as a primary screening tool for microsatellite instability and lynch syndrome in upper gastrointestinal tract cancers. Cancer Epidemiol Biomarkers Prev 2019;28(7): 1246–51.

56. Hempelmann JA, Lockwood CM, Konnick EQ, et al. Microsatellite instability in prostate cancer by PCR or next-generation sequencing. J Immunother Cancer 2018;6(1):29.

57. Le DT, Durham JN, Smith KN, et al. Mismatch repair deficiency predicts response of solid tumors to PD-1 blockade. Science 2017;357(6349):409–13.

58. Konstantinopoulos PA, Ceccaldi R, Shapiro GI, et al. Homologous recombination deficiency: exploiting the fundamental vulnerability of ovarian cancer. Cancer Discov 2015;5(11):1137–54.

59. Pennington KP, Walsh T, Harrell MI, et al. Germline and somatic mutations in homologous recombination genes predict platinum response and survival in ovarian, fallopian tube, and peritoneal carcinomas. Clin Cancer Res 2014;20:764–75.

60. Nik-Zainal S, Alexandrov LB, Wedge DC, et al. Mutational processes molding the genomes of 21 breast cancers. Cell 2012;149:979–93.

61. Decker B, Karyadi DM, Davis BW, et al. Biallelic BRCA2 mutations shape the somatic mutational landscape of aggressive prostate tumors. Am J Hum Genet 2016;98(5):818–29.

62. Abkevich V, Timms KM, Hennessy BT, et al. Patterns of genomic loss of heterozygosity predict homologous recombination repair defects in epithelial ovarian cancer. Br J Cancer 2012;107(10):1776–82.

63. Birkbak NJ, Wang ZC, Kim J-Y, et al. Telomeric allelic imbalance indicates defective DNA repair and sensitivity to DNA-damaging agents. Cancer Discov 2012;2(4):366–75.

64. Telli ML, Timms KM, Reid J, et al. Homologous recombination deficiency (HRD) score predicts response to platinum-containing neoadjuvant chemotherapy in patients with triple-negative breast cancer. Clin Cancer Res 2016;22(15):3764–73.

65. Dong F, Davineni PK, Howitt BE, et al. A BRCA1/2 mutational signature and survival in ovarian high-grade serous carcinoma. Cancer Epidemiol Biomarkers Prev 2016;25(11):1511–6.

66. Davies H, Glodzik D, Morganella S, et al. HRDetect is a predictor of BRCA1 and BRCA2 deficiency based on mutational signatures. Nat Med 2017; 23(4):517–25.

67. Gulhan DC, Lee JJ-K, Melloni GEM, et al. Detecting the mutational signature of homologous recombination deficiency in clinical samples. Nat Genet 2019; 51(5):912–9.

68. Crinò L, Cappuzzo F, Zatloukal P, et al. Gefitinib versus vinorelbine in chemotherapy-naïve elderly patients with advanced non–small-cell lung cancer (INVITE): a randomized, phase II study. J Clin Oncol 2008;26(26):4253–60.

69. Redig AJ, Jänne PA. Basket trials and the evolution of clinical trial design in an era of genomic medicine. J Clin Oncol 2015;33(9):975–7.

70. Darrow JJ, Avorn J, Kesselheim AS. New FDA breakthrough-drug category — implications for patients. N Engl J Med 2014;370(13):1252–8.

71. Kim C, Prasad V. Cancer drugs approved on the basis of a surrogate end point and subsequent overall survival. JAMA Intern Med 2015;175(12):1992.

72. Davis C, Naci H, Gurpinar E, et al. Availability of evidence of benefits on overall survival and quality of life of cancer drugs approved by European Medicines Agency: retrospective cohort study of drug approvals 2009-13. BMJ 2017;359:j4530.

73. Subbiah V, Solit DB, Chan TA, et al. The FDA approval of pembrolizumab for adult and pediatric patients with tumor mutational burden (TMB) ≥10: a decision centered on empowering patients and their physicians. Ann Oncol 2020;31(9):1115–8.

74. Prasad V, Addeo A. The FDA approval of pembrolizumab for patients with TMB >10 mut/Mb: was it a wise decision? No. Ann Oncol 2020;31(9):1112–4.

75. Cerami E, Gao J, Dogrusoz U, et al. The cBio cancer genomics portal: an open platform for exploring multidimensional cancer genomics data: figure 1. Cancer Discov 2012;2(5):401–4.

76. Hauschild A, Grob J-J, Demidov LV, et al. Dabrafenib in BRAF-mutated metastatic melanoma: a multicentre, open-label, phase 3 randomised controlled trial. Lancet 2012;380(9839):358–65.

77. Robert C, Karaszewska B, Schachter J, et al. Improved overall survival in melanoma with combined dabrafenib and trametinib. N Engl J Med 2015;372(1):30–9.

78. Lièvre A, Bachet J-B, Le Corre D, et al. KRAS mutation status is predictive of response to cetuximab therapy in colorectal cancer. Cancer Res 2006; 66(8):3992–5.

79. Lindeman NI, Cagle PT, Aisner DL, et al. Updated molecular testing guideline for the selection of lung cancer patients for treatment with targeted tyrosine kinase inhibitors: guideline from the College of American Pathologists, the International Association for the Study of Lung Cancer, and the Association for Molecular Pathology. Arch Pathol Lab Med 2018;142(3):321–46.

80. André F, Ciruelos E, Rubovszky G, et al. Alpelisib for PIK3CA-mutated, hormone receptor–positive advanced breast cancer. N Engl J Med 2019; 380(20):1929–40.

81. Janku F, Wheler JJ, Naing A, et al. PIK3CA mutation H1047R is associated with response to PI3K/AKT/mTOR signaling pathway inhibitors in early-phase clinical trials. Cancer Res 2013;73(1): 276–84.

82. Janku F, Hong DS, Fu S, et al. Assessing PIK3CA and PTEN in early-phase trials with PI3K/AKT/mTOR inhibitors. Cell Rep 2014;6(2):377–87.

83. Romond EH, Perez EA, Bryant J, et al. Trastuzumab plus adjuvant chemotherapy for operable HER2-positive breast cancer. N Engl J Med 2005; 353(16):1673–84.

84. Piccart-Gebhart MJ, Procter M, Leyland-Jones B, et al. Trastuzumab after adjuvant chemotherapy in HER2-positive breast cancer. N Engl J Med 2005; 353(16):1659–72.

85. Hainsworth JD, Meric-Bernstam F, Swanton C, et al. Targeted therapy for advanced solid tumors on the basis of molecular profiles: results from MyPathway, an open-label, phase IIa multiple basket study. J Clin Oncol 2018;36(6):536–42.

86. Audeh MW, Carmichael J, Penson RT, et al. Oral poly(ADP-ribose) polymerase inhibitor olaparib in patients with BRCA1 or BRCA2 mutations and recurrent ovarian cancer: a proof-of-concept trial. Lancet 2010;376(9737):245–51.

87. Tutt A, Robson M, Garber JE, et al. Oral poly(ADP-ribose) polymerase inhibitor olaparib in patients with BRCA1 or BRCA2 mutations and advanced breast cancer: a proof-of-concept trial. Lancet 2010;376(9737):235–44.

88. Golan T, Hammel P, Reni M, et al. Maintenance olaparib for germline BRCA-mutated metastatic pancreatic cancer. N Engl J Med 2019;381(4): 317–27.

89. de Bono J, Mateo J, Fizazi K, et al. Olaparib for metastatic castration-resistant prostate cancer. N Engl J Med 2020;382(22):2091–102.

90. Mossé YP, Voss SD, Lim MS, et al. Targeting ALK with crizotinib in pediatric anaplastic large cell lymphoma and inflammatory myofibroblastic tumor: a Children's Oncology Group study. J Clin Oncol 2017;35(28):3215–21.

91. Loriot Y, Necchi A, Park SH, et al. Erdafitinib in locally advanced or metastatic urothelial carcinoma. N Engl J Med 2019;381(4):338–48.

92. Abou-Alfa GK, Sahai V, Hollebecque A, et al. Pemigatinib for previously treated, locally advanced or metastatic cholangiocarcinoma: a multicentre, open-label, phase 2 study. Lancet Oncol 2020; 21(5):671–84.

Molecular Pathology of Myeloid Neoplasms
Molecular Pattern Recognition

Sam Sadigh, MD[a], Annette S. Kim, MD, PhD[b],*

KEYWORDS

- Myeloid neoplasms • Mutational patterns • Next-generation sequencing • Clonal hematopoiesis

---

Key points

- Mutations can be used to aid the diagnosis and classification of myeloid neoplasms and are becoming increasingly important in their prognostication and disease monitoring.

- Genetic alterations, predominantly in epigenetic modifiers and splicing complex genes. accumulate with age and produce the underlying background disposition to develop myeloid neoplasms.

- Although many myeloid neoplasms share overlapping patterns of genetic alterations in common pathways, the individual players in those pathways can be quite varied with enrichment of specific genes in different diagnostic entities.

- Clonal architecture can be complex with subclonal events, convergent evolution, and clonal evolution.

- Pediatric myeloid neoplasms follow the same patterns as those in adults but lack a foundation in aging stem cells.

ABSTRACT

Despite the apparent complexity of the molecular genetic underpinnings of myeloid neoplasms, most myeloid mutational profiles can be understood within a simple framework. Somatic mutations accumulate in hematopoietic stem cells with aging and toxic insults, termed clonal hematopoiesis. These "old stem cells" mutations, predominantly in the epigenetic and RNA spliceosome pathways, act as "founding" driver mutations leading to a clonal myeloid neoplasm when sufficient in number and clone size. Subsequent mutations can create the genetic flavor of the myeloid neoplasm ("backseat" drivers) due to their enrichment in certain entities or act as progression events ("aggressive" drivers) during clonal evolution.

OVERVIEW

Myeloid neoplasms encompass a diverse spectrum of hematopoietic malignancies that are all derived from common myeloid progenitor stem cells that accumulate sequential molecular genetic alterations to confer a survival and/or growth advantage. The broad categories are the "chronic" myeloid neoplasms, including myelodysplastic syndromes (MDS), myeloproliferative neoplasms (MPN), MDS/MPN overlap syndromes, and mast

---

[a] Department of Pathology, Brigham and Women's Hospital, 75 Francis Street, Boston, MA 02115, USA;
[b] Department of Pathology, Brigham and Women's Hospital, Harvard Medical School, 75 Francis Street, Boston, MA 02115, USA
* Corresponding author.
E-mail address: askim@bwh.harvard.edu

Surgical Pathology 14 (2021) 517–528
https://doi.org/10.1016/j.path.2021.05.013
1875-9181/21/© 2021 Elsevier Inc. All rights reserved.

cell neoplasms, and the "acute" presentation of myeloid neoplasms that manifests either as "de novo" acute myeloid leukemia (AML) or the leukemic progression of any of the chronic myeloid neoplasms (resulting in secondary AML, s-AML). These main categories, as defined by the World Health Organization monograph on hematopoietic neoplasms (WHO 2017 edition), are summarized in **Fig. 1.**[1] Despite the discrete diagnostic categories, the molecular genetic underpinnings of all these entities are highly overlapping and complex such that no single mutation or set of mutations is entirely specific to an entity. However, the myeloid mutational patterns can be encompassed within a simple framework presented as follows.

PATTERNS ARE ESSENTIAL

Recurring patterns of mutations in myeloid neoplasm are easily recognized and can be much more informative than the specific mutations or specific genes involved. The broad mutational categories include genes involved in epigenetic regulation (both DNA methylation and chromatin modification); the RNA spliceosome complex; signaling pathways; transcriptional regulators; and cohesin complex, with a handful of other genes that are highly recurrent but do not fit into one of these aforementioned categories. **Fig. 2** summarizes these categories with the most commonly mutated genes within each, and the relative frequency that they are reported in the main types of myeloid neoplasms.[2,3]

The myeloid neoplasms all share a common pattern of acquisition of mutations within these pathways, but the individual genes and mutations in those pathways can be quite varied. There is an accumulation of mutations with aging and various toxic exposures, and these "passenger" mutations (typically involving noncoding sequences) do not themselves necessarily lead to pathogenesis. However, mutations within specific genes, in particular genes within the epigenetic and RNA spliceosome pathways, can occur in these aging stem cells, and, with the accumulation of additional alterations and potentially clone size over time, may lead eventually to the development of a myeloid neoplasm. These "founding driver" mutations are thought to be the initiating event in development of myeloid neoplasms. In this fertile soil there is outgrowth of subclonal events, some of which may be "backseat drivers" that may be enriched in specific disease entities; these are mutations that direct the character of a myeloid neoplasm and are often in the cell signaling pathway. Additional accumulation of mutations, the "aggressive driver" mutations, is associated with disease progression or transformation to acute leukemia, typically involving genes in cell signaling and DNA transcription pathways as well as other known progression events such as *TP53*, *SETBP1*, or additional epigenetic gene mutation acquisition. This sequential acquisition of "founding drivers," "backseat drivers," and "aggressive drivers" is schematized in **Fig. 3**, with each mutational category separately color coded. How this schema is manifest in the

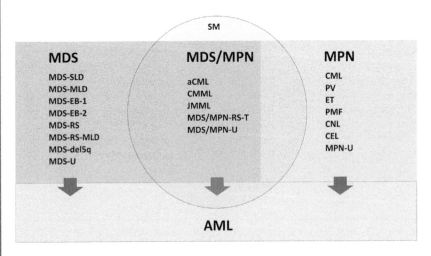

Fig. 1. Schematic of myeloid neoplasms, demonstrating the relative relationships between the chronic myeloid neoplasms (shown on *top, blue, pink, and the overlapping lavender*) and their potential progression to AML (*bottom, green*). In addition, SM can co-occur with any of the other myeloid neoplasms and is represented by the overlying circle. The specific entities recognized by the WHO within the chronic myeloid neoplastic categories are listed in their respective boxes.[1] CEL, chronic eosinophilic leukemia; CNL, chronic neutrophilic leukemia; EB, excess blasts; MLD, multilineage dysplasia; RS, ring sideroblasts; SLD, single lineage dysplasia; T, thrombocytosis; U, unclassifiable.

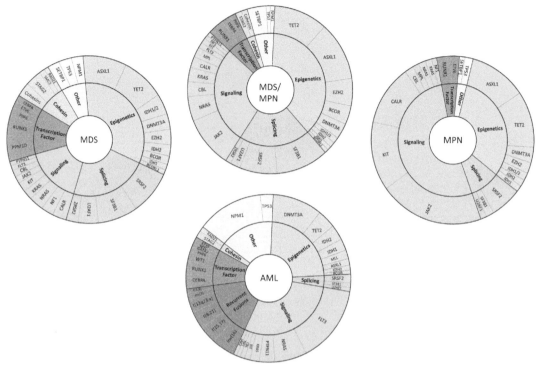

Fig. 2. Relative frequency of mutations in MDS, MDS/MPN, MPN, and AML. These plots emphasize the relative prevalence of mutations in different pathways (epigenetic in *gold*, splicing in *blue*, signal transduction in *green*, transcription factors in *purple*, cohesins in *gray*, and other individual gene categories in *yellow*). These plots do not depict the co-mutational patterns (as might be shown in circos plots) and do not represent absolute numbers. (*Data from* McClure RF, Ewalt MD, Crow J, et al. Clinical Significance of DNA Variants in Chronic Myeloid Neoplasms: A Report of the Association for Molecular Pathology. J Mol Diagn. 2018;20(6):717-737, Papaemmanuil E, Gerstung M, Bullinger L, et al. Genomic Classification and Prognosis in Acute Myeloid Leukemia. N Engl J Med. 2016;374(23):2209-2221.)

precursor states and in specific myeloid neoplasms is discussed as follows.

THE "OLD" STEM CELL AND CLONAL HEMATOPOIESIS

The normal aging process leads to the random acquisition of various "passenger" mutations in hematopoietic stem cells, approximately 14 mutations per year, most in noncoding portions of the genome.[4] However, coding sequences may be involved. When these mutations are identified in individuals with no evidence of a hematologic malignancy (even as young as 30 years old with recent reports of *JAK2* mutations identified in utero[5,6]) and normal peripheral blood counts, it is known as clonal hematopoiesis (CH; also known as CH of indeterminate potential or CHIP). The genes that are recurrently mutated in CH are the same usual suspects as those found in MDS and the rise in CH in these genes parallels the rise in the incidence of MDS.[7–10] In particular, epigenetic

genes such as *DNMT3A*, *ASXL1*, and *TET2*, occur at very high frequency in CH, and appear to be a hallmark of an aged stem cell.[8,10] Spliceosome mutations, such as *SF3B1* and *SRSF2*, tend to occur in an even older population, older than 70, and indicate an even older stem cell.[11] These mutations may confer a survival or fitness advantage in these stem cells allowing their clonal expansion, although recent studies in post–stem cell transplantation (post-SCT) suggest that this effect may be modest.[12]

CH is not benign; there is a robust association with cardiovascular disease as well as risk of developing a hematologic malignancy at a rate of approximately 0.5% to 1.0% per year.[8,13] Patients with cancer who have received certain types of chemotherapy (such as radiotherapy and certain cytotoxic agents, especially topoisomerase II inhibitors and carboplatin) or patients with smoking history have an up to a fourfold increased risk of having CH, and in these patients the CH can be associated with a therapy-related myeloid

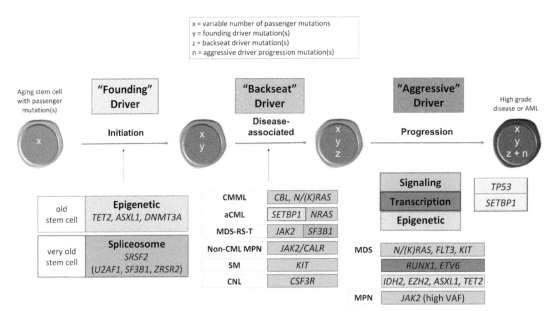

Fig. 3. Schematic of common alterations sequentially acquired in the differentiation and progression of myeloid neoplasms, adapted from McClure et al.[2] These are classified as "passenger," "founding" driver, "backseat" driver, and "aggressive" driver mutations. Below each driver category are listed the most common pathways affected by each type of driver and examples of recurrently mutated genes in these pathways. The epigenetic pathway is colored gold, splicing pathway blue, signal transduction pathway green, and transcription regulation pathway purple. CNL, chronic neutrophilic leukemia; RS-T, ring sideroblasts and thrombocytosis.

neoplasm that is particularly enriched for *PPMID* and other DNA-damage mutations that confer worse prognosis.[14–17]

Of note, CH also can manifest as mosaic chromosomal alterations (copy number variations) in addition to somatic mutations. These have been detected in patients who subsequently developed (therapy-related) myeloid neoplasms and may represent an important, but less well understood component of CH that, in combination with somatic mutations, can result in biallelic targeting of certain genes, such as *TP53*, *TET2*, and *JAK2*.[18–20] In addition, there are rare germline polymorphisms that may predispose the individual to developing CH, including variants in *TERT*, *TET2*, *DNMT3A*, and *JAK2* and in the noncoding region of *HAPLN1* enhancers.[21]

USING MUTATIONS TO DIAGNOSE, PROGNOSTICATE, TREAT, AND MONITOR PATIENTS

Myelodysplastic Syndromes

The MDSs are a group of clonal myeloid neoplasms occurring predominantly in the elderly, defined by ineffective hematopoiesis that results in cytopenia(s) and cytologic dysplasia. To date, with the exception of certain key "MDS-defining" cytogenetic alterations (summarized in **Box 1**)

and a single *SF3B1* hotspot mutation that modifies the threshold for calling ring sideroblasts, the remaining WHO diagnostic criteria for MDS are based solely on morphology. However, approximately 90% of patients with MDS will indeed harbor a pathogenic mutation when tested with a routine clinical next-generation sequencing (NGS) panel, the most frequent of which involve the same epigenetic and spliceosome genes that are also seen in CH (**Fig. 2**).[22] The extensive overlap between these gene sets precludes their use in discriminating between the old stem cell that is the hallmark of MDS and aged stem cells in CH.[23,24] Haferlach and colleagues[22] demonstrated 47 genes that were statistically significantly recurrently mutated in MDS with a median number of 3 mutations per patient.[22] Given frequent biallelic mutations in genes such as *ASXL1* or *TET2*, there are more than 100,000 combinatorial possibilities ($47 \times 47 \times 46$), not to mention the individual variants, numerous subclonal events, genes with rare mutations, cases with even more numerous mutations, and changes over time (clonal evolution). Despite this vast complexity, the overall mutational patterns remain evident, with epigenetic and splicing "founding driver" mutations, varied subclonal architecture, and recurrent patterns of progression "aggressive driver" mutations. Thus, although there are no specific mutations

---

Box 1
Recurrent cytogenetic alterations in myelodysplastic syndromes (MDS)

Unbalanced abnormalities

+8[a]

−7 or del(7q)

−5 or del(5q)

del(20q)[a]

−Y [a]

i(17q) or t(17p)

−13 or del(13q)

del(11q)

del(12p) or t(12p)

del(9q)

idic(X) (q13)

Balanced abnormalities

t(11;16) (q23;p13.3)

t(3;21) (q26.2;q22.1)

t(1;3) (p36.3;q21.1)

t(2;11) (p21;q23)

inv(3) (q21q26.2) or t(3;3) (q21.3;q26.2)

t(6;9) (p23;q34)

[a]Not considered MDS-defining.

Modified from Ref.[1] Data from Swerdlow SH, Campo E, Harris NL, et al. *WHO Classification of Tumours of Haematopoietic and Lymphoid Tissues, Revised 4th Edition.* Lyon, France: International Agency for Research on Cancer; 2017.

---

included in the diagnostic criteria for MDS (with the exception of *SF3B1*), the overall pattern of mutations can support the diagnosis of MDS through establishment of clonality (especially for cases with a normal karyotype) and indicate prognosis through recognition of the clonal evolution patterns.

Disease monitoring and therapy decisions in MDS are also increasingly based on mutational findings. Studies have shown that when mutations were monitored following SCT (either with reduced intensity conditioning or myeloablative conditioning), those patients in whom mutations persisted, even at sub 1% levels, were at risk of progression post-SCT, whereas those who completely cleared their mutations were not.[25] The specific gene that is mutated can also inform transplantation decisions. *TP53* mutations have been associated with abysmal overall survival post-SCT, which may factor into the decision of whether to pursue SCT in these patients. By contrast, although *RAS* mutations were associated with relapse, these

relapses were early and could be overcome with myeloablative SCTs when tolerated.[26]

Mutational Pattern in Myelodysplastic Syndrome Progression to Acute Myeloid Leukemia

MDS prognostication has traditionally been based on clinical criteria and cytogenetic categories; however, mutations can also be used for prognosis in MDS.[2] At a minimum, mutations in the following genes had previously been shown to confer adverse prognosis in MDS: *TP53*, *EZH2*, *ETV6*, *RUNX1*, or *ASXL1*.[27] The Cleveland Clinic has recently incorporated mutations into an online calculator where mutations in 11 genes can be used to modify the prognostic tier of MDS.[28]

Progression in the myeloid neoplasms, as exemplified here by progression from MDS to AML, follows a pattern of accumulation of mutations. Generally, the greater the number of pathogenic mutations, the worse the prognosis and association with progression to AML, providing higher correlation with time to leukemia onset for the patients with poor prognosis than the revised International Prognostic Scoring System.[27,29] These additional "aggressive driver" mutations occur predominantly in genes involved in signal transduction and transcriptional regulation pathways with additional contributions from additional epigenetic genes, and other genes such as *TP53* and *SETBP1*.[30,31] Biallelic lesions in *TP53* (including 2 mutations, mutation/deletion, mutation/copy neutral loss of heterozygosity) are particularly associated with the risk of transformation, although these cases tend to have quieter co-mutational patterns.[32] In many cases, there is a multiplicity of subclonal mutations in signaling and/or transcriptional pathways, often in the same gene or related genes, representing convergent evolution of different subclones through analogous gene mutations and pathways resulting in progression to high-grade disease. Conversely, in AML, the presence of "old stem cell" founding driver mutations in the epigenetic and splicing genes can be used to presume an underlying chronic myeloid neoplasm such as MDS, even if it was not previously diagnosed. In fact, Lindsley and colleagues[31] identified 8 genes (*SRSF2*, *SF3B1*, *U2AF1*, *ZRSR2*, *ASXL1*, *BCOR*, *EZH2*, and *STAG2*) that were 95% specific in the diagnosis of a secondary AML.

Interestingly, pediatric MDS, which can be subcategorized as refractory cytopenia of childhood (low-grade disease) and refractory anemia with excess blasts (high-grade disease) lacks the typical founding drivers (splicing and epigenetic genes) seen in adult MDS, because these patients do not have aged stem cells. Instead, they more commonly have cytogenetic abnormalities, especially chromosomal or q arm level deletions of chromosome 7, as the founding driver aberration. However, as they progress to higher-grade disease and secondary AML, they acquire typical "aggressive driver" mutations in the signaling and transcription pathways, in direct analogy to their adult counterparts.[33]

De Novo Acute Myeloid Leukemia

In addition to serving as the final common destination of MDS and other myeloid neoplasms that transform through genetic progression (secondary AML), AML can also present "de novo." In adult de novo AML, the Cancer Genome Atlas identified 9 classes of mutations.[34] Of these 9 categories, 5 are identical to those described previously in the setting of MDS with separate categories for DNA methylation and chromatin modification pathways, splicing pathway, signal transduction pathway, myeloid transcription regulation, and cohesins, with additional categories of specific transcription factor fusions, *NPM1,* and tumor suppressor genes (*TP53, PHF6*). Of these, in addition to several recurrent translocations (that are not further addressed in this article but may be identified by molecular methods in addition to more standard cytogenetic methods), the WHO specifically recognizes mutations in *NPM1* and biallelic mutations in *CEBPA* (both associated with favorable prognosis in the setting of a normal karyotype and absence of *NPM1* co-mutation with *FLT3* internal tandem duplication [ITD]), with a provisional category of *RUNX1* (associated with adverse prognosis, especially with *ASXL1* co-mutation). Although a number of other gene mutations are mentioned in the WHO, often modifying prognosis, none rise to the level of defining a specific subcategory of AML. The European Leukemia-Net (ELN) has incorporated a number of somatic mutations, in addition to recurrent cytogenetic changes, into their testing recommendations for prognosis, monitoring, and therapy.[35] Specifically, *NPM1*, *FLT3*-ITD, biallelic *CEBPA*, *RUNX1*, *ASXL1*, and *TP53* are used to classify risk in AML with stratification additionally dependent on *FLT3*-ITD allelic ratio (using a cutoff of 0.5 ITD/wild-type allelic ratio to separate *FLT3*-ITD[high] from *FLT3* ITD[low]) as shown in **Table 1**. Notably the presence of *FLT3*-ITD or *KIT* mutations has an adverse effect on the prognosis in core binding factor (CBF) AMLs, t(8;21)-AML and inv(16)-AML, which are otherwise good prognostic subtypes.[36] It has been shown in a very large AML cohort that concomitant mutations in *DNMT3A* and *NPM1* compounded the deleterious effect of *FLT3*-ITD mutations.[3]

Acute Myeloid Leukemia Measurable Residual Disease

Assessment of MRD (measurable residual disease; also known as minimal residual disease) is the ability to detect persistent leukemic disease below the level of 5% morphology-based blast cutoff. There is a growing body of evidence showing the robust utility of NGS-based molecular MRD detection in AML post-therapy prognostication. An early study identified persistent pathogenic mutations (VAFs at least 5%) in half of patients with AML who had achieved morphologic remission (at day 30, post-intensive chemotherapy induction); this group had significantly worse outcomes, with increased risk of relapse, and

Table 1
Genetic risk stratification for acute myeloid leukemia (AML) as published by the European LeukemiaNet in 2017

European LeukemiaNet (ELN) 2017 Guidelines for AML Genetic Risk Stratification		
Risk Category	Genetic Abnormality	More Recent Potential Modifications

Favorable	t(8;21) (q22;q22.1); *RUNX1-RUNX1T1*
	inv(16) (p13.1q22) or t(16;16)
	   (p13.1;q22); *CBFB-MYH11*
	Mutated *NPM1* without *FLT3-ITD* or
	   with *FLT3-ITD*[low]
	Biallelic mutated *CEBPA*
		KIT/FLT3 adverse[b]
		KIT/FLT3 adverse[a]
		Co-occurrence of *NPM1, DNMT3A,*
		   FLT3-ITD adverse[a]

Intermediate	Mutated *NPM1* and *FLT3-ITD*[high]
	Wild-type *NPM1* without *FLT3-ITD* or
	   with *FLT3-ITD*[low] (without adverse-
	   risk genetic abnormalities)
	t(9;11) (p21.3;q23.3); *MLLT3-KMT2A*
	Cytogenetic abnormalities not classified
	   as favorable or adverse	

Adverse	t(6;9) (p23;q34.1); *DEK-NUP214*
	t(v;11q23.3); *KMT2A* rearranged
	t(9;22) (q34.1;q11.2); *BCR-ABL1*
	inv(3) (q21.3q26.2) or t(3;3)
	   (q21.3;q26.2); *GATA2,MECOM(EVI1)*
	−5 or del(5q); 27; 217/abn(17p)
	Complex karyotype, monosomal
	   karyotype
	Wild-type *NPM1* and *FLT3-ITD*[high]
	Mutated *RUNX1*[b]
	Mutated *ASXL1*[b]
	Mutated *TP53*	

[a] Ref.[3]
[b] Adverse prognosis unless co-occurring with a favorable-risk AML subtype.
   Modified from reference[31]. *Adapted from* Dohner H, Estey E, Grimwade D, et al. Diagnosis and management of AML in adults: 2017 ELN recommendations from an international expert panel. *Blood.* 2017;129(4):424-447, with permission.

reduced overall survival.[37] A more recent very large cohort of patients with AML studied at post induction morphologic remission, showed persistent mutations at highly variable rates across genes. Mutations in genes associated with clonal hematopoiesis were very commonly persistent (rates of 78.7% for *DNMT3A*, 54.2% for *TET2*, and 51.6% for *ASXL1*) but did not independently portend adverse prognosis, and are thought to represent nonleukemic clones, or background CH.[38] Mutations in more "aggressive driver" genes, such as the RAS pathway, persisted at lower rates, but were correlated with increased relapse, with this risk independent of allele frequency. The coexistence of CH-related mutations with other mutations was a predictor of relapse. In general, combining multiple molecular MRD markers can increase the ability for effective tracking when complex genetic heterogeneity is present in AML.

Myelodysplastic/Myeloproliferative Neoplasms

The MDS/MPNs are overlap entities with clinical and pathologic features of both MDS and MPNs that mutationally follow a similar pattern to that of MDS, but have frequent "backseat driver" mutations in the RAS signaling pathways.[39,40] Although there are no mutations specified in the diagnostic criteria for chronic myelomonocytic leukemia (CMML) and atypical chronic myeloid leukemia, *BCR-ABL1*-negative (aCML), molecularly these appear to bear a foundation of "old stem cell" mutations: *ASXL1, TET2,* or *SRSF2*. Indeed, 90% of cases of CMML have 1 or more mutations in these 3 founding driver genes with an enrichment of *CBL* mutations and other RAS pathway genes as the "backseat drivers."[40] Similarly, aCML has "old stem cell" drivers, and an enrichment for *SETBP1, ETNK1,* or *NRAS*.[41,42] Genetic progression in both cases is associated with the accumulation of additional "aggressive driver" mutations. The pediatric counterpart of CMML, juvenile myelomonocytic leukemia (JMML), recapitulates the distinction between pediatric and adult MDS. JMML lacks the "old stem cell" pattern and is instead associated with a number of germline disorders, including Noonan syndrome and neurofibromatosis, that contain constitutional mutations in RAS pathway members. JMML may acquire additional mutations in the RAS pathway with common progression mutations including other signaling genes and SETBP1.[43] Finally, MDS/MPN with ring sideroblasts and thrombocytosis (MDS/MPN-RS-T) is a more genetically distinct overlap entity, that includes an SF3B1 mutation in its diagnostic criteria with supportive co-mutations in JAK2 (and less commonly CALR or MPL). The mutational acquisition in MDS/MPN-RS-T can be sequential, with either a more MDS (associated with SF3B1 mutation) or a more MPN (associated with JAK/STAT pathway mutation) initial presentation with subsequent acquisition of the other mutation.

Myeloproliferative Neoplasms

The myeloproliferative neoplasms (MPNs) do not always demonstrate a founding driver of "old stem cell" genes, and may represent a younger stem cell, particularly in chronic myeloid leukemia (CML, driven by BCR-ABL1 translocation and often mutationally very quiet at diagnosis), polycythemia vera (PV; driven by JAK2 activating mutation), and some cases of essential thrombocythemia (ET). Of the non-CML MPNs, primary myelofibrosis (PMF) is the most genomically complex and typically does follow the pattern of founding epigenetic and splicing driver mutations with often numerous subclonal events. As might be expected, this higher mutational burden is associated with adverse outcomes.

In the non-CML MPNs, backseat or founding driver mutations occur in the JAK/STAT pathway, most commonly JAK2 or CALR. The 3 main non-CML MPNs can be characterized as either JAK2-type or CALR-type, the designation of which confers clinical insight. JAK2-mutated cases are associated with thrombosis and erythrocytosis. In addition, there is recurrent acquired copy neutral loss of heterozygosity (CN-LOH) of the JAK2 locus on 9p that occurs often at the time of progression to myelofibrosis or AML. By contrast, CALR types are associated with high platelet counts without the same thrombotic risk seen in JAK2-types, especially type II CALR mutations (5 base pair insertions) that can have extremely high platelet counts (eg, 1–2 million/μL).[44] CN-LOH of CALR is

rare and CALR types tend to have better prognosis. There is no difference between the types with regard to bleeding events, and both can progress to myelofibrosis or AML.[45–47] In rare cases of ET and PMF, JAK2 or CALR is not mutated, but there is activation of the JAK/STAT pathway by an activating mutation of the TPO-receptor, encoded by MPL. In cases with no mutant JAK2, CALR, or MPL (so-called triple-negative MPNs), the "backseat driver" mutation maybe in a rare locus in those genes or in another gene such as NFE2 or SH2B3.[47–51] Because mutant JAK2, CALR, and MPL all act in the same pathway, they are often thought to be mutually exclusive. However, although that is true in a single cell or clone, it is not necessarily true in any individual person in whom more than 1 of these mutations may be seen in separate (sub)clones.[47,48]

The relative temporal acquisition of various mutations may also inform clinical presentation. Those patients who acquire a JAK/STAT pathway mutation initially, as is often the case in PV, tend to be younger with a predominant presentation of erythrocytosis with higher risk of thrombosis and higher apparent JAK2 clone sizes. Those patients who acquire an epigenetic gene mutation first, in keeping with the "old stem cell" phenotype, tend to be older with more effected stem cell compartments.[52]

Mutational profiles in MPNs are increasingly informative in prognostication, in predicting risk of fibrotic progression, transformation to AML, and mortality. Grinfeld and colleagues[49] used mutational data in a large cohort of MPN cases to identify 8 genomic subgroups (with 7 patterns based on driver mutations) that were independent of traditional morphologic categories. Of these, the subgroup with TP53 mutations had abysmal outcomes, and mutations in epigenetic or splicing genes and the RAS pathway were strongly associated with myelofibrosis and a relatively poor prognosis. In fact, the mutation profile was more informative in the prediction of mortality and progression to myelofibrosis than the traditional morphologic category.

Mast Cell Neoplasms

Although mast cell neoplasms are a separate WHO category from the MPNs, they follow the same overall mutational paradigms. Adults typically follow a similar pattern to all other chronic myeloid neoplasms with epigenetic and splicing "old stem cell" founding driver mutations with secondarily acquired "backseat driver" KIT mutations found often exclusively in terminally differentiated mast cells.[53,54] Not surprisingly, these patients frequently have systemic mastocytosis (SM) that may be accompanied by an associated hematologic neoplasm. By contrast, children typically have cutaneous-only mastocytosis with a sole *KIT* mutation present in mast cells without the foundation of an "old stem cell."

SPECIAL TOPICS

Clonal Evolution

As illustrated in the individual disease categories listed previously, clonal evolution is a common phenomenon in myeloid neoplasms and a process in which genetic diversification and selection occurs, both in the form of convergent, as well as divergent evolution. In the former process, separate neoplastic hematopoietic progenitor cells independently acquire mutations in the same genes or within the same pathway that confer a survival or proliferative advantage to the neoplastic progenitors. The resultant myeloid neoplasms therefore frequently have multiple subclones with similar mutational features. A recurrent pathway involved in convergent evolution is the RAS pathway, by which a multiplicity of *RAS* mutations coincides to result in the overall progression phenotype of MDS to secondary AML. This also can be seen with the other "aggressive driver" mutations in the transcription pathway in progression to high-grade disease or secondary AML, as well as in the MPNs in which different subclones may have "mutually exclusive" *JAK2*, *CALR*, or *MPL* "backseat driver" mutations. Divergent evolution is the process of neoplastic progenitors acquiring mutations in different pathways, which occurs under circumstances of the marrow being very promutagenic and leads to the emergence of unrelated or only partially related clones with different mutational profiles.

Use of Peripheral Blood Mutation Screening to Exclude or Predict Myeloid Neoplasms

Although the presence of mutations cannot necessarily distinguish between CH and a bona fide myeloid neoplasm, mutational screening may be very helpful in the workup of cytopenic patients by predicting which patients are unlikely to have or to develop a myeloid neoplasm. A retrospective study examined the diagnostic outcomes of nearly 300 patients with the chief complaint of cytopenia(s) who had peripheral blood mutational testing by a myeloid NGS panel.[55] No pathogenic mutation was found in 72% of these patients, and among these, when their entire workup was completed, only 1% were ultimately diagnosed with a myeloid neoplasm as the cause for their cytopenias. By contrast, in the 28% of patients who did have a pathogenic mutation, 25% were ultimately diagnosed with a concurrent myeloid neoplasm. Clone size and number of mutations were associated with higher risk of diagnosis of a myeloid neoplasm. At 2-year follow-up, from the patients who were not initially diagnosed with a hematologic neoplasm and lacked pathogenic mutations, still only 1% developed a future myeloid neoplasm. In fact, the study demonstrated a 95% negative predictive value (NPV) of NGS mutational screening for a concurrent myeloid neoplasm, with a minimal gene list to achieve this NPV of only 20 genes and 89% NPV achieved by interrogation of only 5 genes (*DNMT3A, TET2, ASXL1, SRSF2,* and *SF3B1*) associated with the aged stem cell. These findings strongly support the use of peripheral blood NGS testing of cytopenic patients to identify those who do not need an invasive and expensive bone marrow biopsy.

Another study followed patients with unexplained cytopenias, demonstrating the value of pathogenic mutations identified in peripheral blood for predicting a future myeloid neoplasm.[56] The positive predictive value (PPV) increased with greater numbers of mutations and higher variant allele frequency (VAFs). Spliceosome genes (*SF3B1, SRSF2, U2AF1*), *JAK2,* and *RUNX1* showed the highest predictive value for future myeloid neoplasms. *TET2, DNMT3A,* and *ASXL1* were much more predictive when co-mutated with other genes (*RUNX1, EZH2, CBL, TP53, NRAS, CUX1,* or *IDH2*) than in isolation. Patients with these high-risk mutational profiles and unexplained cytopenias, which would in the absence of morphologic dysplasia be designated clonal cytopenias of uncertain significance, have the same overall survival as that of low-risk MDS, and should perhaps be regarded as such.

High Concordance of Peripheral Blood and Bone Marrow Next-Generation Sequencing in Myeloid Neoplasms

A recent study with a large cohort of 164 patients with known or suspected hematologic malignancy, compared the performance of NGS mutational testing of paired peripheral blood (PB) versus bone marrow (BM) samples and found very high concordance.[57] There was 88% sensitivity of PB in identifying all BM variants with 99.7% specificity (PPV 95.5% and NPV 99.1%). Most discrepant mutations were shown by manual review to be in fact present in PB, at or near the limit of detection of the assay or in areas with poor coverage. The remaining "BM only" variants (2.8% of all variants) were known leukemic drivers, *NPM1* and *TP53,* and identified in cases of acute leukemias that lacked circulating blasts. This study further supports the role of using PB NGS studies for chronic myeloid neoplasms and for acute leukemias that have circulating disease but emphasizes the importance of BM sampling for evaluation of measurable residual disease in acute leukemias.

Final Thoughts

Although the genetic underpinning of myeloid neoplasms is complex, mutations are often not part of the diagnostic criteria of myeloid neoplasms (in part due to CH). However, mutations can be used as markers of clonality and the pattern of mutations can have significant diagnostic, prognostic, monitoring, and therapy implications. Indeed, the molecular patterns are highly recurrent and overlapping, allowing for a single simple framework of "founding" drivers, "backseat" drivers, and "aggressive" drivers for interpreting mutational patterns in myeloid neoplasms, although the individual mutations and genes can be quite varied. Drivers in the same pathway may be mutually exclusive in a cell but can be found in different subclones. Those subclonal events can show both convergent and divergent evolution with clonal evolution both common and informative. Pediatric neoplasms typically follow the same patterns of "backseat" and "aggressive" drivers without the foundation on an old stem cell. In general, the more driver mutations you have, the worse the prognosis, especially with acquisition of "aggressive" driver mutations. Importantly, for the purposes of ruling in or out a myeloid neoplasm, PB screening has a high NPV and can prevent costly and invasive BM biopsies. For MRD detection, which is increasing in clinical importance in both chronic myeloid neoplasms as well as AML, somatic mutational testing, best performed on BM, is rapidly becoming an important monitoring tool in our armamentarium.

DISCLOSURE

S. Sadigh has nothing to disclose; A.S. Kim consults for LabCorp, Inc. and has received research funding from the Multiple Myeloma Research Foundation.

REFERENCES

1. Swerdlow SH, Campo E, Harris NL, et al. WHO classification of tumours of haematopoietic and lymphoid tissues. Revised 4th edition. Lyon (France): International Agency for Research on Cancer; 2017.
2. McClure RF, Ewalt MD, Crow J, et al. Clinical significance of DNA variants in chronic myeloid neoplasms: a report of the association for molecular pathology. J Mol Diagn 2018;20(6):717–37.
3. Papaemmanuil E, Gerstung M, Bullinger L, et al. Genomic classification and prognosis in acute myeloid leukemia. N Engl J Med 2016;374(23):2209–21.
4. Welch JS, Ley TJ, Link DC, et al. The origin and evolution of mutations in acute myeloid leukemia. Cell 2012;150(2):264–78.
5. Williams N, Lee J, Moore L, et al. Driver mutation acquisition in utero and childhood followed by life-long clonal evolution underlie myeloproliferative neoplasms. Blood 2020;136(Supplement_2). LBA-1-LBA-1.
6. Van Egeren D, Escabi J, Nguyen M, et al. Reconstructing the lineage histories and differentiation trajectories of individual cancer cells in myeloproliferative neoplasms. Cell Stem Cell 2021;28(3):514–23.e9.
7. Cogle CR, Craig BM, Rollison DE, et al. Incidence of the myelodysplastic syndromes using a novel claims-based algorithm: high number of uncaptured cases by cancer registries. Blood 2011;117(26):7121–5.
8. Jaiswal S, Fontanillas P, Flannick J, et al. Age-related clonal hematopoiesis associated with adverse outcomes. N Engl J Med 2014;371(26):2488–98.
9. Genovese G, Kahler AK, Handsaker RE, et al. Clonal hematopoiesis and blood-cancer risk inferred from blood DNA sequence. N Engl J Med 2014;371(26):2477–87.
10. Xie M, Lu C, Wang J, et al. Age-related mutations associated with clonal hematopoietic expansion and malignancies. Nat Med 2014;20(12):1472–8.
11. McKerrell T, Park N, Moreno T, et al. Leukemia-associated somatic mutations drive distinct patterns of age-related clonal hemopoiesis. Cell Rep 2015;10(8):1239–45.
12. Boettcher S, Wilk CM, Singer J, et al. Clonal hematopoiesis in donors and long-term survivors of related allogeneic hematopoietic stem cell transplantation. Blood 2020;135(18):1548–59.
13. Jaiswal S, Natarajan P, Silver AJ, et al. Clonal hematopoiesis and risk of atherosclerotic cardiovascular disease. N Engl J Med 2017;377(2):111–21.
14. Olszewski AJ, Chorzalska AD, Kim AS, et al. Clonal haematopoiesis of indeterminate potential among cancer survivors exposed to myelotoxic chemotherapy. Br J Haematol 2019;186(3):e31–5.
15. Gibson CJ, Lindsley RC, Tchekmedyian V, et al. Clonal hematopoiesis associated with adverse outcomes after autologous stem-cell transplantation for lymphoma. J Clin Oncol 2017;35(14):1598–605.
16. Gillis NK, Ball M, Zhang Q, et al. Clonal haemopoiesis and therapy-related myeloid malignancies in

elderly patients: a proof-of-concept, case-control study. Lancet Oncol 2017;18(1):112–21.

17. Bolton KL, Ptashkin RN, Gao T, et al. Cancer therapy shapes the fitness landscape of clonal hematopoiesis. Nat Genet 2020;52(11):1219–26.

18. Loh PR, Genovese G, Handsaker RE, et al. Insights into clonal haematopoiesis from 8,342 mosaic chromosomal alterations. Nature 2018;559(7714):350–5.

19. Takahashi K, Wang F, Kantarjian H, et al. Copy number alterations detected as clonal hematopoiesis of indeterminate potential. Blood Adv 2017;1(15):1031–6.

20. Gao T, Ptashkin R, Bolton KL, et al. Interplay between chromosomal alterations and gene mutations shapes the evolutionary trajectory of clonal hematopoiesis. Nat Commun 2021;12(1):338.

21. Bick AG, Weinstock JS, Nandakumar SK, et al. Inherited causes of clonal haematopoiesis in 97,691 whole genomes. Nature 2020;586(7831):763–8.

22. Haferlach T, Nagata Y, Grossmann V, et al. Landscape of genetic lesions in 944 patients with myelodysplastic syndromes. Leukemia 2014;28(2):241–7.

23. Steensma DP, Bejar R, Jaiswal S, et al. Clonal hematopoiesis of indeterminate potential and its distinction from myelodysplastic syndromes. Blood 2015;126(1):9–16.

24. Zink F, Stacey SN, Norddahl GL, et al. Clonal hematopoiesis, with and without candidate driver mutations, is common in the elderly. Blood 2017;130(6):742–52.

25. Duncavage EJ, Jacoby MA, Chang GS, et al. Mutation clearance after transplantation for myelodysplastic syndrome. N Engl J Med 2018;379(11):1028–41.

26. Lindsley RC, Saber W, Mar BG, et al. Prognostic mutations in myelodysplastic syndrome after stem-cell transplantation. N Engl J Med 2017;376(6):536–47.

27. Bejar R. Clinical and genetic predictors of prognosis in myelodysplastic syndromes. Haematologica 2014;99(6):956–64.

28. Nazha A, Komrokji RS, Meggendorfer M, et al. A personalized prediction model to risk stratify patients with myelodysplastic syndromes. Blood 2018;132(Supplement 1):793.

29. Greenberg PL, Tuechler H, Schanz J, et al. Revised international prognostic scoring system for myelodysplastic syndromes. Blood 2012;120(12):2454–65.

30. Mossner M, Jann JC, Wittig J, et al. Mutational hierarchies in myelodysplastic syndromes dynamically adapt and evolve upon therapy response and failure. Blood 2016;128(9):1246–59.

31. Lindsley RC, Mar BG, Mazzola E, et al. Acute myeloid leukemia ontogeny is defined by distinct somatic mutations. Blood 2015;125(9):1367–76.

32. Bernard E, Nannya Y, Hasserjian RP, et al. Implications of TP53 allelic state for genome stability, clinical presentation and outcomes in myelodysplastic syndromes. Nat Med 2020;26(10):1549–56.

33. Schwartz JR, Ma J, Lamprecht T, et al. The genomic landscape of pediatric myelodysplastic syndromes. Nat Commun 2017;8(1):1557.

34. Cancer Genome Atlas Research Network, Ley TJ, Miller C, et al. Genomic and epigenomic landscapes of adult de novo acute myeloid leukemia. N Engl J Med 2013;368(22):2059–74.

35. Dohner H, Estey E, Grimwade D, et al. Diagnosis and management of AML in adults: 2017 ELN recommendations from an international expert panel. Blood 2017;129(4):424–47.

36. Roloff GW, Griffiths EA. When to obtain genomic data in acute myeloid leukemia (AML) and which mutations matter. Blood Adv 2018;2(21):3070–80.

37. Klco JM, Miller CA, Griffith M, et al. Association between mutation clearance after induction therapy and outcomes in acute myeloid leukemia. JAMA 2015;314(8):811–22.

38. Jongen-Lavrencic M, Grob T, Hanekamp D, et al. Molecular minimal residual disease in acute myeloid leukemia. N Engl J Med 2018;378(13):1189–99.

39. Savona MR, Malcovati L, Komrokji R, et al. An international consortium proposal of uniform response criteria for myelodysplastic/myeloproliferative neoplasms (MDS/MPN) in adults. Blood 2015;125(12):1857–65.

40. Meggendorfer M, Haferlach T, Alpermann T, et al. Specific molecular mutation patterns delineate chronic neutrophilic leukemia, atypical chronic myeloid leukemia, and chronic myelomonocytic leukemia. Haematologica 2014;99(12):e244–6.

41. Makishima H, Yoshida K, Nguyen N, et al. Somatic SETBP1 mutations in myeloid malignancies. Nat Genet 2013;45(8):942–6.

42. Piazza R, Valletta S, Winkelmann N, et al. Recurrent SETBP1 mutations in atypical chronic myeloid leukemia. Nat Genet 2013;45(1):18–24.

43. Stieglitz E, Taylor-Weiner AN, Chang TY, et al. The genomic landscape of juvenile myelomonocytic leukemia. Nat Genet 2015;47(11):1326–33.

44. Tefferi A, Wassie EA, Guglielmelli P, et al. Type 1 versus Type 2 calreticulin mutations in essential thrombocythemia: a collaborative study of 1027 patients. Am J Hematol 2014;89(8):E121–4.

45. Rumi E, Pietra D, Ferretti V, et al. JAK2 or CALR mutation status defines subtypes of essential thrombocythemia with substantially different clinical course and outcomes. Blood 2014;123(10):1544–51.

46. Guglielmelli P, Pacilli A, Rotunno G, et al. Presentation and outcome of patients with 2016 WHO diagnosis of prefibrotic and overt primary myelofibrosis. Blood 2017;129(24):3227–36.

47. Tefferi A, Barbui T. Polycythemia vera and essential thrombocythemia: 2017 update on diagnosis, risk-stratification, and management. Am J Hematol 2017;92(1):94–108.

48. Lundberg P, Karow A, Nienhold R, et al. Clonal evolution and clinical correlates of somatic mutations in myeloproliferative neoplasms. Blood 2014;123(14): 2220–8.

49. Grinfeld J, Nangalia J, Baxter EJ, et al. Classification and personalized prognosis in myeloproliferative neoplasms. N Engl J Med 2018;379(15): 1416–30.

50. Cabagnols X, Favale F, Pasquier F, et al. Presence of atypical thrombopoietin receptor (MPL) mutations in triple-negative essential thrombocythemia patients. Blood 2016;127(3):333–42.

51. Maslah N, Cassinat B, Verger E, et al. The role of LNK/SH2B3 genetic alterations in myeloproliferative neoplasms and other hematological disorders. Leukemia 2017;31(8):1661–70.

52. Ortmann CA, Kent DG, Nangalia J, et al. Effect of mutation order on myeloproliferative neoplasms. N Engl J Med 2015;372(7):601–12.

53. Jawhar M, Schwaab J, Schnittger S, et al. Molecular profiling of myeloid progenitor cells in multi-mutated advanced systemic mastocytosis identifies KIT D816V as a distinct and late event. Leukemia 2015;29(5):1115–22.

54. Jawhar M, Schwaab J, Schnittger S, et al. Additional mutations in SRSF2, ASXL1 and/or RUNX1 identify a high-risk group of patients with KIT D816V(+) advanced systemic mastocytosis. Leukemia 2016; 30(1):136–43.

55. Shanmugam V, Parnes A, Kalyanaraman R, et al. Clinical utility of targeted next-generation sequencing-based screening of peripheral blood in the evaluation of cytopenias. Blood 2019; 134(24):2222–5.

56. Malcovati L, Galli A, Travaglino E, et al. Clinical significance of somatic mutation in unexplained blood cytopenia. Blood 2017;129(25):3371–8.

57. Lucas F, Michaels PD, Wang D, et al. Mutational analysis of hematologic neoplasms in 164 paired peripheral blood and bone marrow samples by next-generation sequencing. Blood Adv 2020; 4(18):4362–5.

Molecular Pathology of Mature Lymphoid Malignancies

Alisha D. Ware, MD[a,1], Katelynn Davis, MD[a,2],
Rena R. Xian, MD[a,b,*]

KEYWORDS

- B-cell lymphoma • T-cell lymphoma • Hodgkin lymphoma • Molecular pathology
- Next generation sequencing • Fluorescence in situ hybridization

Key points

- Chromosomal and molecular abnormalities are becoming increasingly important in the diagnosis and classification of lymphomas.

- Specific genetic abnormalities have been associated with distinct morphologic and phenotypic findings.

- Particular chromosomal and molecular abnormalities can also inform clinical prognosis and treatment selection in patients with lymphoma.

ABSTRACT

L ymphoid malignancies are a broad and heterogeneous group of neoplasms. In the past decade, the genetic landscape of these tumors has been explored and cataloged in fine detail offering a glimpse into the mechanisms of lymphomagenesis and new opportunities to translate these findings into patient management. A myriad of studies have demonstrated both distinctive and overlapping molecular and chromosomal abnormalities that have influenced the diagnosis and classification of lymphoma, disease prognosis, and treatment selection.

OVERVIEW

Hematologic malignancies are grouped by cell of origin (COO) with the broadest separating myeloid and lymphoid processes. The wealth of basic science, translational and clinical research in myeloid neoplasms has emphasized the clinical utility of ancillary studies. While the diagnosis of lymphoma remains anchored to histopathology and immunophenotyping, the 2017 edition of the *WHO Classification of Tumors of Haematopoietic and Lymphoid Tissues*[1] shows the emerging importance of genetic testing in lymphoid malignancies with the introduction of genetically defined entities and detailed cataloging of molecular findings and their prognostic and treatment implications.

While immunoglobulin and T-cell receptor gene rearrangements have long been used by pathologists to aid in the diagnosis of lymphoma,[2] these do not contribute to lymphoma classification. Recently other techniques, such as fluorescence in-situ hybridization (FISH), single nucleotide polymorphism (SNP) array, and next-generation sequencing (NGS) have become more routine in

[a] Department of Pathology, Johns Hopkins Medical Institutions, Baltimore, MD, USA; [b] Department of Oncology, Sidney Kimmel Comprehensive Cancer Center, Johns Hopkins Medical Institutions, Johns Hopkins School of Medicine, 1812 Ashland Avenue, Suite 200, Baltimore, MD 21205, USA
[1] Present address: 401 North Broadway, Weinberg 2242, Baltimore, MD 21287.
[2] Present address: 600 North Wolfe Street, Pathology Building Room 401, Baltimore, MD 21287.
* Corresponding author. Johns Hopkins School of Medicine, 1812 Ashland Avenue, Suite 200, Baltimore, MD 21205.
E-mail address: rxian1@jhmi.edu

Surgical Pathology 14 (2021) 529–547
https://doi.org/10.1016/j.path.2021.06.001
1875-9181/21/© 2021 Elsevier Inc. All rights reserved.

clinical practice to identify diagnostic and prognostic markers. Some cytogenetic and molecular abnormalities are disease defining, while others show varying degrees of association with a specific entity. Occasionally, the absence of particular abnormalities can have a greater influence on diagnosis than the presence of a nonspecific change.

Herein, we discuss the current genetic landscape of select lymphomas, particularly new entities in the 2017 WHO classification and how these findings can be incorporated into practice. Special care should be taken when interpreting these results, as the clinical and pathologic context remains the cornerstone of a definitive diagnosis and patient management. Key concepts will be highlighted as diagnostic "Pearls and Pitfalls," and illustrative cases underscore the importance of clinicopathologic correlation.

MATURE B-CELL NEOPLASMS

Most lymphomas in the Western hemisphere are B-cell in origin and can be grouped by COO as either germinal center B-cell (GCB) or non-germinal center/activated B-cell (non-GCB/ABC).

B-cell lymphomas will be reviewed based on histologic grade and COO.

LOW-GRADE B-CELL LYMPHOMA WITH GERMINAL-CENTER PHENOTYPE

Follicular lymphoma (FL) is the prototypic GCB low-grade lymphoma usually expressing CD10 and/or BCL6. BCL2 is expressed in most cases, although grade 3 FL may lack BCL2, and even CD10.[1] Translocation t(8;14) (q32;q21), IGH/BCL2, occurs in more than 90% of conventional FL (cFL) but may be absent in high-grade histology and FL variants. Characteristic molecular and cytogenetic abnormalities (Box 1)[1,3–9] found in FL reflect the GCB COO of these tumors. Mutations frequently involve epigenetic regulators, such as EZH2 (~30%),[10] CREBBP, and KMT2D. In 2020, the first targeted agent in lymphoma treatment, tazemetostat, was approved by the Federal Drug Administration for EZH2-mutated FL.[11]

Follicular Lymphoma Variants with Low-Grade Histology

These FL variants share GCB phenotype and low-grade histology with cFL but show clinical,

---

Box 1
Cytogenetic/molecular abnormalities in FL

Aberrancy (frequency)

Rearrangements

    t(14;18) (q32;q21) IGH-BCL2 (90%)[a]

    BCL6 rearrangements or 3q27 abnormalities (5%–15%)[b]

    t(8;14) (q24;q32) MYC-IGH (rare)[c]

Mutations

    EZH2

    CREBBP

    KMT2D

    RRAGC (~17%)

    TP53[c]

    TNFRSF14

    CDKN2A[c]

    MYC[c]

    STAT6[d]

Copy Number Abnormalities (CNA)

    Deletion of chromosomes 1p (including TNFRSF14)[d,e], 6q, 10q, 17p

    Gains of chromosomes 1, 6p, 7, 8, 12q, X, 18q

[a] Indistinguishable from IGH/MALT1 by conventional cytogenetics. [b] Seen in tFL. [c] Implicated in transformation to DLBCL. [d] Highly enriched in diffuse variant of FL. [e] Common in all forms of FL.

histologic, or genetic differences. In situ follicular neoplasia (ISFN) and duodenal-type FL differ from cFL based on histology and absence of nodal disease, respectively. Both express BCL2 and have *IGH/BCL2* rearrangements.[1] Diffuse variant of FL also demonstrates low-grade histology but shows unusual microfollicular growth with variable expression of BCL2. While these lymphomas have a mutational profile similar to cFL, near-uniform mutation of *STAT6* and conspicuous absence of *IGH/BCL2* appears to be defining features.[1,3–5] All these variants are associated with favorable prognosis, particularly ISFN.

Follicular Lymphoma Variants with High-Grade Histology

These FL variants share GCB phenotype and high-grade histology with cFL but show clinical, histologic, or genetic differences. Testicular FL (tFL) lacks BCL2 expression and t(14;18); *BCL6* rearrangements and/or abnormalities involving chromosome 3q27 may be found.[1] Pediatric-type FL (ptFL) presents predominantly in the head and neck and may be seen in both pediatric and adult populations. Similar to tFL, these tumors lack BCL2 expression and t(14;18). Mutations of *TNFRSF14* or deletion 1p (*TNFRSF14*) occur at a rate similar to cFL. However, ptFL has a different molecular profile with enrichment for mitogen-activated protein kinase pathway mutations and absence of mutations involving epigenetic regulators.[12,13] Although histologic grade is high in both variants, both are associated with a favorable prognosis.[1]

Pearls and Pitfalls

When encountering a GCB phenotype lymphoma with sites of presentation and histologies suggestive of an FL variant, such as diffuse, testicular, or pediatric-type, FISH studies must be performed to exclude *IGH/BCL2*, as these variants are partly defined by absence of t(14;18). Should an *IGH/BCL2* be detected, then a cFL diagnosis should be assigned with the corresponding grade. As tFL and ptFL are histologically high-grade, yet clinically indolent, distinction from grade 3 cFL is paramount. NGS studies may also reveal characteristic mutational profiles that support one of these diagnoses.

LOW-GRADE B-CELL LYMPHOMA WITH NON-GERMINAL-CENTER PHENOTYPE

Non-GCB B-cell lymphomas originate from mantle-zone cells, ABCs, marginal zone cells, or cells with plasmacytic differentiation.[14] Pre-GC mature B-cell lymphomas include most mantle cell lymphoma (MCL),[15] many chronic lymphocytic leukemia/small lymphocytic lymphoma (CLL/SLL),[16] and a small subset of hairy cell leukemia (HCL).[17] These neoplasms are histologically low-grade, and classification is mainly guided by immunophenotype. Many of these lymphomas show perturbed B-cell receptor signaling and can be treated with Bruton tyrosine kinase (BTK) inhibitors. Other lymphomas in this group have disease-defining mutations with corresponding targeted agents.

Mantle Cell Lymphoma

MCL is a CD5+ lymphoma that expresses Cyclin-D1 (>95%) and SOX11 (>90%) and lacks CD200. The hallmark genetic abnormality is t(11;14) (q13;q32), *CCND1/IGH*, although other abnormalities may also be found (**Box 2**).[1,18–22] Pathologic evaluation is crucial to disease prognosis, as leukemic non-nodal MCL and in situ mantle cell neoplasia are clinically indolent, but blastoid and pleomorphic variants are clinically aggressive. Genetic abnormalities also aid in prognostication: complex karyotype[23] and *MYC* rearrangements[24] are associated with poor prognosis. MCL shows abnormal BTK pathway signaling and can be treated with a variety of BTK inhibitors, which is also effective in CLL/SLL and O-umlaut Waldenstrom macroglobulinemia. Patients being treated with BTK inhibitors may develop drug resistance, which is often demonstrated as mutations in *BTK* and *PLCG2*.[25]

Chronic Lymphocytic Leukemia/Small Lymphocytic Lymphoma

CLL/SLL is a CD5+ lymphoma that expresses CD23, CD200, and LEF1 and lacks Cyclin-D1 and SOX11 expression and t(11;14) translocation.[1] A variety of genetic abnormalities have been associated with CLL/SLL (**Box 3**)[1,22,26–29] that have both diagnostic and prognostic implications. *IGHV* hypermutation status has long been evaluated, as a mutated status is associated with good prognosis, but unmutated status is associated with poor prognosis.[16] Del13q14.3 (*RB1*) is the most common cytogenetic abnormality (**Fig. 1**) and is associated with favorable outcomes when present as an isolated finding.[26] Although a small subset of lymphoplasmacytic lymphoma (LPL) may demonstrate *RB1* loss,[30] this is not typically present in isolation. Deletion 11q (*ATM* and *BIRC3*), deletion 17p (*TP53*), and *NOTCH1* mutations are associated with adverse outcomes.[26,27]

Box 2
Cytogenetic/molecular abnormalities in MCL

Aberrancy (frequency)

  Rearrangements

    t(11;14) (q13;q32) *CCND1/IGH* (>95%)[a]

    t(8;14) (q24;q32) *MYC/IGH*, variant *MYC* translocations (rare)[c]

    CCND2 translocations with *IGH*, *IGK*, or *IGL* (50% of *CCND1*-negative MCL)

    BCL6 (3q27) translocations (rare)[d]

  Mutations

    ATM (40%–75%)[f]

    CCND1 (~35%)[e]

    KMT2D (~14%)[f]

    NOTCH1 (5%–12%)[f]

    NOTCH2 (<10%)[f]

    TP53 [g]

    BMI1 [g]

    CDK4 [g]

    RB1[g]

    CDKN2A[g]

    CDKN2C [g]

  CNA

    Amplification of *BCL2* (18q21)

    Gains of chromosomes 3q26 (31%–50%), 7p21 (16%–34%), 8q24 (*MYC*, 16%–36%), 12 (~25%)[b]

    Loss of chromosomes 1p13 to 31 (29%–52%), 6q23 to 27 (*TNFAIP3*, 23%–38%), 9p21 (*CDKN2A*, 18%–31%), 11p22 to 23 (*ATM*, 21%–59%), 13q14 to 34 (43%–51%), 13q11 to 13 (22%–55%), 13q14 to 34 (43%–51%), 17p13 (*TP53*%, 21%–45%)

    Copy neutral LOH (~60%)

[a] Variant translocations with *IGK* or *IGL* are rarely reported. [b] Usually seen with other genetic aberrations. [c] Aggressive clinical course. [d] Associated with BCL6 expression. [e] Usually seen in *IGHV*-mutated cases. [f] Reported only in association with SOX11+ MCL. [g] Associated with highly proliferative variants of MCL.

Hairy Cell Leukemia and Hairy Cell Leukemia Variant

HCL is a CD5-negative lymphoma with characteristic cytoplasmic projections and expresses CD11c, CD103, CD25, and CD123; annexin A1; and cyclin-D1 (**Fig. 2**).[1] There are a variety of clinical, pathologic, immunophenotypic, and genetic abnormalities (**Table 1**)[1,31,32] that distinguish HCL and hairy cell leukemia variant (HCL-v), although the absence of *BRAF* p.V600E is required for the diagnosis of HCL-v. *BRAF* p.V600E mutations are found in nearly all HCL, and BRAF inhibitors are frequently used in relapsed/refractory HCL.[33] HCL-v often show mutated *IGHV* and deletion of chromosome 11q22 (*ATM*).

Marginal Zone Lymphoma and Lymphoplasmacytic Lymphoma

Marginal zone lymphoma (MZL) and LPL (O-umlaut Waldenstrom macroglobulinemia) are CD5-negative lymphomas that have significant morphologic and immunophenotypic overlap, particularly in nodal and marrow presentations, although they are relatively genetically distinct (**Table 2**).[1,34–37] While the associated immunoglobulin expression may be IgM in MZL, non-IgM expression should help exclude LPL.[1] A molecular marker that has become key in this differential consideration is *MYD88* p.L265P: greater than 90% of LPL carry this mutation, whereas only rare cases of MZL have this mutation. Extranodal MZL of mucosa-

---

Box 3
Cytogenetic/molecular abnormalities in CLL/SLL

Aberrancy (frequency)

CNA

Deletion of chromosomes 13q14.3 (*RB1*) (~50%)[a], 11q (*ATM* and *BIRC3*)[b], 17p (*TP53*)[b], 6q21 and 14q.

Gains of chromosomes 12 (trisomy or partial trisomy 12q13) (~20%), 2p and 8q24 (*MYC*)

Rearrangements

t(14;18) (q32;q21) *IGH/BCL2* (~2%)

t(14;19) (q32;q13) *IGH/BCL3* (rare)

Mutations

Mutated *IGHV* (50%–70%)[a]

NOTCH1 (frequently seen with trisomy 12)[b]

SF3B1[b]

TP53[b]

ATM[b]

BIRC3[b]

POT1

MYD88 (rare)

[a] Associated with favorable prognosis, particularly isolated del 13q14.3. [b] Associated with poor prognosis.

---

associated lymphoid tissue (MALT lymphoma) has a unique cytogenetic profile, including frequent rearrangements in *MALT1* or *IGH*.

Pearls and Pitfalls

When the differential diagnosis includes MZL and LPL, the identification of *MYD88* mutation supports a diagnosis of LPL. However, infrequent *MYD88* mutations have been reported in splenic, nodal, and extranodal MZL and even CLL/SLL (see Fig. 2). Using MYD88 to ascertain a diagnosis becomes even more challenging in the setting of an unusual immunophenotype, such as CD5+ MZL and atypical CLL/SLL. In addition, if a high-grade process cannot be excluded based on morphology, detection of *MYD88* may not represent a low-grade lymphoma, but rather a large B-cell lymphoma, as *MYD88* mutations are found in many non-GCB diffuse large B-cell lymphoma.

AGGRESSIVE B-CELL LYMPHOMA WITH PREDOMINANTLY GERMINAL-CENTER PHENOTYPE

Burkitt Lymphoma and Burkitt-like Lymphoma with 11q Aberration (BLL)

Burkitt lymphoma (BL) and Burkitt-like lymphoma with 11q aberration (BLL) are both GCB lymphomas

with exceptionally high Ki-67 proliferation rates, uniform MYC expression, and absence of BCL2 expression. The main distinction between these two related entities is the presence/absence of *MYC* rearrangements, typically t(8;14) (q24;q32) *MYC/IGH*, among other findings (**Table 3**).[38–41] In addition, mutations in *TCF3* and/or *ID3* are found in most BL, and Epstein Barr virus (EBV)-status may be associated with unique mutational profiles.[41] Aside from the absence of *MYC* rearrangements, BLL shows gains and/or losses of the terminus of 11q,[1] most readily detected by SNP microarray.

Diffuse Large B-cell Lymphoma, Not Otherwise Specified

Diffuse large B-cell lymphoma, Not Otherwise Specified (DLBCL, NOS) is subtyped by immunophenotype as either GCB or non-GCB/ABC, with GCB accounting for ~42% of cases.[42] Although DLBCL is not predominantly GCB in phenotype, it is frequently considered in the differential for all aggressive B-cell lymphomas. GCB and non-GCB DLBCL have distinct genetic profiles that reflect their COO (**Table 4**).[1,43,44] GCBs often have mutations in *EZH2*, *GNA12*, *SIPR2*, *TNFRSF14*, and *CREBBP*, whereas ABCs often have mutations in *CARD11*, *MYD88*, *CD79B*, and *CDKN2A*. *MYD88* mutations are found in most

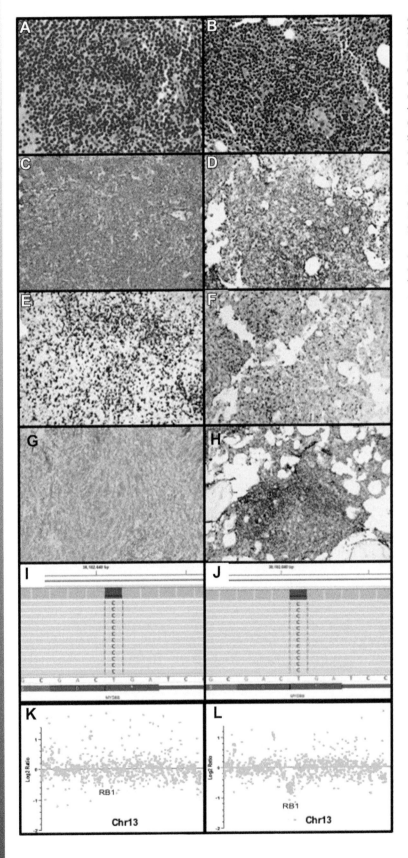

Fig. 1. An unusual case of CLL/SLL with *MYD88* mutation. H&E (400x) of bone marrow involved by (*A*) LPL and (*B*) CLL. The LPL expresses strong CD20 (*C*) and is negative for CD5 (*E*) and IgM (*G*), while the CLL expresses variable CD20 (*D*), weak CD5 (*F*), and strong IgM (*H*). NGS showed *MYD88* p.L265P in both LPL (*I*) and CLL (*J*), with loss of 13q (*RB1*) in CLL (*L*), but not in LPL (*K*). The long-standing clinical history of an indolent lymphoma with a typical CLL/SLL immunophenotype, del 13q and absence of significant gammopathy supported a diagnosis of CLL/SLL despite the presence of *MYD88* mutation.

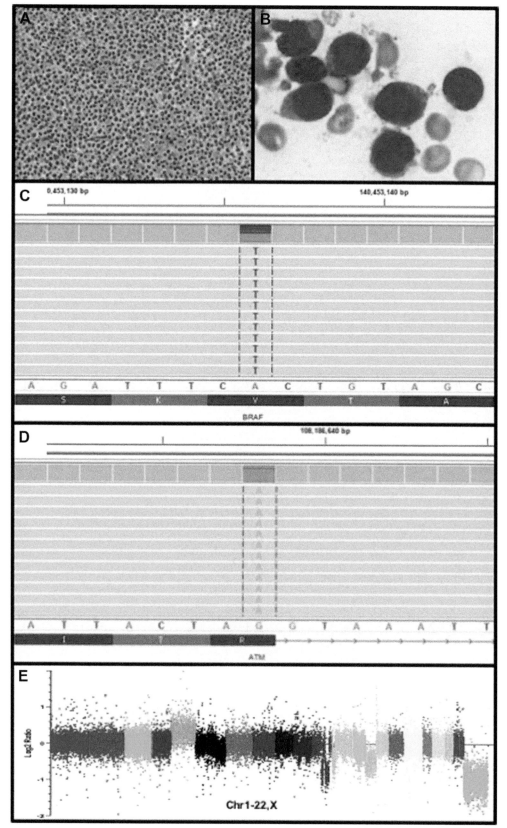

Fig. 2. HCL with *BRAF* p.V600E mutation and deletion 11q22 (*ATM*). H&E (400x) of bone marrow involved by (*A*) HCL. Aspirate smear (1000x) showing (*B*) small atypical lymphocytes with cytoplasmic projections. Peripheral blood NGS showed (*C*) *BRAF* p.V600E (variant allele frequency [VAF] 41.88%) mutation and (*D*) *ATM* p.R2032K (VAF 87.68%). Whole genome copy number plot (*E*) showed +5, partial −11q (inclusive of *ATM*), −14, and –X in this male patient. While deletion 11q22 (*ATM*) are associated with HCL-v, and not HCL, the presence of a *BRAF* mutation along with other typical clinical and pathologic characteristics supported a diagnosis of HCL.

Table 1
Cytogenetic/molecular abnormalities in HCL and HCL-v

Aberrancy (Frequency)—HCL	Aberrancy (Frequency)—HCL-v
Mutations	Mutations
BRAF p.V600E (nearly all cases)	TP53 (seen in IGHV-unmutated cases)
Mutated IGHV (>85%)	MAP2K1
	Mutated IGHV (~67%)
CNA	CNA
Deletion chr7q	Deletion of chr11q22 (ATM)
Numerical aberrations of chr5	

primary CNS lymphoma, which are usually ABC.[38] These molecular differences have led to proposed genetic classifications of DLBCL that further divides this heterogeneous disease.[44]

High-Grade B-cell Lymphoma with MYC and BCL2 and/or BCL6 Rearrangements and High-Grade B-cell Lymphoma, NOS

High-grade B-cell lymphoma (HGBL) can be similar in morphology to DLBCL, NOS (**Fig. 3**), or BL, although blastoid or lymphoblastoid morphology has been reported. This is a highly aggressive lymphoma with a poor response to conventional DLBCL chemotherapy and requires higher intensity chemotherapy.[45] Thus, distinguishing HGBL from DLBCL is of critical clinical importance. This is usually done by demonstrating co-occurring rearrangements involving BCL2 and/or MYC, BCL6 and/or MYC, or exceedingly rarely rearrangements involving all three loci ("triple hit lymphoma"). Rare cases that lack these rearrangements but still show high-grade morphology and a markedly elevated proliferation index may be categorized as HGBL, NOS. Although most HGBLs show a GCB phenotype, a significant proportion with MYC and BCL6 rearrangements are non-GCB.[1] These tumors may also show mutations in TP53, MYD88, and ID3, among other abnormalities (**Box 4**).[1,45–47]

Pearls and Pitfalls

Although most HGBLs are GCB phenotype, a subset may be non-GCB/ABC, particularly those with MYC and BCL6 rearrangements. Clinical testing algorithms that only perform FISH for high-grade GCB lymphomas may miss these latter cases. Testing of all large B-cell lymphoma for these loci will improve accurate identification of HGBL.

AGGRESSIVE B-CELL LYMPHOMA WITH PREDOMINANTLY NON-GERMINAL-CENTER PHENOTYPE

Large B-cell Lymphoma with IRF4 Rearrangement

Large B-cell Lymphoma (LBCL) with IRF4 rearrangement is a rare tumor most commonly seen in pediatric populations involving Waldeyer's ring or head and neck lymph nodes and has a favorable prognosis.[1,48,49] While this lymphoma has an ABC phenotype with strong expression of MUM1/IRF4 and BCL6, some cases express partial CD10 and BCL2, raising the possibility of an unusual ptFL.[1,48] FISH is the preferred method to detect IRF4 rearrangements. However, these breakpoints may be cryptic leading to a false-negative FISH result. Additional rearrangements may involve BCL6, and some cases also show loss of 17p (TP53).[1,48–50]

ALK-Positive Large B-cell Lymphoma

ALK-positive LBCL shows a sinusoidal growth pattern with granular ALK expression, which correlates with t(2;17) (p23;q23), CLTC/ALK, or a variant ALK translocations. Pan-B-cell antigens and CD30 are typically negative or only present in a subset of cells, but there is strong expression of plasmacytic markers. Activation of the STAT3 pathway is frequently seen.[1,51]

Plasmablastic Lymphoma

Plasmablastic lymphoma (PBL) may show variable morphology including immunoblastic or plasmacytic differentiation. Pan-B-cell antigens are usually negative, but plasmacytic markers are positive. Distinct from ALK + LBCL, EBV is found in 60% to 70% of PBL, although HHV8 is absent. MYC translocations are seen in ~50%, which portend a worse outcome and are associated with EBV positivity.[1,52–54]

MATURE T-CELL AND NATURAL KILLER CELL NEOPLASMS

T-cell and natural killer cell (NK-cell) lymphomas represent a minority of lymphomas in the Western hemisphere. T-cell lymphoma can be grouped into different COOs based on expression of CD4 and CD8, for example, CD4+, CD8+, CD4+/CD8+, and CD4-/CD8-. Unlike B-cell lymphoma, T-cell lymphomas are less uniform with respect to COO and can be highly variable within a single entity. As pan T-cell antigen (eg, CD2, CD3, CD5, and CD7) loss defines phenotypic abnormalities, diagnosis is far more challenging. Identification of molecular and cytogenetic abnormalities can greatly

Table 2
Cytogenetic/molecular abnormalities in LPL and MZL

Aberrancy (Frequency)—LPL	Aberrancy (Frequency)—MZL

Mutations
  MYD88 p.L265P (>90%)
  CXCR4 (S338X or frameshift mutations, ~30%)
  ARID1A (17%)
  TP53
  CD79B
  KMT2D
  MYBBP1A
  Mutated *IGHV*
	Mutations
	  IGHV3 and *IGHV4* family members
	  IGHV1-69[a]
	  NOTCH2 (20%–25%)
	  KMT2D
	  PTPRD
	  KLF2
	  MYD88 p.L265P (rare)

CNA
  Deletion 6q (>50% of bone
    marrow-based cases)
  Trisomy 4 (20%), 3 and 18
  Deletion 17p and 11q
	CNA
	  Gains of chromosomes 3, 12 and 18
	  Deletion of chromosome 6q23–24

	Aberrancy (frequency)—MALT lymphoma

	Rearrangements
	  t(11;18) (q21;q21) *BIRC3/MALT1*
	    • Lung (31%–53%) > Intestine
	      (12%–56%) > Stomach (6%–26%)
	  t(14;18) (q32;q21) *IGH/MALT1*
	  t(3;14) (q32;q21) *IGH/FOXP1*
	  t(1;14) (p22;q32) *IGH/BCL10*

	CNA
	  Trisomy 3
	    • Stomach (11%)
	    • Intestine (75%)
	    • Ocular adnexa/orbit (38%)
	    • Salivary gland (55%)
	    • Lung (20%)
	    • Skin (20%)
	    • Thyroid (17%)
	  Trisomy 18
	    • Stomach (6%)
	    • Intestine (25%)
	    • Ocular adnexa/orbit (13%)
	    • Salivary gland (19%)
	    • Lung (7%)
	    • Skin (4%)

	Mutations
	  TNFAIP3 (15%–30%)
	  MYD88 p.L265P (6%–9%)

[a] Seen in cases associated with hepatitis C virus infection.

aid in the recognition of lymphoma, but molecular subtyping is not currently recommended. T-cell lymphomas will be reviewed based on leukemic versus nodal presentations.

T-CELL LYMPHOMAS WITH LEUKEMIC MANIFESTATIONS

T-cell Large Granular Lymphocytic Leukemia and Natural Killer-Cell Leukemia

Large granular lymphocytic leukemia is characterized by a persistent increase in circulating large granular lymphocytes (LGLs) that can have an effector T-cell phenotype, or infrequently an NK-cell phenotype.[1] Activating *STAT3* mutations in the SH2 domain, usually in codons p.Y640 or p.D661, are seen in ~33% of T-cell large granular lymphocytic leukemia (T-LGLL). *STAT5B* SH2 domain mutations have rarely been described and may portend a worse prognosis.[55]

Aggressive NK-cell leukemia is a highly aggressive disease, in which neoplastic cells may resemble LGLs. EBV expression (85%–100%)[1] can aid in the differential diagnosis, but mutational

Table 3
Cytogenetic/molecular abnormalities in BL and BLL

BL	BLL
CNA	CNA
t(8;14) (q24;q32) *MYC/IGH* [a]	Gains of chromosomes 11q23.2–23.3,
t(2;8) (p12;q24) *MYC/IGK*	12q13.11–24.32, 7q34-ter
t(8;22) (q24;q11) *MYC/IGL*	Loss of chromosomes 11q24.1-ter,
Gains of chromosomes 1q (*MDM4*), 7, 12	13q32.3–34
Loss of chromosomes 6q, 13q32–34, 17p	Complex karyotype
Mutations	Mutations
Mutated *IGHV*	*GNA13*
TCF3 (70%)[b]	*ETS1*
ID3 (70%)[b]	
CCND3	
TP53	
RHOA	
SMARCA4	
ARID1A	
IGLL5	
BACH2	
SIN3A	
DNMT1	
MYD88	

[a] Most frequent abnormality.
[b] More common in sporadic than endemic BL.

Table 4
Cytogenetic/molecular abnormalities in DLBCL, GCB, and non-GCB

GCB DLBCL	Non-GCB/ABC DLBCL
Mutations	Mutations
EZH2	*CARD11*
GNA12	*MYD88*
S1PR2	*CD79B*
TP53[d]	*TP53*[d]
NOTCH2[d]	*NOTCH1*[d]
SPEN	*NOTCH2*[d]
DTX1	*SPEN*
TNFAIP3	*DTX1*
BCL10	*TNFAIP3*
PRKCB	*BCL10*
CCND3	*PRKCB*
CXCR5	*CCND3*
TNFRSF14	*CXCR5*
CREBBP	*CDKN2A*[d]
EP300	*ETV6*
KMT2D	*BTG1/BTG2*
STAT6 [e]	*TRAF3*

(continued on next page)

Table 4 (continued)	
GCB DLBCL	**Non-GCB/ABC DLBCL**
SOCS1	
CNA	CNA
Gains/amplification of chromosomes 2p16, 8q24 (*MYC*)	Gains of chromosome 3q27[d]
Deletion of chromosome 1p36	Gains/amplification of chromosome 8q24 (*MYC*)
Deletion of chromosome 10q23	Gains of chromosome 11q23–24
	Gains of chromosome 18q21
	Deletion of chromosome 6q21
	Deletion of chromosome 9p21[d]
Gene Rearrangements in GCB and ABC DLBCL	
t(14;18) (q32;q21.3) *IGH/BCL2* (20%–30%, GCB > ABC)[d]	
BCL6 rearrangement (30%, ABC > GCB)[e]	
MYC rearrangement (GCB = ABC)[a,b,d]	
TBL1XR rearrangement (GCB)	
CD274 rearrangement[c]	
PDCD1LG2 rearrangement[c]	

[a] Associated with a complex karyotype.
[b] If associated with *BCL2* and/or *BCL6* rearrangements, reclassify as HGBL.
[c] More common in primary testicular DLBCL.
[d] Worse prognosis.
[e] Favorable prognosis.

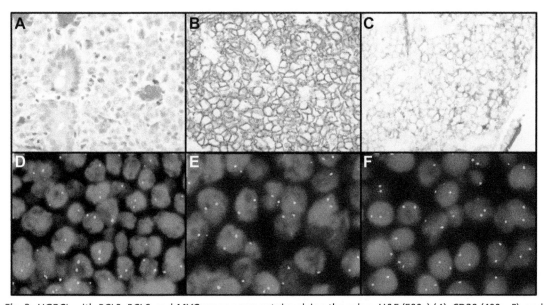

Fig. 3. HGBCL with *BCL2*, *BCL6*, and *MYC* rearrangements involving the colon. H&E (500x) (*A*), CD20 (400x, *B*), and CD10 (400x, *C*) stains. FISH studies showed rearrangements of *MYC* (*D*), *BCL2* (*E*), and *BCL6* (*F*).

Box 4
Cytogenetic/molecular abnormalities in HGBL

Aberrancy (frequency)

Cytogenetic Abnormalities

MYC (8q24) rearrangement[a,b]

With BCL2 (18q21) rearrangement[b,c]

With BCL6 (3q27) rearrangement

Complex karyotype

Mutations

TP53

MYD88

ID3

---

[a] 65% of MYC rearrangements occur with an immunoglobulin partner (IGH > IGK or IGL); other partners include 9p13, BCL6/3q27, or others. [b] MYC rearrangement or amplification with BCL2 amplification may be seen in HGBL, NOS[c] >95% of MYC/BCL2 double-hit lymphomas are GCB.

---

studies are of limited utility because the same STAT3 and STAT5B mutations may be seen. Mutations in TP53, TET2, CREBBP, and KMT2D have also been reported.[1,56–59]

T-cell Prolymphocytic Leukemia

T-cell prolymphocytic leukemia (T-PLL) is predominantly CD4+, although some are double positive or CD8+. The neoplastic cells do not resemble LGL but can be highly convoluted resembling adult T-cell leukemia/lymphoma (ATLL) (**Fig. 4**). TCL1-positivity is seen in greater than 90% of cases and is associated with TCL1A rearrangements.[1] Mutations in JAK/STAT pathway, including STAT5B, and other cytogenetic abnormalities are frequently seen in T-PLL (**Box 5**).[1,60,61]

Adult T-cell Leukemia/Lymphoma

ATLL is a predominantly CD4+ lymphoma driven by human lymphotropic virus (HTLV) infection. The lymphoma cells have highly convoluted and multilobed nuclei referred to as "flower cells",[1] which may also be seen in other T-cell lymphomas. Aside from demonstration of HTLV in serum or in tumor tissue, ATLL may be associated with CD28 rearrangement or other abnormalities (**Box 6**).[1,62–64]

Pearls and Pitfalls

T-cell/NK-cell lymphomas with a leukemic presentation may show significant morphologic and phenotypic overlap. Although STAT3 mutations are the most common genetic abnormality identified in T-LGLL, STAT5B mutations have also been found. Mutations in STAT3 or STAT5B are also found in other T-cell lymphomas. Neither STAT3 nor STAT5 mutations are specific for T-LGLL and should not be used to subclassify T-cell lymphomas. Definitive diagnosis requires clinicopathologic correlation.

ANGIOIMMUNOBLASTIC T-CELL LYMPHOMA AND OTHER PERIPHERAL T-CELL LYMPHOMA

Angioimmunoblastic T-cell Lymphoma and Other Nodal Lymphomas of T Follicular Helper Cell Origin

Angioimmunoblastic T-cell lymphoma (AITL) is the most common and well-described entity within the group of T follicular helper cell (TFH) lymphomas (**Fig. 5**). All these lymphomas have a TFH phenotype, including CD4-expression and expression of other TFH markers (eg, CD10, CXCL13, ICOS, BCL6, and PD1). As these tumors originate from the same COO, mutational and cytogenetic findings are highly overlapping (**Table 5**).[1,65–68] DNMT3A and TET2 are frequently mutated all TFH lymphomas, although IDH2 mutations appear specific for AITL. Not only are DNMT3A and TET2 mutations very common in myeloid diseases, including clonal hematopoiesis and clonal cytopenia,[69] rare cases of AITL and myeloid neoplasms harboring the same mutations have also been reported[70] suggesting a common origin. Given significant molecular overlap, genetic abnormalities must be interpreted in the clinical and pathologic context.

Peripheral T-cell Lymphoma, Not Otherwise Specified

Peripheral T-cell lymphoma, NOS, is a diagnosis of exclusion. These tumors show a wide range of morphologic and immunophenotypic features. GATA3 gene expression profile (GEP), TBX21 GEP in the setting of cytotoxic T-cell phenotype, and mutations in MLL (or KMT2A), MLL2 (or KMT2D), KDM6A, TET2, or DNMT3A are associated with adverse prognosis (see **Table 5**).[1,65–68]

Fig. 4. T-PLL involving bone marrow and blood with distinct molecular profiles. (A) H&E (400x) of bone marrow. (B) Wright's stain of blood (1000x) at relapse. Two STAT5B mutations were seen in the original bone marrow (C), p.V712E, variant allele frequency [VAF] 21%; (E) p.N642H, VAF 10%), but only one was reported in the blood (D, p.V712E, VAF 0.2%; (F) p.N642H, VAF 12%). Whole genome copy number plot of the bone marrow (G) and peripheral blood (H) showing complex and shared abnormalities, and new partial -5q and -12p, and –Y in the blood of this male patient (yellow arrows). The remaining focal gains represent known artifacts.

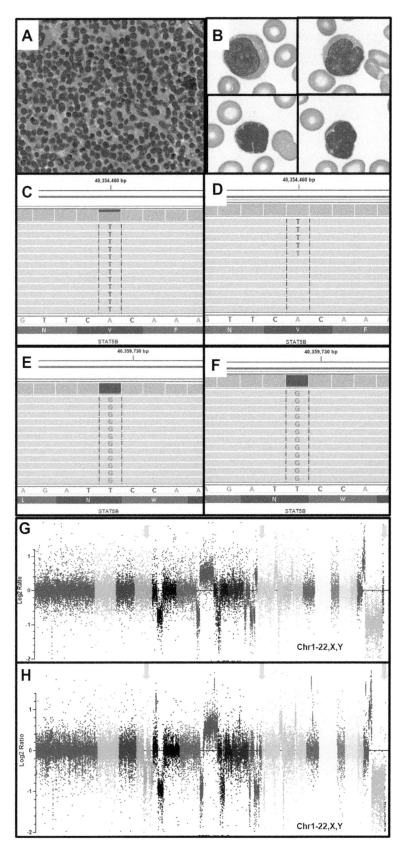

Box 5
Cytogenetic/molecular abnormalities in T-PLL

Aberrancy (frequency)

  Cytogenetic Abnormalities

    inv(14) (q11q32) *TCL1A/TRA* or *TCL1B/TRA* (80%)[a]

    t(14;14) (q11;q32) *TCL1A/TRA* or *TCL1B/TRA* (10%)[a]

    t(X;14) (q28;q11) *TRA/MTCP1*[a,b]

    Chromosome 8 abnormalities (70%–80%)

      idic(8) (p11)

      t(8;8) (p11–12;q12)

      Trisomy 8q

    Gains in 8q24 (*MYC*)

    Amplification of chromosome 5p

    Loss of chromosomes 11q23 (*ATM*), 12p13 or 22q

    Chromosome 6 abnormalities

  Mutations

    JAK3 (30%–42%)[c]

    JAK1 (8%)[c]

    STAT5B (21%–36%)[a,c]

    EZH2 (rare)

    BCOR (rare)

[a] Poor prognosis. [b] MTCP1 is homologous to TCL1A/B. [c] Usually mutually exclusive.

Box 6
Cytogenetic/molecular abnormalities in ATLL

Aberrancy

  Mutations

    CREB

    HBZ

    CCR4

    CCR7

    PLCG1

    PRKCH

    VAV1

    IRF4

    FYN

    CARD11

    STAT3

    TP53

    TP73

  Cytogenetic Abnormalities

    CTLA4/CD28 rearrangement

    ICOS/CD28 rearrangement

    Loss of chromosome 9p21.3

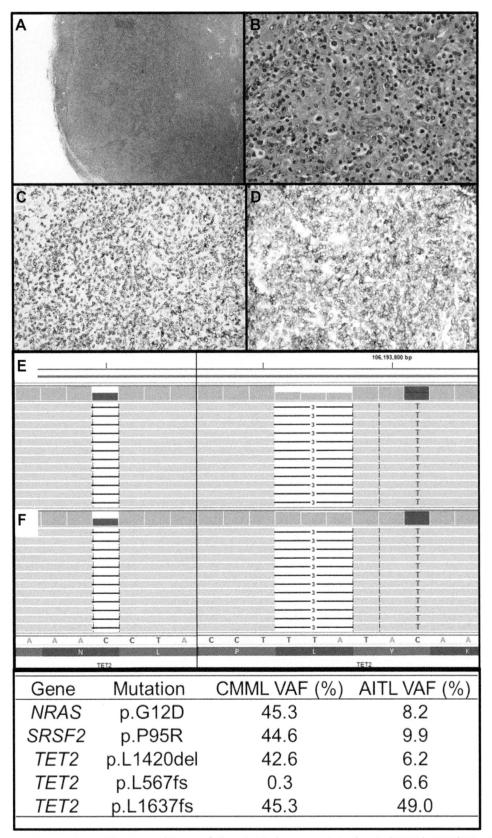

Gene	Mutation	CMML VAF (%)	AITL VAF (%)
NRAS	p.G12D	45.3	8.2
SRSF2	p.P95R	44.6	9.9
TET2	p.L1420del	42.6	6.2
TET2	p.L567fs	0.3	6.6
TET2	p.L1637fs	45.3	49.0

Fig. 5. AITL in a patient with a 3-year history of Chronic Myelomonocytic Leukemia (CMML). H&E (200x, *A* and 400x, *B*) of AITL with CD5 (*C*) and PD-1 (*D*) expression. NGS showed all previously detected mutations present in the CMML. All showed reduced variant allele frequency (VAF), including *TET2* p.L1420del (*F*), except for a germline *TET2* p.L1637 fs (*E*). Given low VAFs in the AITL specimen, mutations are all ascribed to admixed clonal myeloid cells, as opposed to lymphoma (bottom panel).

Table 5
Cytogenetic/molecular abnormalities in AITL and other TFH lymphoma, as compared to PTCL, NOS

AITL/TFH Lymphomas	PTCL, NOS
Cytogenetic Abnormalities	Cytogenetic Abnormalities
Trisomy 3 (rare), 5 (rare) and 21	Complex karyotype
Gain of chromosomes X, 22q, 19, 11q13	
Loss of chromosomes 6q, 13q	
CTLA4/CD28 rearrangement	
t(5;9) (q33;q22) *ITK/SYK*[b]	
Mutations	Mutations
Clonal T-cell receptor rearrangement (75%–90%)	GATA3 gene expression profile[c]
Clonal immunoglobulin rearrangement (25%–30%)	TBX21 gene expression profile[d]
IDH2[a]	*VAV1*
TET2	*MLL2* (or *KMT2D*)[c]
DNMT3A	*KDM6A*[c]
RHOA	*MLL* (or *KMT2A*)[c]
FYN	*TET2*[c]
PLCG1	*DNMT3A*[c]
CD28	*RHOA*
	EP300
	CREBBP
	SETD2
	TP53

[a] Specific for AITL.
[b] Specific for follicular T-cell lymphoma (FTCL).
[c] Adverse outcome.
[d] If cytotoxic phenotype, then adverse outcome.

Pearls and Pitfalls

When TFH phenotype lymphomas are encountered, and sequencing studies are pursued to identify characteristic mutations, special consideration must be given to cell type(s) contributing to these mutations. As genes typically mutated in TFH lymphomas are also commonly mutated in myeloid processes, a myeloid origin must be considered if mutations in *DNMT3A*, *TET2*, or *IDH2* are found in the lymphoma specimen. Variant allele frequencies can help in the estimation of clonal cell content, which should be correlated with tumor cellularity based on immunohistochemistry. In particularly challenging cases, an uninvolved peripheral blood or bone marrow specimen may also need to be sequenced to exclude the possibility of clonal myeloid process.

SUMMARY AND FUTURE DIRECTIONS

As we gain a greater understanding of the genetic landscape of lymphoid malignancies, the molecular/cytogenetic findings are becoming increasingly important in the classification of these diseases, as is now the case for myeloid neoplasms. The diagnostic utility of genetic abnormalities has been demonstrated for B-cell lymphomas with the increasing number of genetically defined entities. Prognostic and therapeutic utility of genetic abnormalities are highly variable and disease-specific. As our understanding of the biology and mechanisms of lymphoid malignancies continue to evolve, molecular findings hold great potential to inform future clinical and pathologic practice.

CLINICS CARE POINTS

- Genetic findings are becoming increasingly important in the diagnosis and treatment of lymphoid malignancies.
- There can be significant overlap in the genetic landscape of lymphoid neoplasms.
- Care must be used in interpreting results of molecular tests when diagnosing lymphomas.

DISCLOSURE

The authors have nothing to disclose. This work was supported in part by the Sidney Kimmel Comprehensive Cancer Center grant from the National Institutes of Health (P30CA006973; R.X.X.).

REFERENCES

1. Swerdlow S, Campo E, Harris NL, et al. WHO classification of tumours of haematopoietic and lymphoid tissues. Revised 4th ed. International Agency for Research on Cancer (IARC); 2017.

2. Nikiforova MN, Hsi ED, Braziel RM, et al. Detection of clonal IGH gene rearrangements: summary of molecular oncology surveys of the College of American Pathologists. Arch Pathol Lab Med 2007;131(2): 185–9.

3. Xian RR, Xie Y, Haley LM, et al. CREBBP and STAT6 co-mutation and 16p13 and 1p36 loss define the t(14;18)-negative diffuse variant of follicular lymphoma. Blood Cancer J 2020;10(6):69. https://doi.org/10.1038/s41408-020-0335-0.

4. Zamò A, Pischimarov J, Horn H, et al. The exomic landscape of t(14;18)-negative diffuse follicular lymphoma with 1p36 deletion. Br J Haematol 2018; 180(3):391–4. https://doi.org/10.1111/bjh.15041.

5. Nann D, Ramis-Zaldivar JE, Müller I, et al. Follicular lymphoma t(14;18)-negative is genetically a heterogeneous disease. Blood Adv 2020;4(22):5652–65. https://doi.org/10.1182/bloodadvances.2020002944.

6. Carbone A, Roulland S, Gloghini A, et al. Follicular lymphoma. Nat Rev Dis Primers 2019;5(1):83. https://doi.org/10.1038/s41572-019-0132-x.

7. Sugimoto T, Watanabe T. Follicular Lymphoma: The Role of the Tumor Microenvironment in Prognosis. J Clin Exp Hematop 2016;56(1):1–19. https://doi.org/10.3960/jslrt.56.1.

8. Devan J, Janikova A, Mraz M. New concepts in follicular lymphoma biology: From BCL2 to epigenetic regulators and non-coding RNAs. Semin Oncol 2018;45(5–6):291–302. https://doi.org/10.1053/j.seminoncol.2018.07.005.

9. Agostinelli C, Akarca AU, Ramsay A, et al. Novel markers in pediatric-type follicular lymphoma. Virchows Arch 2019;475(6):771–9. https://doi.org/10.1007/s00428-019-02681-y.

10. Bödör C, Grossmann V, Popov N, et al. EZH2 mutations are frequent and represent an early event in follicular lymphoma. Blood 2013;122(18):3165–8.

11. Hoy SM. Tazemetostat: first approval. Drugs 2020; 80(5):513–21.

12. Louissaint A, Schafernak KT, Geyer JT, et al. Pediatric-type nodal follicular lymphoma: a biologically distinct lymphoma with frequent MAPK pathway mutations. Blood 2016;128(8):1093–100.

13. Schmidt J, Gong S, Marafioti T, et al. Genome-wide analysis of pediatric-type follicular lymphoma reveals low genetic complexity and recurrent alterations of TNFRSF14 gene. Blood 2016;128(8): 1101–11.

14. Mlynarczyk C, Fontán L, Melnick A. Germinal center-derived lymphomas: The darkest side of humoral immunity. Immunol Rev 2019;288(1):214–39. https://doi.org/10.1111/imr.12755.

15. Orchard J, Garand R, Davis Z, et al. A subset of t (11; 14) lymphoma with mantle cell features displays mutated IgVH genes and includes patients with good prognosis, nonnodal disease. Blood 2003; 101(12):4975–81.

16. Hamblin TJ, Davis Z, Gardiner A, et al. Unmutated Ig VH genes are associated with a more aggressive form of chronic lymphocytic leukemia. Blood 1999; 94(6):1848–54.

17. Forconi F, Sozzi E, Cencini E, et al. Hairy cell leukemias with unmutated IGHV genes define the minor subset refractory to single-agent cladribine and with more aggressive behavior. Blood 2009; 114(21):4696–702.

18. Cheah CY, Seymour JF, Wang ML. Mantle Cell Lymphoma. J Clin Oncol 2016;34(11):1256–69. https://doi.org/10.1200/JCO.2015.63.5904.

19. Cortelazzo S, Ponzoni M, Ferreri AJM, et al. Mantle cell lymphoma. Crit Rev Oncol Hematol 2020;153: 103038. https://doi.org/10.1016/j.critrevonc.2020.103038.

20. Ruan J. Molecular profiling and management of mantle cell lymphoma. Hematol Am Soc Hematol Educ Program 2019;2019(1):30–40. https://doi.org/10.1182/hematology.2019000011.

21. Nadeu F, Martin-Garcia D, Clot G, et al. Genomic and epigenomic insights into the origin, pathogenesis, and clinical behavior of mantle cell lymphoma subtypes. Blood 2020;136(12):1419–32. https://doi.org/10.1182/blood.2020005289.

22. Puente XS, Jares P, Campo E. Chronic lymphocytic leukemia and mantle cell lymphoma: crossroads of genetic and microenvironment interactions. Blood 2018;131(21):2283–96. https://doi.org/10.1182/blood-2017-10-764373.

23. Greenwell IB, Staton AD, Lee MJ, et al. Complex karyotype in patients with mantle cell lymphoma predicts inferior survival and poor response to intensive induction therapy. Cancer 2018;124(11): 2306–15.

24. Hu Z, Medeiros LJ, Chen Z, et al. Mantle Cell Lymphoma With MYC Rearrangement. Am J Surg Pathol 2017;41(2):216–24.

25. Hershkovitz-Rokah O, Pulver D, Lenz G, et al. Ibrutinib resistance in mantle cell lymphoma: clinical, molecular and treatment aspects. Br J Haematol 2018; 181(3):306–19. https://doi.org/10.1111/bjh.15108.

26. Hallek M. Chronic lymphocytic leukemia: 2020 update on diagnosis, risk stratification and treatment. Am J Hematol 2019;94(11):1266–87. https://doi.org/10.1002/ajh.25595.

27. Fabbri G, Dalla-Favera R. The molecular pathogenesis of chronic lymphocytic leukaemia. Nat Rev Cancer 2016;16(3):145–62. https://doi.org/10.1038/nrc.2016.8.

28. Crassini K, Stevenson WS, Mulligan SP, et al. Molecular pathogenesis of chronic lymphocytic leukaemia. Br J Haematol 2019;186(5):668–84. https://doi.org/10.1111/bjh.16102.

29. Gaiti F, Chaligne R, Gu H, et al. Epigenetic evolution and lineage histories of chronic lymphocytic leukaemia. Nature 2019;569(7757):576–80. https://doi.org/10.1038/s41586-019-1198-z.

30. Nguyen-Khac F, Lambert J, Chapiro E, et al. Chromosomal aberrations and their prognostic value in a series of 174 untreated patients with Waldenström's macroglobulinemia. Haematologica 2013; 98(4):649.

31. Durham BH, Getta B, Dietrich S, et al. Genomic analysis of hairy cell leukemia identifies novel recurrent genetic alterations. Blood 2017;130(14):1644–8. https://doi.org/10.1182/blood-2017-01-765107.

32. Angelova EA, Medeiros LJ, Wang W, et al. Clinicopathologic and molecular features in hairy cell leukemia-variant: single institutional experience. Mod Pathol 2018;31(11):1717–32. https://doi.org/10.1038/s41379-018-0093-8.

33. Maitre E, Cornet E, Troussard X. Hairy cell leukemia: 2020 update on diagnosis, risk stratification, and treatment. Am J Hematol 2019;94(12):1413–22. https://doi.org/10.1002/ajh.25653.

34. Wang W, Lin P. Lymphoplasmacytic lymphoma and Waldenström macroglobulinaemia: clinicopathological features and differential diagnosis. Pathology 2020;52(1):6–14. https://doi.org/10.1016/j.pathol.2019.09.009.

35. Spina V, Rossi D. Molecular pathogenesis of splenic and nodal marginal zone lymphoma. Best Pract Res Clin Haematol 2017;30(1–2):5–12. https://doi.org/10.1016/j.beha.2016.09.004.

36. Spina V, Khiabanian H, Messina M, et al. The genetics of nodal marginal zone lymphoma. Blood 2016;128(10):1362–73. https://doi.org/10.1182/blood-2016-02-696757.

37. Pileri S, Ponzoni M. Pathology of nodal marginal zone lymphomas. Best Pract Res Clin Haematol 2017;30(1–2):50–5. https://doi.org/10.1016/j.beha.2016.11.001.

38. Lauw MIS, Lucas CG, Ohgami RS, et al. Primary Central Nervous System Lymphomas: A Diagnostic Overview of Key Histomorphologic, Immunophenotypic, and Genetic Features. Diagnostics (Basel) 2020;10(12). https://doi.org/10.3390/diagnostics10121076.

39. Panea RI, Love CL, Shingleton JR, et al. The whole-genome landscape of Burkitt lymphoma subtypes. Blood 2019;134(19):1598–607. https://doi.org/10.1182/blood.2019001880.

40. Wagener R, Seufert J, Raimondi F, et al. The mutational landscape of Burkitt-like lymphoma with 11q aberration is distinct from that of Burkitt lymphoma. Blood 2019;133(9):962–6. https://doi.org/10.1182/blood-2018-07-864025.

41. Grande BM, Gerhard DS, Jiang A, et al. Genome-wide discovery of somatic coding and noncoding mutations in pediatric endemic and sporadic Burkitt lymphoma. Blood 2019;133(12):1313–24.

42. Hans CP, Weisenburger DD, Greiner TC, et al. Confirmation of the molecular classification of diffuse large B-cell lymphoma by immunohistochemistry using a tissue microarray. Blood 2004; 103(1):275–82. https://doi.org/10.1182/blood-2003-05-1545.

43. Pham-Ledard A, Beylot-Barry M, Barbe C, et al. High frequency and clinical prognostic value of MYD88 L265P mutation in primary cutaneous diffuse large B-cell lymphoma, leg-type. JAMA Dermatol 2014;150(11):1173–9. https://doi.org/10.1001/jamadermatol.2014.821.

44. Schmitz R, Wright GW, Huang DW, et al. Genetics and Pathogenesis of Diffuse Large B-Cell Lymphoma. N Engl J Med 2018;378(15):1396–407. https://doi.org/10.1056/NEJMoa1801445.

45. Ennishi D, Jiang A, Boyle M, et al. Double-Hit Gene Expression Signature Defines a Distinct Subgroup of Germinal Center B-Cell-Like Diffuse Large B-Cell Lymphoma. J Clin Oncol 2019;37(3):190–201. https://doi.org/10.1200/JCO.18.01583.

46. Scott DW, King RL, Staiger AM, et al. High-grade B-cell lymphoma with MYC and BCL2 and/or BCL6 rearrangements with diffuse large B-cell lymphoma morphology. Blood 2018;131(18):2060–4. https://doi.org/10.1182/blood-2017-12-820605.

47. Huang W, Medeiros LJ, Lin P, et al. MYC/BCL2/BCL6 triple hit lymphoma: a study of 40 patients with a comparison to MYC/BCL2 and MYC/BCL6 double hit lymphomas. Mod Pathol 2018;31(9):1470–8. https://doi.org/10.1038/s41379-018-0067-x.

48. Grimm KE, O'Malley DP. Aggressive B cell lymphomas in the 2017 revised WHO classification of tumors of hematopoietic and lymphoid tissues. Ann Diagn Pathol 2019;38:6–10. https://doi.org/10.1016/j.anndiagpath.2018.09.014.

49. Quintanilla-Martinez L, Sander B, Chan JK, et al. Indolent lymphomas in the pediatric population: follicular lymphoma, IRF4/MUM1+ lymphoma, nodal marginal zone lymphoma and chronic lymphocytic leukemia. Virchows Arch 2016;468(2):141–57. https://doi.org/10.1007/s00428-015-1855-z.

50. Ramis-Zaldivar JE, Gonzalez-Farré B, Balagué O, et al. Distinct molecular profile of IRF4-rearranged large B-cell lymphoma. Blood 01 2020;135(4): 274–86. https://doi.org/10.1182/blood.2019002699.

51. Jiang XN, Yu BH, Wang WG, et al. Anaplastic lymphoma kinase-positive large B-cell lymphoma:

Clinico-pathological study of 17 cases with review of literature. PLoS One 2017;12(6):e0178416. https://doi.org/10.1371/journal.pone.0178416.

52. Jaffe ES. Navigating the cutaneous B-cell lymphomas: avoiding the rocky shoals. Mod Pathol 2020;33(Suppl 1):96–106. https://doi.org/10.1038/s41379-019-0385-7.

53. Castillo JJ, Reagan JL. Plasmablastic lymphoma: a systematic review. ScientificWorldJournal 2011;11:687–96. https://doi.org/10.1100/tsw.2011.59.

54. Ambrosio MR, Mundo L, Gazaneo S, et al. MicroRNAs sequencing unveils distinct molecular subgroups of plasmablastic lymphoma. Oncotarget 2017;8(64):107356–73. https://doi.org/10.18632/oncotarget.22219.

55. Barilà G, Calabretto G, Teramo A, et al. T cell large granular lymphocyte leukemia and chronic NK lymphocytosis. Best Pract Res Clin Haematol 2019;32(3):207–16. https://doi.org/10.1016/j.beha.2019.06.006.

56. Nicolae A, Ganapathi KA, Pham TH, et al. EBV-negative Aggressive NK-cell Leukemia/Lymphoma: Clinical, Pathologic, and Genetic Features. Am J Surg Pathol 2017;41(1):67–74. https://doi.org/10.1097/PAS.0000000000000735.

57. Huang L, Liu D, Wang N, et al. Integrated genomic analysis identifies deregulated JAK/STAT-MYC-biosynthesis axis in aggressive NK-cell leukemia. Cell Res 2018;28(2):172–86. https://doi.org/10.1038/cr.2017.146.

58. Tang YT, Wang D, Luo H, et al. Aggressive NK-cell leukemia: clinical subtypes, molecular features, and treatment outcomes. Blood Cancer J 2017;7(12):660. https://doi.org/10.1038/s41408-017-0021-z.

59. Dufva O, Kankainen M, Kelkka T, et al. Aggressive natural killer-cell leukemia mutational landscape and drug profiling highlight JAK-STAT signaling as therapeutic target. Nat Commun 2018;9(1):1567. https://doi.org/10.1038/s41467-018-03987-2.

60. Matutes E. The 2017 WHO update on mature T- and natural killer (NK) cell neoplasms. Int J Lab Hematol 2018;40(Suppl 1):97–103. https://doi.org/10.1111/ijlh.12817.

61. Staber PB, Herling M, Bellido M, et al. Consensus criteria for diagnosis, staging, and treatment response assessment of T-cell prolymphocytic leukemia. Blood 2019;134(14):1132–43. https://doi.org/10.1182/blood.2019000402.

62. Kataoka K, Iwanaga M, Yasunaga JI, et al. Prognostic relevance of integrated genetic profiling in adult T-cell leukemia/lymphoma. Blood 2018;131(2):215–25. https://doi.org/10.1182/blood-2017-01-761874.

63. Kogure Y, Kataoka K. Genetic alterations in adult T-cell leukemia/lymphoma. Cancer Sci 2017;108(9):1719–25. https://doi.org/10.1111/cas.13303.

64. Mehta-Shah N, Ratner L, Horwitz SM. Adult T-Cell Leukemia/Lymphoma. J Oncol Pract 2017;13(8):487–92. https://doi.org/10.1200/JOP.2017.021907.

65. Heavican TB, Bouska A, Yu J, et al. Genetic drivers of oncogenic pathways in molecular subgroups of peripheral T-cell lymphoma. Blood 2019;133(15):1664–76. https://doi.org/10.1182/blood-2018-09-872549.

66. Lunning MA, Vose JM. Angioimmunoblastic T-cell lymphoma: the many-faced lymphoma. Blood 2017;129(9):1095–102. https://doi.org/10.1182/blood-2016-09-692541.

67. Iqbal J, Amador C, McKeithan TW, et al. Molecular and Genomic Landscape of Peripheral T-Cell Lymphoma. Cancer Treat Res 2019;176:31–68. https://doi.org/10.1007/978-3-319-99716-2_2.

68. Marchi E, O'Connor OA. The rapidly changing landscape in mature T-cell lymphoma (MTCL) biology and management. CA Cancer J Clin 2020;70(1):47–70. https://doi.org/10.3322/caac.21589.

69. Sperling AS, Gibson CJ, Ebert BL. The genetics of myelodysplastic syndrome: from clonal haematopoiesis to secondary leukaemia. Nat Rev Cancer 2017;17(1):5.

70. Couronné L, Bastard C, Bernard OA. TET2 and DNMT3A mutations in human T-cell lymphoma. N Engl J Med 2012;366(1):95–6.

Moving?

Make sure your subscription moves with you!

To notify us of your new address, find your **Clinics Account Number** (located on your mailing label above your name), and contact customer service at:

Email: journalscustomerservice-usa@elsevier.com

800-654-2452 (subscribers in the U.S. & Canada)
314-447-8871 (subscribers outside of the U.S. & Canada)

Fax number: 314-447-8029

**Elsevier Health Sciences Division
Subscription Customer Service
3251 Riverport Lane
Maryland Heights, MO 63043**

*To ensure uninterrupted delivery of your subscription, please notify us at least 4 weeks in advance of move.

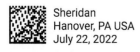

Sheridan
Hanover, PA USA
July 22, 2022